The Midwives of Seventeenth-Century London

This book is the first comprehensive and detailed study of early modern midwives in seventeenth-century London. Until quite recently, midwives, as a group, have been dismissed by historians as being inadequately educated and trained for the task of child delivery. *The Midwives of Seventeenth-Century London* rejects these claims by exploring the midwives' training in an unofficial apprenticeship and their licensing by the Church. Dr. Evenden also offers an informed depiction of the midwives in their socioeconomic context by examining a wide range of seventeenth-century sources. This expansive study recovers the names of almost twelve hundred women who worked as midwives in and about London. It also brings to light details about midwives, their spouses, families, and associates in the setting of twelve London parishes.

Doreen Evenden is an associate professor of history at Mount Saint Vincent University, Halifax, Nova Scotia. Dr. Evenden's doctoral thesis that developed into this book was awarded the Canadian Historical Association prize for the best doctoral thesis on a non-Canadian topic in 1991. She is the author of *Popular Medicine in Seventeenth-Century England* (1988) and contributor to *The Art of Midwifery* (1993). Dr. Evenden has also been published in *Medical History* (1998).

T0275624

Cambridge Studies in the History of Medicine

Cambridge History of Medicine

Edited by

CHARLES ROSENBERG, Professor of History and Sociology of Science, University of Pennsylvania, and COLIN JONES, University of Warwick

Continued on pages following the Index

The Midwives of Seventeenth-Century London

DOREEN EVENDEN

Mount Saint Vincent University

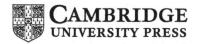

CAMBRIDGE
UNIVERSITY PRESS

CAMBRIDGE UNIVERSITY PRESS
Cambridge, New York, Melbourne, Madrid, Cape Town, Singapore, São Paulo

Cambridge University Press
The Edinburgh Building, Cambridge CB2 2RU, UK

Published in the United States of America by Cambridge University Press, New York

www.cambridge.org
Information on this title: www.cambridge.org/9780521661072

First published 2000
This digitally printed first paperback version 2006

A catalogue record for this publication is available from the British Library

Library of Congress Cataloguing in Publication data
Evenden, Doreen.
The midwives of seventeenth-century London / Doreen Evenden.
p.   cm. – (Cambridge studies in the history of medicine)
Includes bibliographical references and index.
ISBN 0-521-66107-2 (hc)
1. Midwives – England – London – History – 17th century.
2. Obstetrics – England – London – History – 17th century.
3. Obstetricians – England – London – History – 17th century.
4. n-uk-en.   I. Title.   II. Series.
RG950.E94   1999
618.2'09421'09032 – dc21   99-26518
                                                      CIP

ISBN-13 978-0-521-66107-2 hardback
ISBN-10 0-521-66107-2 hardback

ISBN-13 978-0-521-02785-4 paperback
ISBN-10 0-521-02785-3 paperback

To the midwives of all times and places whose names will never be known.

CONTENTS

Contents

TABLES AND FIGURES

Tables

Figures

ACKNOWLEDGEMENTS

This study of seventeenth-century midwives had its genesis more than a decade ago when I set off for London on a quest for information about female medical practitioners. I was not particularly interested in midwives as I shared many of the prevailing misconceptions about early modern midwives and also believed that there was nothing more to discover about them. That was about to change upon my arrival at the manuscript section of London's Guildhall Library.

Initially, then, to Jim Alsop for insisting that I take at least a "quick look" at midwives, and who continued to provide scholarly guidance and direction, and to the efficient and welcoming staff at the Guildhall Library, must go a sincere "thank you." As my search widened, the resources of other archives were tapped, and I am also deeply indebted to the archivists and librarians of the Corporation of London Record Office, London Metropolitan Archives (formerly the Greater London Record Office), the Public Record Office, Lambeth Palace Library, and, back home, McMaster University Library in Hamilton, Ontario. Special thanks as well to the Bodleian Library, Oxford, for permission to make extensive use of Ms. Rawl. D 1141, to the Marta Danylewycz Memorial Fund for support in the early stages of my research in London archives, and to Mount St. Vincent University for assistance with expenses incurred by publication.

I was sustained throughout the long months away from family by the friendship, encouragement, and generosity of many, but I am particularly grateful to Jacky Cox, Gill and Tim Clark, Joan Anderson and Ian Jamieson, Clare Rider, Barbara Hanawalt, Hilary Marland, Mike Adams, Linda Hayner, and the late Trudy Stein.

Finally, there are my four children who, unintentionally, allowed me the experience of childbirth. These occasions, along with my first career as a registered nurse, have, I believe, permitted me to read seventeenth-century sources relating to midwives with a heightened sensitivity. Beyond that, Nancy and Steven both read and commented on parts of the manuscript, Peter gave assistance with translation, and John read and edited a draft of the entire manuscript.

My sincere thanks to everyone who helped in ways both big and small and whose names I have forgotten to include.

Doreen A. Evenden
August 1998
Plympton, Nova Scotia

ABBREVIATIONS

BL	British Library
CLRO	Corporation of London Record Office
CRO	Cumbria Record Office
GLRO	Greater London Record Office (now London Metropolitan Archives)
GL	Guildhall Library
LPL	Lambeth Palace Library
PRO	Public Record Office
RCOG	Royal College of Obstetricians and Gynaecologists
VL	Victoria Library

Note: For purposes of this study the new year will commence on January the first.

INTRODUCTION

The identity of midwives has traditionally been shrouded in anonymity, but nowhere more so than in the bustling seventeenth-century metropolis of London. Frequently nameless in the records of their own parishes, who were these faceless women who moved so silently about their tasks, participants in that human drama which touched the lives of London's richest and poorest citizens alike? In a city flooded with migrants who were cut off from home ties, the London midwife's role assumed even greater significance as a timeless symbol of the past, present, and future, and as a bridge between the long-time resident and the newcomer who shared the universal experience of childbirth.[1]

Until recently, perceptions of seventeenth-century English midwives have largely been shaped by the uncritical acceptance of accounts written by male midwives such as Percival Willughby, and very little attempt has been made to reconstruct their lives.[2] As a result, the stereotypical early modern English midwife has been portrayed as ignorant, incompetent, and poor. Although it is a portrait which scholarship from the past decade is now revising, there is still some way to go.[3] The single most influential source in the historiography of English midwifery has been Willughby's compilation of some 200 midwifery cases selected from his own forty-year practice. Willughby's seventeenth-century manuscript was not published until 1863, but from that time up to the present, it has continued to play a major role in informing historians' views of English early modern midwifery.

---

1 A. L. Beier and Roger Finlay have suggested that "isolation and insecurity" might have had considerable impact on the large migrant population. "Introduction: The Significance of the Metropolis," A. L. Beier and Roger Finlay, eds., *London 1500–1700* (London: Longman, 1986), 20.
2 Percival Willughby, *Observations in Midwifery* (H. Blenkinsop, 1863; reprint ed., Wakefield: SR publishers, 1972).
3 David Harley, "Ignorant Midwives – a persistent stereotype," *The Society for the History of Medicine Bulletin* 28 (June 1981): 6–9. For an example of how historians of women's history have been influenced by the stereotype, see Hilda Smith, "Gynaecology and Ideology in Seventeenth-century England," Bernice A. Carroll, ed., *Liberating Women's History* (Urbana, Ill.: University of Illinois Press, 1976): 109–113. David Cressy also notes the lingering misconceptions despite recent reappraisals of early modern midwives. David Cressy, *Birth, Marriage and Death: Ritual, Religion and the Life-Cycle in Tudor and Stuart England* (Oxford and N.Y.: Oxford University Press, 1997), 59.

The earliest historians of English midwifery were physicians whose accounts were inevitably weighted in favour of the male professionals.[4] Working within the context of the late nineteenth century, J. H. Aveling, M.D. reflected his era's bias against female practitioners as well as its antiquarian style of historical writing. Aveling drew heavily on Willughby and the accounts of a few male practitioners. As a result, his comments about seventeenth- and eighteenth-century midwifery embodied the contemporary view of women's incapacity to assimilate scientific knowledge as well as an acceptance of their exclusion from institutions of higher learning.[5] Aveling introduced his influential account, *English Midwives, Their History and Prospects* (1872) with the following statement:

I am not standing up to plead the cause of women as obstetricians, because I think, if there is one occupation for which they are less fitted than another, it is that of attending the emergencies of obstetric practice.[6]

Aveling mentioned a few royal midwives as well as midwife and author Jane Sharpe, and the political and highly visible Elizabeth Cellier, but reserved most of his praise for male practitioners William Harvey (who he says "was the first to rescue English midwifery from its age of darkness"), Peter Chamberlen, William Sermon, and the legendary Willughby.[7] Aveling took great pains to point out the academic and professional qualifications of the four men and concluded:

. . . these self-constituted instructors of midwives were men of high social and medical position. Had they considered the study and practice of midwifery beneath their dignity,

4 This historiographical pattern is not uniquely English. Medical historians, in particular, have been taken to task by the scholar of continental Europe, M. Wiesner, for adopting a blanket judgement of midwives as "superstitious and bungling" while ignoring the bizarre practices of many physicians. Merry E. Wiesner, "Early Modern Midwifery: A Case Study," Barbara A. Hanawalt, ed., *Women and Work in Pre-Industrial Europe* (Bloomington: Indiana University Press, 1986), 94. For examples of medical treatments of the day, see Doreen Evenden Nagy, *Popular Medicine in Seventeenth-century England* (Bowling Green: Bowling Green State University Press, 1988), 43–53. Simon Schama has commented on the way in which two doctors were responsible for the "bad press" given to seventeenth-century midwives in the Netherlands. Simon Schama, *The Embarrassment of Riches* (New York: Alfred A. Knopf, 1987), 526. It is an image which is undergoing revision; see Hilary Marland, ed. *The Art of Midwifery* (London: Routledge, 1993) and David Cressy, n.3 above.

5 For Victorian attitudes toward women, higher education, and the professions, see Josephine Kamm, *Hope Deferred: Girl's Education in English History* (London: Methuen, 1965); Martha Vicinus, *Independent Women: Work and Community for Single Women 1850–1920* (Chicago: University of Chicago Press, 1985); Enid Moberley Bell, *Storming the Citadel: the rise of the woman doctor* (London: Constable, 1953).

6 James H. Aveling, *English Midwives, Their History and Prospects* (London, 1872: reprint ed., London: Hugh K. Elliott Ltd., 1967), "Introduction," vi.

7 Aveling, 35. It is highly unlikely that Harvey's work, *De Generatione Animalium* (London,1651), which was based on experiments with fertilized hen's eggs, had any direct bearing on the practice of midwifery, particularly in the seventeenth century. However, Jonathan Sawday has portrayed Harvey's role as key in the masculinization of scientific knowledge and the theory of male generation. Jonathan Sawday, *The Body Emblazoned* (London: Routledge, 1995), 238–43. William Sermon was the author of *The Ladies Companion or the English Midwife* (London, 1671). See also Smith, 105. For other discussions of royal midwives, see Harvey Graham, *Eternal Eve* (New York: Doubleday, 1951) and M. Carter, "The Royal Midwives," *Midwives Chronicle* 90 (1977): 300–1.

how disastrous would it have been to English mothers, and who can say how much longer the dark ages of midwifery would have continued in this country.[8]

Ten years later, Aveling published his tribute to the Chamberlen family, inventors of the midwifery forceps, which were described by Aveling as "this most benificent of instruments."[9] Aveling's description is indicative of the positive light in which he viewed the "scientific" advances being made by a small group of male practitioners of midwifery. It is worth noting, however, that Jonathan Sawday in his recent fascinating study of renaissance (blazon) poetry and anatomy texts, has concluded that the appropriation of medical knowledge (including that relating to childbirth) by male practitioners in the seventeenth century was motivated by anything but the altruistic motives attributed to them by writers such as Aveling.[10] Moreover, Aveling and the practitioners whom he applauds give no hint of how their expertise in child delivery was acquired.

Following Aveling, medical personnel published midwifery studies which, again, found their inspiration in the earlier studies about male midwives and adhered to the narrow perspective of biographical writing. In their studies of midwifery, physicians continued to espouse a patronizing stance toward female midwives while describing male practitioners in heroic terms. As late as 1975, a member of the medical profession adopted the customary stance: "Nevertheless the 17th and 18th centuries saw considerable advances in obstetric knowledge by male obstetricians who were called man-midwives, and they recognized the importance of teaching midwives."[11] More recently, an award-winning essay about an eighteenth-century male midwife traced the linear ascent of childbirth from "the hands of the unskilled sixteenth-century midwife to those of the trained accoucheur, or man midwife, and finally to those of the physician *skilled in the art of healing.*"[12]

---

8 Aveling, 46.

9 James H. Aveling, *The Chamberlens and the Midwifery Forceps* (London: J.&.A. Churchill, 1882; reprint ed. AMS, 1985), ix. It is a viewpoint which has persisted, in some quarters, up to the present. See Adrian Wilson, *The Making of Man-midwifery* (Cambridge, Mass.: Harvard University Press, 1995), 71. This study, however, will challenge the validity of this assumption for the seventeenth century in particular.

10 Sawday sees the male practitioners' activities as motivated by their desire to control and dominate female sexuality, one aspect of which was exclusion of women from the realm of "scientific" knowledge. Sawday, 230–56.

11 Humphrey Arthure, "Early English Midwifery," *Midwife, Health Visitor & Community Nurse* 2 (June 1975): 187. We have uncovered little or no evidence of male surgeons or physicians who instructed midwives in the seventeenth century. See also the account of Dr. Tate, "Celebrated Midwives of the 17th and Beginning of the 18th Centuries," *St Thomas's Hospital Gazette* 5 (no.3 1895): 33–6; Herbert Spencer, *The History of British Midwifery from 1650–1800* (London: John Bale, Sons & Danielson, 1927). I will argue that men midwives were taught by midwives who were then relegated to an inferior role.

12 An Osler Gold Medal was awarded to Steven A. Brody for "The Life and Times of Sir Fielding Gould: man midwife and master physician," *Bulletin of the History of Medicine* 52 (1978): 228–50. The emphasis is mine in order to draw attention to the fact that medical doctors have generally considered pregnancy and childbirth an illness which demands medical attention in all cases, a position which was not held by seventeenth-century women and their midwives.

In the 1960s, Thomas Forbes, an early historian of medicine, began to publish on the subject of midwifery. Forbes perpetuated the stereotypes, which had originated with Willughby via Aveling, although he also began to introduce limited archival evidence.[13] A study of English obstetrics and gynaecology covering the years 1540–1740, published in 1982, once more relied primarily on published works by Willughby (whose casebook documented selected cases from his seventeenth-century practice in Derby and London) as well as other male practitioners who wrote, for the most part, in the prescriptive vein.[14] Willughby's records reflected the author's self-proclaimed competence, frequently at the expense of midwives whom he variously characterized as ignorant, poor, or perpetrators of torture. His overall perception was that the routine work of midwifery should be carried out by women and, more important for this study, that London midwives, as a group, were more competent and better trained than most country midwives.[15] Despite this concession, Willughby saw himself as having superior knowledge of "nature's secrets" and, according to Elizabeth Harvey, in so doing, usurped the midwife from her authoritarian role in matters relating to childbirth.[16]

Adrian Wilson's 1982 study of seventeenth-century childbirth and midwifery incorporated archival sources such as visitation records and testimonial certificates from the diocese of Norwich, but Willughby's observations loom large in the author's conclusions.[17] Wilson's recent examination of the emergence of the male

---

13 Forbes has included reproductions of eight midwives' testimonials which he has mistakenly identified as midwives' licences. Thomas Rogers Forbes, *The Midwife and the Witch* (New York: AMS Press, 1966), following 144. Donna Snell Smith cites six testimonials in "Tudor and Stuart Midwifery" (Ph. D. dissertation, University of Kentucky, 1980), 96.

14 Audrey Eccles, *Obstetrics and Gynaecology in Tudor and Stuart England* (London: Croom Helm, 1982). Eccles' study, which explored Tudor and Stuart midwifery and gynaecology, did not challenge the testimony of a few male midwives and practitioners whose selective reporting of a relatively small number of midwife-assisted labours and deliveries, which turned out badly, left unacknowledged the work of many competent women whose practice involved thousands of deliveries each year where no mishap occurred to mother or child. The resulting view of midwives and women's own experience of childbirth is a distorted one. It also promotes the image of male superiority in theory and technique. See also Alice Clark, *Working Life of Women in the Seventeenth Century* (London: Frank Cass and Co. Ltd., 1919; reprint ed., Fairfield, N.J.: Augustus M. Kelly, 1978), 281; Robert Michel, "English Attitudes Towards Women 1640–1700," *Canadian Journal of History* 13 (April 1978): 36–60.

15 Willughby, vi, 45, 73, 239. While Willughby practised almost forty years in Derby, his London practice was limited to the years 1656–60.

16 Elizabeth Harvey, *Ventriloquized Voices: Feminist Theory and English Renaissance Texts* (London: Routledge, 1992), 92.

17 Adrian Wilson, "Childbirth in seventeenth and eighteenth-century England" (Ph. D. dissertation University of Sussex, 1983). An overview of the history of midwives by Jean Towler and Joan Bramall, *Midwives in History and Society* (London: Croom Helm, 1986) devotes little more than one short chapter to seventeenth-century midwives. In her important pioneering study of interprofessional rivalry, Jean Donnison synthesised much of the work of earlier historians, including Forbes. It reflects Willughby's values and depreciates midwives' training, while at the same time crediting the early male midwives and surgeons with "*advances* in operative obstetrics" (emphasis mine) a mind set which this study will challenge. Jean Donnison, *Midwives and Medical Men: A History of Inter-Professional Rivalries and Women's Rights* (London: Heinemann, 1977), 8, 10.

midwife, while ameliorating, to some extent, earlier critical views of female midwives, continues to embrace the implicit acceptance of male midwives as suppliers of services which were superior to those of traditional midwives.[18] Relying heavily on publications by and selective case records of the male midwives themselves, it also fails to acknowledge the midwife as the repository of expertise in child delivery she was, a repository upon which the male midwife drew until his own skills were honed and he could assume the mantle of "expert."

Before the 1993 publication of a collection of essays, edited by Hilary Marland, began the revisionary process, major studies on the topic of Tudor–Stuart midwifery have, in the main, accepted the image of the (female) midwife who lacked any verifiable training and carried out her work with minimal competence.[19] Marland, more recently, has also explored the influence of the Sairey Gamp stereotype in producing negative perceptions of early modern midwives.[20] These earlier and negative traditional views of midwives have, unfortunately, been reflected in the work of social historians whose works of synthesis necessarily rely on earlier specialized studies such as those by Forbes.[21]

In the main, then, the historiography of midwifery has been dominated by a viewpoint restricted not only by the inherent biases of the male midwife, but also by the paucity of archival sources which historians have employed in their studies of seventeenth-century midwifery.[22] In order to break free of this stereotype, for this study of seventeenth-century London midwives, a methodology was adopted which utilized an abundance of archival sources in the hope that a more representative view of this important group of women would emerge. This book is the product of these archival explorations.

18 Isobel Grundy previously noted that Wilson's perspective "assumes the non-existence of skilled women," Isobel Grundy, "Sarah Stone: Enlightenment Midwife," Roy Porter, ed., *Medicine in the Enlightenment* (Amsterdam: Rodopi, 1995), 129. For an example of a midwife whose knowledge surpassed that of the doctors see Wendy Perkins, *Midwifery and Medicine in Early Modern France: Louise Bourgeois* (Exeter: University of Exeter Press, 1996), 111–12.

19 My own essay on London midwives was included in this book and began the revisionary process relating to this particular group of women. Doreen Evenden, "Mothers and their midwives in seventeenth-century London," Marland, ed., *The Art of Midwifery*, 9–26. David Harley's short paper on English provincial midwives, published in 1981, also attempted to revise traditional views of midwives, n.3, above. More recently, David Cressy's fine study *Birth, Marriage and Death* acknowledges the unfair treatment which historians in general have accorded English midwives in Tudor and Stuart England.

20 Hilary Marland, " 'Stately and dignified, kindly and God-fearing': midwives, age and status in the Netherlands in the eighteenth century," Hilary Marland and Margaret Pelling, eds., *The Task of Healing: Medicine, religion and gender in England and the Netherlands 1450–1800* (Rotterdam: Erasmus, 1996), 273–4.

21 Lawrence Stone, *Family, Sex and Marriage in England, 1500–1800* (Harmondsworth, Middlesex: Penguin, 1979), 64; Keith Thomas, *Religion and the Decline of Magic* (Harmondsworth, Middlesex: Penguin, 1971), 15. Thomas cites one of Willughby's most graphic vignettes in condemnation of an unnamed midwife's practices. Ralph A. Houlbrooke, *The English Family 1450–1700* (London: Longman, 1984), 129.

22 David Harley has also noted the "contempt of an earlier generation of medical historians" in depicting early modern midwives. David Harley, "English Archives, Local History, and the Study of Early Modern Midwifery," *Archives* 21 (92, October 1994): 152.

As a result of my research, I have concluded that licensed London midwives served lengthy informal apprenticeships in which the educational experience was entirely of a practical nature.[23] Similarly, women of all social classes, who were never licensed, witnessed and participated in community childbirth and, in some cases, became skilled in midwifery.

In order to set the scene for this study, which is based mainly on archival evidence, a brief sampling of printed material available to the seventeenth-century midwife in London demonstrates its character and limitations.[24] Literate midwives and other female attendants were able to utilize written medical information, but it is questionable to what extent this was either necessary or perceived as helpful when put to the test of the actual childbirth process. Certainly there existed not only a market for midwifery tracts but for a steady stream of medical works. Many of these claimed to have been written for midwives in particular and women in general, but they were only of value to the minority of women (including midwives) who were literate.[25]

EARLY MODERN MIDWIFERY TEXTS

The standard early work *The Birth of Mankind or the Woman's Book* first appeared in English translation in 1540.[26] The English edition was a translation of Rosselin's *Rosengarten* which was published in 1513 in Strassburg. Although the author, who was the City Physician of Worms, cites only classical sources, he had obviously sought the advice of midwives and women in compiling his manual, which was used by the well-trained midwives of Nuremberg in the late medieval and early modern periods.[27] The second and all subsequent editions bore the name of physician Thomas Raynald who, according to a recent analysis of textbooks of the period, probably lacked any personal experience of midwifery.[28] The prologue, addressed to "women readers," expressed its intent to assist women in understanding their own anatomy as well as conception, childbearing, and the

23 The first recorded program of instruction for midwives by a midwife which included lectures on anatomy and the use of instruments, in addition to the customary experiential teaching, would not come until the end of the eighteenth century. Margaret Stephen, *The Domestic Midwife* (London, 1795).

24 For an overview of seventeenth-century obstetrical literature, which includes most of the popular authors of the period, see Eccles, chapter 1, "English Obstetrical Textbooks Before 1740."

25 David Cressy, *Literacy and the Social Order* (Cambridge: Cambridge University Press, 1980), 147. Particularly around mid-century (when a number of midwifery publications appeared), Cressy estimates that less than 22% of women could sign their names and thus possessed, by his definition, "full literacy."

26 E. Rosselin, *The Byrth of Mankynde*, trans. Thos. Raynald (London, 1540); D'Arcy Power, "The Birth of Mankind or the Woman's Book: A Bibliographical Study," *The Library* Fourth Series, 8 (June 1927): 1–33. A recent investigation has discovered the existence of a manuscript on midwifery in English which preceded the *Birth of Mankind* by almost a hundred years. The original manuscript may have been written or translated from Latin by a woman. Beryl Rowland, *Medieval Woman's Guide to Health* (Kent: The Kent State University Press, 1981), xvi.

27 Wiesner, 100.   28 Eccles, 12.

nursing of infants.[29] This extremely popular book underwent a number of editions, the last printing appearing in 1654. The first edition was dedicated to Katherine Howard, wife of Henry VIII. In the second edition, Raynald augmented the prologue with the observation that literate women could take the book to deliveries for the edification and instruction of the presiding midwife. His advice may or may not have been followed in the seventeenth century, but it would have had limited practical value in view of the traditionally darkened chambers in which women of the period were "brought to bed."[30]

Whether or not midwives actually availed themselves of midwifery literature which might have been of value to their practice, there was the perception in some quarters that they did. According to a seventeenth-century pamphlet: "midwives sometimes have a midwives' book out of which they get their knowledge."[31] Elizabeth Harvey has found a darker side to the publication of midwifery books in the vernacular in the late sixteenth and early seventeenth centuries. She sees these books as early evidence of invasive male activity which would take them into a space previously profoundly female and presided over by midwives.[32] Harvey's argument is supported by the observation that the literature of childbirth found its main market in male readers, both professional and lay.[33]

In 1612, a translation of the French work by the physician Jacques Guillimeau, entitled *Child Birth or the Happie Deliverie of Women*, made its appearance.[34] Guillimeau acknowledged female control of the birthing process when he explained why women preferred midwives for their deliveries: ". . . Necessitie (the mistresse of Arts) hath constrained women to learn and practice Physicke, *one with another* (for reasons of modesty)."[35] Guillimeau's contribution was notable in that it contained the first description of podalic version to appear in English.[36]

---

29 In her "Introduction," Wendy Arons presents a different, less altruistic view of the author's motivation. Wendy Arons, trans., *When Midwifery Became the Male Physician's Province: The Sixteenth Century Handbook "The Rose Garden for Pregnant Women and Midwives, Newly Englished"* (Jefferson, N.C. and London: McFarland & Co. Inc., 1994).

30 Donnison, 7; Power, 4; Wilson, "The ceremony of childbirth and its interpretation," Valerie Fildes, ed., *Women as Mothers in Preindustrial England* (London and New York: Routledge, 1990), 73.

31 BL E 112, 61. From the pamphlet of an unlicensed London female medical practitioner. By the end of the eighteenth century, midwives' literacy was assumed and the pupils of one midwife-teacher were expected to compile a pocket-sized book of lecture notes which they could carry to deliveries. Stephen, 4.

32 Elizabeth Harvey, 79. See also Gail Kern Paster, *The Body Embarrassed: Drama and the Disciplines of Shame in Early Modern England* (Ithaca: Cornell University Press, 1993), 188; Sawday, especially chapter 8, "Royal Science."

33 Cressy, *Birth*, 38.

34 Jacques Guillimeau, *Child-Birth or the Happie Deliverie of Women* (London, 1612; reprint ed., Amsterdam: Theatrum Orbis Terrarum, 1972).

35 Guillimeau, 80. Emphasis mine.

36 Eccles, 12. Guillimeau, 152. Paré had earlier described this manoeuvre where the infant's foot was grasped and used to turn the child in utero in cases of malpresentation. Objections have been raised to Paré's being credited with inventing podalic version on the grounds that peasant midwives, in particular, would have had the opportunity to observe the births of animals and could

In 1617, Peter Chamberlen (a member of the previously mentioned Chamberlen family) proposed a scheme whereby London midwives would be incorporated into an association directly under his personal control. His efforts failed but his son, Dr. Peter Chamberlen, revived the plan in 1634. Some ten years after the rejection of this second attempt (supposedly intended to educate the midwives), Chamberlen published a diatribe against the midwives and physicians who had blocked his scheme.[37] The midwives rejected Chamberlen on the grounds that they had a far better knowledge of midwifery (based on practical experience) than Chamberlen. Yet Chamberlen's defence of himself and his vitriolic attack on midwives, whom he labelled "femal-Arbiters of Life and Death," reveals – despite his stated aims – no plan for implementing the so-called "education" of midwives, or affords any practical information for practising midwives.[38]

In 1651, the radical proponent of medical reform, Nicholas Culpeper, published *A Directory for Midwives* which bewailed the lack of educational opportunities for midwives.[39] There is no questioning Culpeper's genuine concern regarding the midwives' exclusion from formal education, but not only does Culpeper fail to appreciate the practical knowledge of midwives, he has, again, offered little or nothing by way of information which would be of use during child delivery. This was not surprising since, by his own admission, he had no personal experience of the process.[40] Culpeper points out the futility of midwives' approaching the monopolistic College of Physicians for assistance in upgrading their education since the physicians are interested only in making money. He suggests instead that the midwives pray for godly enlightenment in their work.

In 1656, four midwives published *The Compleat Midwife's Practice*. Two of the authors have been tentatively identified as Dina Ireland of St Brides, licensed in 1638, and Catherine Turner of St Martin in the Fields, licensed in 1632. It is obvious that, like other midwifery treatises of the period, there had been borrowing from and editing of earlier authors. But in the "Preface" the women explain why they have written the treatise:

It is high time, there being already published many Treatises of this kind, for us to discharge our consciences. . . . we have perused all that have been in this nature in English and find them strangely deficient, so crowded with unnecessary notions and dangerous mistakes,

have learned how to intervene in this way. See Bonnie Anderson and Judith Zinsser, *A History of their Own: Women in Europe from Prehistory to the Present* (New York: Harper and Row, 1988), 107. For a good description of the various techniques, including podalic version, for delivering malpresentations, see Wilson, *Man-midwifery*, 20, 21.

37 Wilson, *Man-midwifery*, 32; Peter Chamberlen, *A Voice in Rhama: or, The Crie of Women and Children* (London, 1646).
38 Aveling, *The Chamberlens*, 34–60, gives an account of this affair.
39 Nicholas Culpeper, *A Directorie for Midwives: or a Guide for Women, In their Conception, Bearing and Suckling their Children* (London, 1651). See chapter 4 for information about Culpeper's wife who was widowed at the age of 29 and subsequently became a midwife.
40 Eccles, 13.

that we thought it fit to give warning of them, that for the future the unfortunate practicers may prevent the *almost guilt* of the crying sin of murder.[41]

The women (who describe themselves as "practitioners") are critical of various works, especially Culpeper's which they find "the most desperately deficient of all."[42] On the other hand, they note that their treatise has the "approbation and good liking of sundry the most-knowing [female] Professors of midwifery now living in the City of London, and other places." This treatise contains a wealth of practical advice for the pregnant woman: how much sleep she needed (nine hours a night maximum); frequency of intercourse during pregnancy (none for the first four months); exercise (moderate for eight months, increased in the ninth month but no riding in coaches the last three months).[43]

There are the usual more technical details regarding the correction of malpresentations in which the midwife is firmly identified as the operator. In the gravest of obstetrical situations, the presence of a surgeon is acknowledged, but it is clear that the midwife will be working with him, if not actually guiding him through various procedures to deal with emergencies such as haemorrhage. A section containing a dozen or so personal case studies highlights the observed malpractice of several male midwives.[44] Written in language which was accessible to women of the period, and containing discussions which focused on peculiarly female concerns (both of client and practitioner), this small book written by and for midwives contained more valuable, practical information for childbearing women and their midwives than any number of treatises by male authors of the mid-century.[45] The treatise is all the more remarkable given the constraints placed upon women as authors or authorities in the early modern period and the resulting predominance of male-dictated prescriptive publications.[46]

De Morbeis Foeminis (The Womans Counsellour) by Massarius was translated into English in 1657. Addressed to midwives and those intending to be midwives and typical of much of the pamphlet literature of the period, it promised much, but delivered nothing instructive to women on the topic of midwifery.[47]

41 T.C., I.D., M.S., T.B., *The Compleat Midwifes Practice, In the most weighty and high Concernments of the Birth of Man* (London, 1656), "Preface." There are parallels in this work with that of Margaret Cavendish who also used women's knowledge of domestic matters to broaden their scientific horizons. Sawday, 253. In view of Sawday's arguments, it was extremely courageous of these four women to venture into the field of publication at this particular time.
42 Ibid., "Preface."   43 Ibid., 56–9.
44 There is a discussion of the place of, and hazards in, using a male midwife. T.C. et al., 125–6.
45 Eccles notes an "almost identical" work published in 1659 by "C.R." Eccles, 13. The author is, in all probability, a midwife, possibly Rachel Coles of St Martin in the Fields who was licensed in 1662, but who had many years of experience as a midwife at the time of her licensing. GL MS 10,116/2.
46 Hence the use of initials or, in some cases, anonymity of authorship for women writers. See Suzanne W. Hull, *Chaste, Silent and Obedient: English Books for Women 1475–1640* (San Marino: Huntington Library, 1982), 133–7, for a discussion of the male as instructor and author.
47 A. Massarius, *De Morbeis Foeminis. The Womans Counsellour or the Feminine Physitian.* Trans. R.T. (London, 1657).

Dr. William Sermon published *The Ladies Companion or the English Midwife* in 1671. Much of Sermon's treatise is a virtual paraphrase of the above midwives' publication of 1656, *Compleat Midwife's Practice*, especially those sections relating to the actual conduct of labour and delivery.[48] Sermon's work is not aimed as specifically at female practitioners. This is evident in the more general nature of his directions for such things as the preparation of liniment or in his language when he talks of how short the umbilical cord should be cut.[49] Sermon's inclusion of material obviously intended for midwives could well have been an attempt to disclose to male midwives, surgeons, and physicians, the way that a normal delivery should be managed. Aside from the parts taken from the midwives' publication, Sermon's work is typical of the medical literature of the day (both lay and professional) which was an untidy mixture of Galenic or humoral theory, superstition, and, in a few cases, common sense.[50] It has been dismissed as primarily designed to advertise Sermon's cathartic and diuretic pills and, indeed, Sermon's main qualification seems to have been his cure of the Duke of Albermarle who had suffered from dropsy.[51]

The best known seventeenth-century textbook on midwifery written by a woman was published in London in 1671.[52] Jane Sharp, its author, had been a midwife for more than thirty years. As a literate individual, with at least a basic level of education, she stressed that a midwife needed practical as well as theoretical knowledge, but accepted the fact that women could not aspire to the educational opportunities which were afforded to men.[53] Sharp believed that publications such as her *Midwives Book* would help to rectify what she perceived as the deficiencies in midwives' training, although she went to great lengths to

---

48 William Sermon, *The Ladies Companion or the English Midwife* (London, 1671).

49 The midwives' receipt for liniment supplies details like cutting the capon or goose grease "into little pieces," and melting them in an "earthenware dish." T.C. et al., 58. Elizabeth Harvey has noted that the prefaces to midwifery books reveal that male translators were aiming at a far wider audience than midwives. Indeed, in one instance from the year 1637, the translator seems to be suggesting that with the better information he is providing, male midwives could make more money. Harvey, 89, 91.

50 Despite Harvey's discoveries about the circulatory system, the medical theory based on body "humours" (blood, bile, urine, and phlegm), and associated with the ancients such as Galen, still held sway in the seventeenth century.

51 Eccles, 14.

52 For a discussion of Sharp's text as a critique of male medical knowledge, see Eve Keller, "Mrs Jane Sharp: midwifery and the critique of medical knowledge in seventeenth-century England," *Women's Writing*, vol. 2 (no. 2, 1995): 101–11. See also Helen King " 'As if None Understood the Art that Cannot Understand Greek': The Education of Midwives in Seventeenth-Century England," Vivian Nutton and Roy Porter, eds., *The History of Medical Education in Britain* (Amsterdam: Rodopi, 1995), 184–98.

53 Like many other experienced midwives, Jane Sharp almost certainly passed on her skills and knowledge to a family member, possibly her daughter or more likely, her daughter-in-law. In keeping with the practice of several midwives who remembered an associate in their wills, midwife Anne Parrott of St Clement Danes left a small bequest to "Sarah Sharpe the daughter of Jane Sharpe." GL MS 9172/88.

stress that practical skill was more important in the final analysis.[54] Described as containing "much good sense," like other medical and midwifery treatises of the period, it was marred by superstition.[55]

Sharp has been criticised for her seeming unawareness of podalic version, but this was a shortcoming which was shared by most of the midwifery authors of the period.[56] Moreover, one of the foremost advocates of podalic version in theory, Percival Willughby, seldom used the manoeuvre in practice, possibly because of a perceived danger to the life of the mother.[57] The famous early seventeenth-century French midwife, Louise Bourgeois, described podalic version in her first book of *Observations diverses* in 1609, and English translations appeared later in the century. The four midwives, whose treatise of 1656 included some of Bourgeois's writings, recommend podalic version in specific situations.[58] Although experienced midwives had undoubtedly acquired expertise in emergencies involving malpresentation, Bourgeois's book as well as the London midwives' publication provided literate midwives with a reliable confirmation of the technical aspects of the manoeuvre.[59]

In 1680, C.R. published *The Complete Midwives Practice Enlarged*. Its introduction bore the initials of five other individuals; at least four of the five were, in all likelihood, midwives from St Martin in the Fields. Rachel Coles, Jane Davis, Mary Stuart, and Margaret Hall were all licensed in 1662.[60] In addition to the customary rehashing of available midwifery treatises, it too has included information by "the Queen of France's midwife" and contains homely advice which sets it apart from the male-authored treatises. Not only is the principal purported author (Coles) a midwife, she mentions that her daughter is also a midwife.[61]

Two translations of Mauriceau's work produced by Hugh Chamberlen have been judged to be the first "satisfactory" English textbooks on the topic of midwifery but they did not appear until 1673 and 1683.[62] However, there is no

54 Jane Sharp, *The Midwives Book* (London, 1671; reprint ed. New York: Garland Publishing, Inc., 1985), 2–5. Although Sharp began practising in the years when ecclesiastical licensing was interrupted, unlike at least some other venerable midwives, to our knowledge, she did not acquire a license in the Restoration period. Like so many other midwives, she may have been widowed and remarried, her licence having been issued at the time of her first marriage.

55 Donnison, 15.

56 Eccles seems to believe that since Paré's work on podalic version appeared in translation in 1612, the midwife should have known about it. Indeed, Sharp does describe different malpresentations and how they could be corrected, but her descriptions are very brief so that what may be a description of podalic version (201), is not adequately explained. Perhaps midwife Sharp felt that any experienced midwife would know what to do in the various situations which she described very matter-of-factly (199–204). For a brief appraisal of Sharp's work, see Elaine Hobby, *Virtue of Necessity* (London: Virago Press, 1988), 185–7.

57 Wilson, "Childbirth," 293.

58 The midwives describe a number of malpresentations, but in only two cases recommend what can be described as podalic version: for knee presentations and in the delivery of twins. T.C. et al., 122, 126. They also describe cephalic version, to be used in a number of situations.

59 Wendy Perkins, *Midwifery and Medicine*, 25.   60 GL MS 10,116/1.

61 C.R., *The Complete Midwives Practice Enlarged* (London, 1680).

62 Eccles, 14. Eccles has not taken the treatise by the four midwives into account in her evaluation.

way of assessing their impact, if any, on the quality of midwifery practised in the last quarter of the seventeenth century in England's capital.

At the end of the century, John Pechey, M.D. published *Compleat Midwife's Practice Enlarged—Containing a Perfect Directory or Rules for Midwives and Nurses*.[63] Intended to instruct midwives, critical of previously published works, and purportedly endorsed by practitioners long dead, Pechey's treatise continued to propagate the errors typical of the period in his work which was obviously "borrowed" from earlier authors.[64] He advocated, for example, that a *placenta praevia* should be "cut off" by the midwife, a manoeuvre which would have resulted in instant death for the infant.[65] Pechey, moreover, ridiculed the advice of midwives who urged their clients to eat a good diet in the postpartum period to compensate for blood lost at the time of delivery since he considered what was lost "unnecessary blood."[66]

Despite his obvious bias against many midwives, especially those in the country, Percival Willughby's writings contained useful observations on the work of child delivery. At least four manuscript copies of Willughby's treatise were produced, but inasmuch as the work was not published until the nineteenth century, the information about his practical experience could not have been widely disseminated before that time.[67]

We cannot say with certainty what practising midwives actually read about midwifery, although the four midwives who published the treatise for their colleagues in 1656 noted that they were writing not only out of the experience of the English, but also from the experience of "the most accomplisht and absolute Practicers among the French, Spanish, Italian and other nations."[68] This would indicate a remarkable awareness, not only of English midwifery publications, but also of those originating on the continent.[69]

With a medical profession still in the thrall of Galenic, Aristotelian, and Hippocratic teachings and whose anatomical dissections were limited by widespread

---

63 John Pechey, *Compleat Midwife's Practice Enlarged* (London, 1698).

64 Although Pechey acknowledged Mayerne, Chamberlen, and Culpeper (who died in 1654), parts of the treatise are drawn almost word for word from the work of William Sermon (see above).

65 Pechey, 131. This is the condition where the placenta is situated over the internal orifice of the uterus.

66 Ibid., 148. Another example of the way in which midwives' common sense advice was devalued by doctors was reported by the Rev. John Ward. He noted that midwives who urged their clients to obtain exercise by walking in the last two months of pregnancy (to facilitate labour and delivery) were belittled by the doctors. Rev. John Ward, *Diary of the Rev. John Ward A.M.: Vicar of Stratford-on-Avon 1648–79*, C. Severn, ed. (London: Henry Colborn Pub., 1839), 255. For examples of the early twentieth-century common-sense midwifery practices of a highly successful North American midwife, see Onnie Lee Logan, as told to Katherine Clark, *Motherwit: An Alabama Midwife's Story* (New York: E. P. Dutton, 1989).

67 John L. Thornton, "The First Printed English Edition of 'Observations in Midwifery By Percival Willughby (1596–1685),' " *Practitioner* 208 (1972): 296.

68 T.C. et al., "Preface."

69 Their claims gain credibility from the inclusion of the work of renowned French midwife Louise Bourgeois.

prejudices against the practice, seventeenth-century midwives received little or no practical help from the male medical professionals.[70] Throughout the century, midwives clearly relied, for the most part, on oral traditional knowledge conveyed through their own network and frequently through a close association with a senior midwife, who, in some cases was their mother. This traditional knowledge supplemented what their own eyes, minds, and hands taught them about the process of childbirth.[71]

THE SUBJECTS OF THE STUDY

This study, which focuses on the midwives of London, examines their licensing under the auspices of the Church of England, their system of training, their clients, and their social and economic world.[72] Extensive use was made of ecclesiastical records, churchwardens' accounts, vestry minutes, tithe rolls, tax records (such as lay subsidy, hearth tax assessments, and the 1695 "marriage duty" act), as well as wills.[73] Midwives' case and account books, seventeenth-century diaries, and published material were also scrutinised. In particular, the midwives' testimonial certificates were intensively analysed in an attempt to recover the lives of hundreds of women from anonymity and to redress the inequities imposed by neglect and selective reading of only a few seventeenth-century sources. The archival evidence of, and about, these female practitioners and their clients as individuals plays a key role in the history of early modern English midwifery.[74] It is a social history of midwives of a particular and important metropolis and cannot be taken as representative of midwives outside its confines. Moreover, the technical details of midwifery are difficult to retrieve since most midwives left no records about what they actually did for patients. Midwifery and giving birth were women's business and women kept their secrets. In Chapter 3, however, there is a reconstruction of

70 Eccles, 23–5. For the continuing difficulties faced by anatomists in the eighteenth and nineteenth centuries, Peter Linebaugh, "The Tyburn Riot against the Surgeons," D. Hay, et al., *Albion's Fatal Tree* (London: Pantheon Books, 1975), 65–117; Ruth Richardson, *Death, Dissection and the Destitute* (Harmondsworth: Penguin, 1989).
71 Helen King has concluded that midwifery texts were not only useless, they were expendable in view of the practical training which London midwives enjoyed. King, " 'As if none understood the Art,' " 191. Cressy has come to very similar conclusions. Cressy, *Birth*, 36.
72 Willughby acknowledged that London midwives had different standards of training and performance from those of provincial midwives. Willughby, 45, 73, 239.
73 For a discussion of churchwardens' accounts, vestry minutes, and other parish ecclesiastical records, see W. E. Tate, *The Parish Chest* (Cambridge: University Press, 1946).
74 As a case in point which demonstrates the need for such a study, a recent attempt to reconstruct childbirth from the mother's point of view was based on standard sources, written, in the main, by men. Adrian Wilson, "Participant or patient? Seventeenth-century childbirth from the mother's point of view," Roy Porter, ed., *Patients and Practitioners: Lay Perceptions of Medicine in Pre-Industrial Society* (Cambridge: Cambridge University Press, 1985), 129–44. Roy Porter, in particular, has been critical of the way in which social historians of medicine have neglected the patient's viewpoint in their studies. For Porter's contribution toward rectifying the imbalance, see Roy and Dorothy Porter, *In Sickness and in Health: the British Experience 1650–1850* (London: Fourth Estate, 1988). See also his introduction to *Patients and Practitioners*.

the midwife's role in the birthing chamber. Similarly, this study does not attempt to assess the merits of midwives by analysing estimated case loads or maternal death rates. For the most part, the sources do not lend themselves to methodologies which address such concerns, although some conclusions will be drawn about infant mortality as it relates to an anonymous midwife's late seventeenth- and early eighteenth-century practice.[75]

Aside from Quakers, there is only limited evidence about London midwives of other religious persuasions. As a result, the study concentrates on midwives licensed under the aegis of the Church of England.[76] When Thomas Taylor, the minister of St Olave Silver Street, supplied Mary Taylor with a testimonial statement in 1661, he stressed the fact that she was "no papist," indicating the Church's stance that Roman Catholics should be excluded from licensing.[77] There is no record of the licensing of Elizabeth Cellier, the highly visible seventeenth-century midwife and author who was a convert to Catholicism.[78] Recusant wives,

---

75 Adrian Wilson has been a strong proponent of attempting to establish annual case loads in order to assess not only the ability, but the essence of the "typical" early modern midwife. However, the idea of a "typical" midwife whose identity is tied solely to the number of deliveries which she carries out per year is unhelpful; the endeavour is also fraught with problems, some of which have been pointed out by B. and J. Boss in "Ignorant Midwives – a Further Rejoinder," *The Society for the Social History of Medicine* Bulletin 33 (December 1983): 71. The Bosses were responding to Adrian Wilson, "Ignorant Midwives – a Rejoinder," *The Society for the Social History of Medicine* Bulletin 32 (June 1983): 48. As an example of the pitfalls bedevilling such manipulations, see Wilson's attempts to establish annual delivery rates for male midwife William Giffard. Wilson has made a number of suppositions or guesses about Giffard's incomplete records, enabling him to arrive at annual delivery rates of "perhaps 80–90 per year." On the other hand, Wilson did not attempt to make any such allowances for a female midwife whose domestic responsibilities almost certainly led to career interruptions, but whose annual rate of delivery in many years was considerably higher than the "only about 23 births per year" with which Wilson credits her. Conclusions based on this type of juggling must be viewed as profoundly flawed. See Wilson, *Male-midwifery*, 94, 35, 43: n.89. For a discussion of mortality in childbed, see B. M. Willmott Dobbie, "An Attempt to estimate the true rate of maternal mortality, sixteenth to eighteenth centuries," *Medical History* 26 (1982): 79–90; R. Schofield, "Did the Mothers really die?", L. Bonfield, ed., *The World We Have Gained* (Oxford: Basil Blackwell, 1986), 231–60. Schofield concludes that the risk to the mother while higher than today, was not as high as previously believed, 260. For an earlier estimate of maternal mortality, see Thomas R. Forbes, *Chronicle from Aldgate* (New Haven and London: Yale University Press, 1971), 106. On infant mortality, see Roger Schofield and E. A. Wrigley, "Infant and child mortality in England in the late Tudor and early Stuart Period," Charles Webster, ed., *Health, Medicine and Mortality in the Sixteenth Century* (Cambridge: Cambridge University Press, 1979), 61–95.

76 The late Miss E. R. Poyser, archivist of the Westminster Diocesan Archives in London, had no knowledge of any records which would cast light upon seventeenth-century recusant midwives. Anne Giardina Hess has worked on Quaker records for her study which concentrates mainly on rural midwives. Ann Giardina Hess, "Community Case Studies of Midwives from England and New England c. 1650–1720" (Ph.D. dissertation, Cambridge University, 1993). Quaker birth records, while naming the midwife, do not contain the rich information found in the London testimonials used for this study of midwives licensed by the Church of England.

77 GL MS 10,116/1.

78 The fact that Cellier was thrice married could also be a reason that no record of her licensing was found, but she never describes herself as a "licensed midwife" as did most of the women who had obtained licences. For an interesting perspective on Cellier, see Helen King, "The politick midwife: models of midwifery in the work of Elizabeth Cellier," Hilary Marland, ed., *Art of Midwifery,*

among the most ardent defenders of the Roman Church, strongly resisted engaging a midwife sworn to uphold the tenets of the Church of England.[79] In at least one instance in the sixteenth century, a "papist" midwife was granted a bishop's licence to practise midwifery, but the circumstances appear to have been unusual.[80]

There is the occasional mention of a Quaker midwife in personal papers of the period such as the diary of the wife of Dr. Francis Turner, Dean of Windsor in 1678, or the Verney family records which refer to a skillful Quaker midwife who was paid fees of £5, £10, and £20 by Edmund Verney for deliveries, but who refused traditional gifts from godparents on religious grounds.[81] Although Quaker midwives living in London are not the central concern of this study, which draws largely upon licensing records generated by the Church of England, in Chapter 3, evidence from Quaker records will demonstrate unexpected connections between Quaker mothers and London midwives licensed by the Church of England.[82]

115–30. See also J. Elise Gordon, "Mrs. Elizabeth Cellier – 'the Popish Midwife' of the Restoration," *Midwife, Health Visitor & Community Nurse*, 2 (May 1975): 139. For a full description of the "popish plot" and Cellier's role, see J. C. H. Aveling, *The Handle and the Axe: The Catholic Recusants in England from Reformation to Emancipation* (London: Blond and Briggs, 1976), 204–21.

79 John Bossy, *The English Catholic Community 1570–1850* (London: Darton, Longman and Todd, 1975); Marie B. Rowlands, "Recusant Women 1560–1640," Mary Prior, ed., *Women in English Society 1500–1800* (London: Methuen, 1985), 149–80. The stillborn child of a Catholic gentlewoman delivered by a midwife who was a vicar's wife became the unfortunate subject of a tract published in 1646 under the title *A Declaration of a strange and wonderful Monster*. The woman's alleged defence of her recusancy was blamed for the fact that the child was reportedly born without a head. R. C. Richardson, *Puritanism in north-west England* (Manchester: Manchester University Press, 1972), 166–7.

80 Aveling, *English Midwives*, 19. Jane Scarisbrycke in West Derby was the midwife in question. Apparently many recusant gentlewomen "assisted poor women in child bed." The Countess of Arundel, for example, assisted a poor vagrant female who gave birth in the "cage" (a structure for confining felons in full public view) on the busy thoroughfare between Hammersmith and London. Rowlands, 164. For the description of a sixteenth- and early seventeenth-century recusant gentlewoman, Dorothy Lawson, who lived in the country and ministered to the sick and needy, see Sister Joseph Damien Hanlon, "These be But Women," Charles H. Carter, ed., *From the Renaissance to the Counter Reformation* (New York: Random House, 1965). Despite the wealth of information in Boulton's recent study of Southwark, the question of who delivered the women of the wealthy and influential Catholic Montague family remains a tantalizing enigma. Jeremy Boulton, *Neighbourhood and Society: A London suburb in the Seventeenth Century* (Cambridge: Cambridge University Press, 1987), 266. Later in the century, there is evidence that midwives from the City on occasion travelled to Southwark to deliver women, but such a large and growing population must have also demanded midwifery services from midwives who lived in the area. Bossy's maps of the distribution of Roman Catholics indicate that they were relatively sparsely settled in the London area, which leads to the conclusion that there were correspondingly fewer popish midwives in London compared with the provinces.

81 Unfortunately Mrs. Turner did not survive the delivery. Rev. Edward Lake, *Diary of the Rev. Edward Lake (1641–1704)* (Camden Miscellany ser.1 Vol.39, 1847; reprint New York: Johnson Reprint Corporation), 22. Frances P. Verney and M. M. Verney, *The Verney Memoirs*, vol. 2 (London: Longmans, Green and Co., 1925), 277.

82 A local study of rural Quaker midwives has revealed similarities with non-Quaker midwifery practice, Ann Giardina Hess, "Midwifery practice among the Quakers in southern rural England in the late seventeenth century," Marland, ed., *The Art of Midwifery*, 49–76.

Seventeenth-century clergy might hope to persuade Quaker midwives to apply for an ecclesiastical licence, but Benjamin Younge, rector of Enfield, described Quakers as "stubborn and infractory" when confronted with the requirement of a midwifery licence.[83] On the other hand, Quaker women were not reluctant to call on the services of competent licensed London midwives outside their own religious persuasion, and conforming and nonconforming midwives attended deliveries together as circumstances dictated.

Despite the prominent role assigned by historians to events connected to the civil war years, its impact on the lives of London midwives left few traces. Certainly, no fighting took place in London or its suburbs, and the civilian population was left largely undisturbed. Even so, the civil war was perceived in some quarters as affecting midwives' practises, as evidenced by the handbill in the form of a "petition" reputedly submitted by the midwives of London to Parliament in 1643. In it, they demanded that the war be stopped because their business was suffering with so many husbands called away at the behest of the military.[84] Aside from dealing with a few individual instances where the war touched the lives of midwives, no evidence has come to our attention that the actual work of child delivery was affected by the events of the war years.[85]

In what follows a picture of seventeenth-century London midwives will emerge that takes into account their training in a well-developed, albeit unofficial, system of apprenticeship under senior midwives. Within this system, most women had many years of practical experience as deputy midwives before obtaining an ecclesiastical licence. Licensing depended not only on proof of character and church attendance, but also on competence. Indeed, there is evidence to support the argument that competence was more important than moral rectitude in the minds of many, including at least some church officials. The stereotype of the poor and inadequate midwife will disappear. London midwives were economically viable and generally of the middle class. Some were married to gentlemen as well as professional men. A number were wealthy widows while others were married to men of substance who held positions of the highest responsibility in their respective parishes. Undoubtedly, there were midwives at work in London who lacked the qualifications required for licensing, and others who were qualified, but not

83 GL MS 10,116/9.

84 Anon., *The Midwives Just Petition* (London, 1643). Generally considered to be a parody, there may be a germ of truth in the pamphlet.

85 See Christopher Durston, *The Family in the English Revolution* (Oxford: Basil Blackwell, 1989), 111–18, for speculation about the effect of the war and midwives' ability to carry out their work. One delivery affected by war-time conditions was the birth of Princess Henrietta at Exeter. The Queen was en route to Cornwall and embarkation for France. She was attended by John Hinton, physician-in-ordinary to the King and who, in all likelihood, had no experience of child delivery. Sir John Hinton, *Memoirs of Sir John Hinton, Physitian in ordinary to His Majesties Person* (London: T. Bentley, 1814), 18. Although the practice of midwifery was not affected by the events of the civil war, the licensing process was. See Chapter 1, n. 1.

motivated to apply for licences. As the ensuing chapters will show, these were in the minority.

Settled parish poor were entitled to the services of accredited midwives, and the transient poor could take comfort in the fact of the midwife's oath, which bound her to serve the poor as well as the rich. I do not believe that the midwives examined in this study were an élite amongst London midwives, but that London was a special, and in many ways remarkable, urban centre which had the good fortune to be served by a force of respected and well-trained midwives. No such claims are posited for midwives outside its general confines, although studies of provincial midwives have demonstrated striking similarities as well as differences.[86]

SOURCES AND METHODOLOGY

This investigation of seventeenth-century London midwives began with a search of ecclesiastical records to uncover the names of women who had been granted licences by the Church of England to practise midwifery. The registers of both the Bishop of London and the Archbishop of Canterbury, and testimonial certificates from the jurisdictions of London, Canterbury, and the Peculiar of the Deanery and Chapter of St Paul contain evidence central to this study of seventeenth-century London midwives. The registers of the diocese of London and the archdiocese of Canterbury are the only surviving records which provide evidence of midwifery licensing during the first four decades of the seventeenth century. The names of midwives who were licensed in the diocese of London are scattered throughout the Vicar General's records pertaining to the business of the consistory courts. Commencing in 1607 and ending in 1641, the names of at least 170 women who were licensed as midwives in this jurisdiction appear. Despite suggestions that licensing of London midwives did not commence until the second decade of the century, the names of some sixteen women who were licensed in the diocese of London in the years 1607–10 have been recorded.[87] The registers of Archbishops Abbott and Laud have disclosed another twenty London midwives who were licensed in the years covered by the registers of 1611–45.[88]

The quality of the evidence in both sets of registers from the early decades of the century is variable. For the first fifteen or twenty years, the clerks were relatively careful about transferring evidence from the midwives' testimonial certificates (which no longer survive) into the registers. The entries include the

---

86 See the work of Ann Giardina Hess and David Harley, for example.
87 Wilson, "Childbirth," 62; GLRO DL/C 339/9–167, passim.
88 We have not included in this figure the half dozen or so women from Kent, Dorset, and Hertfordshire who were licensed in this jurisdiction because no evidence has been uncovered that they practised in London. Lambeth Palace Library, Registers of Archbishop George Abbott (1611–33) vols.1–3, Archbishop William Laud (1633–45) (no vol. no.). The last recorded pre-civil war midwifery license was issued in this jurisdiction in 1637.

names of the six women who were giving sworn evidence of the midwife's competence and sometimes included their husbands' occupations, the names of church officials, and information about senior midwives and associates. In some cases, useful information of a qualitative nature has been included, such as a midwife's age and the association with a senior midwife for training purposes. Toward the end of the second decade, there are signs of carelessness in the recording process.[89] Despite various omissions and the limitations they impose upon quantification, these early entries are useful in identifying a substantial number of early modern midwives who would otherwise go unrecognized. In some cases, midwives who were licensed in this early period have been identified as still active in the Restoration years; in at least one case, a matriarchal link between three generations of midwives has been established.

The absence of documentary evidence for the period 1642–60 is in keeping with a complete breakdown in the ecclesiastical licensing process during the civil war period, a breakdown which extended until the period of episcopal restoration. The last midwifery licence recorded before the hiatus was that issued to Mary Hubbard of St Brigid's parish in January 1641.[90] Hubbard's licence is followed by several blank pages in the register, presumably indicative of a break in the licensing process. The next recorded licence was that granted to Elizabeth Dowke of the parish of St Bartholomew the Great by the chancellor Richard Chaworth in January 1661.[91] Although Elizabeth Cellier, London midwife, wrote in 1688 that midwives were examined and licensed at "Chirurgeon's Hall" during the hiatus in ecclesiastical licensing, the extant records of the Barber-Surgeon's Company offer no support for Cellier's allegation.[92]

For the period after the Restoration, there is valuable documentary evidence in the form of both registers and testimonials. In the diocese of London, there are 439 surviving midwives' testimonial certificates for the years 1661–99. Only 164 of these midwives, however, are found in the bishops' and archbishops' registers for the period. The 275 names which have not been entered were victims of a faulty process whereby information received by the court apparently did not reach the recording clerks.[93] In 1669, for example, the testimonial certificates of eight

---

89 Occasionally, the midwife's parish has been left out or only three clients' names were shown. By 1624, in some cases, merely the customary heading with the midwife's name and parish appears with the body of the text omitted. In 1627, 1628, and 1629, lapses again occur, with only the midwife's name and in some, but not all, cases the parish appearing. In 1633, there are more examples of unfinished entries where the text trails off and space has been left for more information which, unfortunately, has never been added.

90 GLRO MS DL/C/344/97v.   91 GLRO MS DL/C/344/121.

92 Elizabeth Cellier, *To Dr. – an answer to His Queries, Concerning the Colledg of Midwives* (London, 1688). Cellier's tract is dated January 16, 1687, which was the old style of dating. I am grateful to Ian Murray, archivist at Barber-Surgeons' Hall, London, for searching their records.

93 We can be confident that it was a defect in the recording procedure and not the failure of the court to issue a licence which resulted in the discrepancy between registers and testimonials because, in almost all of the 275 cases, the chancellor himself or his surrogate has clearly written

women are plainly identified as having been licensed by the abbreviation "lic.," followed by the signature of Chancellor Thomas Exton, but none of their names appear in the Vicar General's register.[94]

Similarly, a comparison between the testimonial certificates preserved at Lambeth Palace Library and the archbishops' registers shows that twelve of the sixty-one women whose testimonials are extant from the years 1669–1700 are not recorded as licensed midwives in the register. Once again, in every case, their testimonial certificates are clearly signed by the chancellor (in five cases by Thomas Exton) as an indication that they have been sworn before him as midwives.[95] Surprisingly, a number of London parishes failed to yield the name of a single midwife throughout the century. (See Appendices H and I.)

A total of 521 testimonial certificates from the period 1661–1700 forms a major source for observations about the licensing, training, and clientele of seventeenth-century London midwives. In addition to the midwives recorded in registers and testimonial certificates, visitation records disclosed the names of other midwives practising in London in the seventeenth century. Court depositions, diaries, letters, and biographies have also revealed the names of London midwives, swelling the list to almost 1,200 names (and still growing) from which a "directory" of London midwives has been compiled. This directory contains the name of the midwife and her spouse, the year of licensing (or first reference), and the parish of residence (see Appendix I).[96]

In order to "flesh out" the formal ecclesiastical records which form the basis for a recreation of the socioeconomic lives of London midwives, a smaller group of midwives was selected as candidates for a prosobiographical methodology. This core group, drawn from 11 of the 97 intramural parishes and 1 of the 13 extramural parishes and representing a broad spectrum of demographic, economic, and social attributes, became the focus of a more intensive search for wills, tax levies,

---

on the testimonial certificate the date which the women (both midwives and clients) appeared before him and were sworn, in the same way as he has done for the 164 names which were registered.

94 GL MS 10,116/6. Additional proof of an unreliable system of recording lies in the fact that no midwives' licences were recorded at all for thirteen years within the periods 1664–1668, 1671–1672, and 1680–1685, and yet there are dozens of surviving testimonials from these years, all duly signed by the chancellor and noting that licences were issued.

95 Two of these are from locations some distance from London, one from an unnamed parish, one from St Sepulchre in 1666, well before the other testimonials which have been preserved, and one from St Sepulchre in 1679 whose testimonials were apparently lost. Five names appear in the registers for whom no testimonials survive. For the twenty testimonials from the Peculiar of the Deanery and Chapter of St Paul, 1664–98, we have no register for comparison but, once again, believe them to be a reliable source about licensed midwives in view of the evidence, not only from the jurisdictions of London and Canterbury, but because they bear the signature of a court official in all but one or two cases and it is unlikely that the testimonials of women who failed to receive their licences would be preserved.

96 The directory provides a basic reference aid, and is similar in concept to John Raach, *A Directory of English Country Physicians 1603–1643* (London: Dawsons of Pall Mall, 1962).

and information contained in other parish records such as churchwardens' accounts and vestry minutes. The result is a brief biography for each of seventy-six midwives.[97] The parish became the organizing unit for this segment of the study and parishes were chosen according to size and wealth. (See Table I.1: Core Parishes.)[98] The parish's location within the City itself influenced not only the size, but the wealth of the parish, and parishes included in this study lie close to the centre of the City as well as at the periphery to the east, west, north, and south. (See Figure I.1: Map of Selected Parishes.)[99]

Aside from the usual difficulties besetting the historian attempting to bring seventeenth-century society to life, midwives of the period present particular problems. These arise in many cases from the very ubiquity of the work in which they were engaged. Although records of the parish such as vestry minutes and churchwardens' accounts contain valuable information about midwives in their professional role, they seldom give the midwife's name; she was usually identified, as "the midwife." Married women rarely appeared on tithe or tax rolls under their own names; fortunately, we have identified the names of many men who were married to midwives. Because midwifery was not organized into a craft guild or company, and midwives never became citizens and freemen of the City, few midwives designated themselves by occupation for purposes of a census or for taxation. For example the "marriage duty" Act of 1695, generally regarded as a reliable, if incomplete, late seventeenth-century source, lists only one midwife – this at a time when licensing records and testimonials show that there were at least 123 midwives licensed by the Bishop of London alone in the years 1685–1700.[100] A comprehensive study of a large suburban London parish in the seventeenth century listed 123 occupational and social categories, but failed to acknowledge the existence of a single midwife in a period which saw the area's population

97 The quality of biography varies from midwife to midwife. Jeremy Boulton has attempted the same type of reconstruction for one seventeenth-century Boroughside inhabitant and points out the difficulties in attempting record linkage over a long period of time such as we have attempted in this study. Boulton, 7,8.
98 A balance had to be struck between a suitable number of midwives and the quality of existing parish records. Important parish records were missing for some parishes which boasted goodly numbers of midwives nicely distributed across the century; conversely, superb records survived for parishes in which no trace of a midwife had been found. Having made the accommodation between numbers of midwives and availability of records, other factors were considered to ensure that the core group was as representative as possible, displaying a wide range of socioeconomic and demographic features. Categories were adapted from Tai Liu, *Puritan London: A Study of Religion and Society in the City Parishes* (Newark, N.J.: University of Delaware Press and Associated University Presses, 1986), 23–43.
99 Emrys Jones, "London in the Early Seventeenth Century: An Ecological Approach," *London Journal* 6 (1980): 123–33. Jones's study encompasses the work of Vance and Sjoberg and, more recently, Valerie Pearl.
100 Roger Finlay, *Population and Metropolis: the Demography of London 1580–1650* (Cambridge: Cambridge University Press, 1981), 73. D. V. Glass, *London Inhabitants Within the Walls 1695* (London: London Record Society 1972), 226.

Table I.1. *Core Parishes*

Parish	Size	Socioeconomic category
Intramural		
Allhallows the Less	ii	poor
St Andrew Wardrobe	iv	poor
St Anne Blackfriars	iv	poor
St Bartholomew by the Exchange	ii	mixed (poor predominate)
St Ethelburgha	iii	poor
St Gregory by St. Pauls	iv	rich
St John the Baptist	iii	rich
St Katherine Coleman	iii	poor
St Martin Outwich	i	mixed (wealthy predominate)
St Mary Aldermanbury	ii	rich
St Olave Silver Street	iii	poor
Extramural		
St Dunstan in the West	iv	rich

Note: Group i: parishes with no more than 50 tithable houses; group ii: parishes with about 60–100 tithable houses; group iii: parishes with about 100–200 tithable houses; group iv: parishes with more than 200 tithable houses.
Source: All of the foregoing categories were adapted from Tai Liu, *Puritan London: A Study of Religion and Society in the City Parishes* (Newark, N.J.: University of Delaware Press and Associated University Presses, 1986), 23–43.

more than treble from that of the mid-sixteenth century.[101] Historians generally have failed to acknowledge the special skills and status of seventeenth-century midwives with the result that midwives have been lumped together with nurses and other lay practitioners in general studies, making it impossible to identify midwives as such.[102] More recently, however, Peter Earle's study of London inhabitants based on court depositions has uncovered information relating to more than twenty women described as midwives. Earle has also recognized that London midwifery was a "high status" occupation.[103]

101 Boulton, 59, 184–6. This neglect of midwives is typical of occupational analyses of the period, but more problematic in this study where the practice of "churching" Southwark mothers (in which the midwife traditionally played an active role) receives considerable attention. Boulton, 276–9.
102 For example, Charles Webster, *Health, Medicine and Mortality in the Sixteenth Century* (Cambridge: Cambridge University Press, 1979), 182–3, 235; Margaret Pelling, "Occupational Diversity: Barber-surgeons and the Trades of Norwich, 1550–1640," *Bulletin of the History of Medicine* 56 (1982): 508.
103 Peter Earle, *A City Full of People: Men and Women of London 1650–1750* (London: Methuen, 1994), 119, 120. Four of the women had ecclesiastical licences and one was probably a nonconformist.

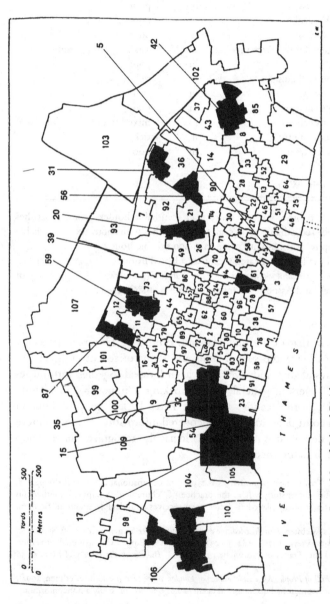

Figure I.I. *Map of Selected Parishes*

5. Allhallows the Less   20. St Bartholomew by the Exchange   42. St Katherine Coleman   39. St John Baptist

15. St Andrew Wardrobe   35. St Gregory by St Paul's   56. St Martin Outwich   87. St Olave Silver Street

17. St Anne Blackfriars   31. St Ethelburga   59. St Mary Aldermanbury   106. St Dunstan in the West

Source: Adapted with kind permission from Tai Liu. *Puritan London: A Study of Religion and Society in the City Parishes*. Newark: University of Delaware Press and Associated Presses, 1986.

In summary, this study will address in turn the themes of ecclesiastical licensing of midwives, the system of unofficial apprenticeship in which London midwives trained, the midwives' clients, the social world of the larger population of London midwives and, in greater depth, the socioeconomic circumstances of midwives in twelve selected parishes. In addition to a directory containing information about almost 1,200 midwives (Appendix I), appendices will present documentary evidence relating to ecclesiastical licensing, as well as copies of a midwife's estate inventory. Aside from the chapter on ecclesiastical licensing, a topic which has received attention from a number of historians, the remaining chapters will move into virtually uncharted waters in an attempt to redress the injustices created by many centuries of neglect and misunderstanding.

1

Ecclesiastical Licensing of Midwives

Licensing of midwives was the responsibility of the Church of England throughout the seventeenth century, with the exception of the years 1641–61 when the Church's authority collapsed along with the breakdown of the monarchical regime. Ecclesiastical licensing of midwives was reinstated with surprising alacrity less than nine months after the Book of Common Prayer was restored to usage, and at least six women from London and its suburbs were licensed by the Church in January 1661.[1] Although the ecclesiastical licensing process continued outside of London until the last decades of the eighteenth century, within the capital itself the system was obsolete by the end of the 1720s.[2]

The English system of ecclesiastical control of midwifery licensing set it apart from its counterparts on the continent. In France, where Henry III introduced legislation regulating the midwives of Paris and vicinity in 1560, midwives were subject to the composite authority of Church and State as well as local governing bodies.[3] Italian midwives in the seventeenth century, while under ecclesiastical control by parish priests supported by synodal injunctions, were not issued formal licences on a national level.[4] The majority of Spanish midwives were supervised by physicians throughout the seventeenth and the first half of the eighteenth centuries[5] while Germany favoured municipal control of mid-

1 GL MS 10,116/1; J. R. Tanner, *English Constitutional Conflicts of the Seventeenth Century 1603–1689* (Cambridge: University Press, 1928), 225. Consistory Court records for London housed at the GLRO indicate that they resumed their responsibilities in 1669.
2 Donnison, 22. Donnison notes that a midwifery licence was issued in Peterborough in 1818 (Donnison, 206, n.6). John Guy states that in theory, the bishops could have granted licences until 1873. John Guy, "The Episcopal Licensing of Physicians, Surgeons and Midwives," *Bulletin of the History of Medicine* 56 (1982): 537.
3 Richard Petrelli, "The Regulation of French Midwifery during the *Ancien Regime,*" *Journal of the History of Medicine and Allied Sciences* 26 (1971): 277.
4 Nadia Maria Filippini, "The Church, the State and childbirth: the midwife in Italy during the eighteenth century," Marland, ed., *The Art of Midwifery,* 159, 162. Filippini points out that in Venice as early as 1624, an official licence was issued to qualified midwives.
5 Teresa Ortiz, "From hegemony to subordination: midwives in early modern Spain," Marland, ed., *The Art of Midwifery,* 96–9. Ortiz points out that occasionally a priest, rather than a physician, controlled the midwives' work.

wives.[6] The Netherlands also favoured town control with the instruction and regulation of midwives carried out at the local level by the middle of the seventeenth century.[7] The Church of England, with thousands of parishes throughout the realm, possessed the necessary bureaucratic framework and was to be the sole licensing authority for the licensing of midwives for more than two hundred years.

ORIGINS OF LICENSING

Historians have generally theorized that the practice of licensing midwives by church authorities was legitimized by the legislation of Henry VIII in 1512, which regulated the practice of medicine and surgery.[8] But midwives were not mentioned in the act and the date when the church first began to issue midwifery licences, and by what authority, remains uncertain.[9] The frequently cited oath administered to Eleanor Pead by the Archbishop of Canterbury in 1567, more than fifty years after Henry's first legislation for the regulation of practitioners, has generally been accepted by historians as the earliest proof of the licensing of midwives.[10] Richard Fitzjames, Bishop of London, however, licensed at least three London midwives in the years 1506–22.[11] Evidence from the continent suggests that the Church's involvement with the licensing of midwives began long before Henry the VIII's legislation regulating the practice of medicine and surgery.[12] Whatever its date of inception, historians have speculated about a mounting interest in enforcing the licensing of midwives in the early Stuart period and have gone so far as to claim that licensing of midwives was most strictly enforced during the Laudian years of the 1630s. Archival sources, however, fail to support the latter view.[13]

Historians of early modern midwifery have traditionally posited five reasons for

6 Wiesner, "Early Modern Midwifery," 95–9; Merry E. Wiesner, "The midwives of south Germany and the public/private dichotomy," Marland, ed., *The Art of Midwifery*, 80–4; Petrelli, 277; Nina Gelbart, "Midwife to a nation: Mme du Coudray serves France," Marland, ed., *The Art of Midwifery*, 133.

7 Hilary Marland, "The *'burgerlike'* midwife: the *stadsvroedvrouw* of eighteenth-century Holland," Marland, ed., *The Art of Midwifery*, 192; M. J. Van Lieburg and Hilary Marland, "Midwife Regulation, Education, and Practice in the Netherlands during the Nineteenth Century," *Medical History* 33 (1989): 298.

8 Gibson, *Codex Juris Ecclesiastici* 2 (Oxford: Clarendon Press, 1761), 1098, 1321; Wilson, "Childbirth," 44; Forbes "Regulation," 237; Donnison, 6.

9 John Guy points out that the bishops were not authorised by either canon or statute law to grant midwifery licences. "Episcopal Licensing," 537.

10 Forbes, *The Midwife and the Witch*, 145; Donnison, 6; Towler and Bramall, 56.

11 J. Harvey Bloom and R. Rutson James, *Medical Practitioners in the Diocese of London, Licensed under the Act of 3 Henry VIII, C.11* (Cambridge: Cambridge University Press, 1935), 84.

12 Guy, 538.

13 Wilson, "Childbirth," 62; Margaret Pelling, "Medicine and Sanitation," John F. Andrews, ed., *William Shakespeare: His World. His Work. His Influence* (New York: Scribner, 1985), 81.

the Church's interest in midwives: its concerns relating to the rite of baptism (a position suggested by ecclesiastical historians); its preoccupation with sorcery; its anxiety over the question of bastardy; the association of midwifery with medicine (which became the responsibility of the Church with regard to licensing in 1512); and, finally, its wish to ensure that midwives were competent to carry out their work in child delivery.[14] In addition, recusancy has been blamed for the Church's desire to regulate midwives, the group which found itself in the best position to ensure that newborns were baptised into the "true faith" of the Church of England.[15] The most widely accepted of the foregoing theories has been that the Church was primarily interested in the moral suitability and ability of midwives to carry out the ceremony of baptism.[16] As recently as 1982, baptism was cited as the main reason for ecclesiastical licensing, and this view is shared by a number of historians of midwifery.[17] Working against this argument, however, is evidence of post-Reformation changes in the medieval conviction that the soul of an unbaptised child was damned. As early as 1560, the catechism explained that baptism with water was only a seal or confirmation that the child of Christian parents had already been received by God.[18] With that in mind, it seems unlikely that ecclesiastical licensing of midwives was undertaken primarily out of a concern with baptism of newborn infants who were unlikely to survive. This view receives support from David Cressy's exploration of the rite of baptism which traces the

14 Wilson, "Childbirth," 41–6. For discussions of bastardy and parish concerns, see W. E. Tate, *The Parish Chest* (Cambridge: University Press, 1946), 213–20; Peter Laslett et al., eds., *Bastardy and its Comparative History* (Cambridge, Mass.: Harvard University Press, 1980). On the penalty for women giving birth to a bastard see Robert H. Michel, "English Attitudes Towards Women, 1640–1700," *Canadian Journal of History* 13 (April 1978): 58. Ecclesiastical historians support the view that baptism was the primary reason for licensing, but have not ventured a date for its inception. Aveling, *Midwives*, 7.

15 Guy, 539.

16 Although an older study of French midwifery adopted the view that the Roman Catholic Church in France similarly selected pious rather than experienced women to act as official midwives, Jacques Gélis' recent study of childbirth in early modern France indicates that childbearing women looked for other qualities in the women whom they (not the Church) chose as their midwives. Gélis describes a process where patience, skill, and dexterity were the qualities prized by women choosing prospective midwives. Gélis, 103. For the traditional argument regarding the moral but inept midwife, see Petrelli, 290.

17 See Edward Shorter, *A History of Women's Bodies* (New York: Basic Books, 1982), 41; Thomas R. Forbes, "The Regulation of London Midwives in the Sixteenth and Seventeenth Centuries," *Medical History* 8 (1964): 235–44; and *The Midwife and The Witch*, 141; Graham, 175; Schnucker, 639–40; R. W. Johnstone, *William Smellie : The Master of British Midwifery* (Edinburgh and London: E. & S. Livingstone Ltd., 1952), 30; E. H. Carter, *The Norwich Subscription Books* (London: Thos. Nelson and Sons Ltd., 1937), 134; Guy, 538–9. Although the licensing of midwives in seventeenth-century Nuremberg was a civic responsibility, the ability to baptise newborns was a concern of both City fathers and Church officials. See Wiesner, "The midwives of south Germany," 85–6, 106–7, for a discussion of their changing role in emergency baptisms. For examples from parish registers of midwives who baptised newborns, J. Charles Cox, *The Parish Registers of England* (Totawa, N.J.: E. P. Publishing, Ltd., 1974), 56–8.

18 Houlbrooke, 130.

ambivalent stance of the Church regarding emergency baptism as well as the declining role of the midwife in administering the rite, particularly by the post-Restoration period.[19]

Closely allied to the baptismal function, in the opinion of historians, was the concern that the midwife might engage in witchcraft and place in jeopardy the soul of the unbaptised infant.[20] The myth of the midwife as witch, however, has finally been demolished in a recent scholarly study by David Harley who argues that by accepting the evidence of demonologists instead of examining early modern sources, historians have erroneously perpetuated the "myth" linking midwifery and witchcraft.[21] Despite a lack of evidence regarding the origins of their licensing, another major study of early modern midwifery has concluded that the legal licensing of midwives was instigated as an extension of the licensing of medical practitioners, as well as a concern for the competence of midwives.[22] This present study, however, focuses on how the licensing system worked, rather than on its origins, and how it touched the lives of midwives residing in London, whose experience of licensing might differ from that of their sisters living in the provinces.

OATHS AND ARTICLES RELATING TO THE MIDWIFE'S OFFICE

Despite widespread acceptance that the Church's concern focused narrowly on ecclesiastical concerns, it is noteworthy that the opening sentence of a sixteenth-century midwife's oath emphasises the "cunning" (or intelligence, ability, and skill) as well as the knowledge which the midwife should bring to her task (see Appendix A).[23] This early midwifery oath also sets forth other demands: The midwife must make her services available without qualification to both rich and poor women;[24] she must report truthfully information involving suspected bastardy; she will never "switch" infants; she will not engage in sorcery; she will not use instruments or mutilate the fetus; she will use the correct form of baptism

---

19 Cressy, *Birth*, 122–3. Aveling, a nineteenth-century historian of childbirth, has asserted that baptism by midwives was practised only until the beginning of the seventeenth century, but Cressy gives an example for London from the year 1635. Aveling, *Midwives*, 6.

20 See Forbes, "Regulation," 141 and "Midwifery and Witchcraft," *Journal of the History of Medicine and Allied Sciences* 16 (1962): 264–82; Keith Thomas, *Religion*, 308.

21 David Harley, "Historians as Demonologists: The Myth of the Midwife-witch," *Social History of Medicine* 3 (April 1990): 1–27.

22 Wilson, "Childbirth," 61.

23 SOED defines cunning in this way. See Appendix A for a copy of the oath administered to Eleanor Pead in 1567. For an example of the oath which seventeenth-century French midwives swore, see J. Gélis, M. Laget, and M. F. Morel, *Entrer dans la Vie: Naissances et enfances dans la France Traditionelle* (Paris: G. Julliard, 1978), 78.

24 Although the oath does not explicitly require it, midwives also attended women who were suffering from contagious diseases. The testimonial of a midwife licensed in 1706 notes that she attended not only rich and poor, "or in what condition soever they were either the smallpox or any other lawfull distemper." GL MS 10,116/16.

(including the use of clean water); and notify the curate of any baptisms she has performed.[25]

Another midwife's oath dating from the middle of the seventeenth century appears to have been the oath administered to candidates who applied in a metropolitan court – probably that of the Bishop of London (see Appendix B).[26] It is a much more complex oath which reflects at least ten concerns of the licensing authorities, four of which are related to the midwives themselves rather than to the practice of midwifery. Interestingly, these ten concerns do not appear in the Canterbury oaths. To her promise not to aid in procuring abortions, nor to extort an unreasonable fee, she must add her promises to maintain patient confidentiality while carrying out her work openly and to ensure that any child who dies in childbirth is buried in a secure place. She must also make sure that she is not a party to any child being baptised as a recusant or in any faith outside of the Church of England.[27] But the portions of the oath which pertain to the midwife's relations with her peers are the features which are of the greatest significance for this study. The midwives are to report other midwives whose practices do not conform with the standards set forth (as above); they are to treat other licensed midwives with respect and cooperation; they are to report unlicensed midwives; they are to ensure that any women who act as their deputies should be competent in the practice of midwifery as well as being of good character; in difficult deliveries, as in the earlier oath, the midwife is forbidden to mutilate or kill the child to expedite delivery, but must instead call in "other midwifes and expert women in that facultie and use their advice and counsell in that behalfe." The "secrets" of the birthing chamber are to be kept from men who are only to be admitted in case of emergency.[28] The final section of the oath mentions the rite of baptism, but only involves the midwife to the extent that she must report any child who was not baptised into the faith of the Church of England.[29] The Church appears by mid-century to be attempting not only to enforce licensing of midwifery practise;[30] it is also acknowledging the midwives' control and expertise in child delivery by granting them the sole responsibility for

25 The ambivalence of the Church with regard to the use of charms is illustrated by the fact that an eagle stone (a hollow stone supposedly found in an eagle's nest) was one of the prized possessions of Canterbury Cathedral in the 1670s. It was in frequent use, available to neighbourhood women, but in the care of Dean Bargrave's wife. Thomas Forbes, "Midwifery and Witchcraft," 273. Jane Sharp refers to their use in removing a dead fetus, but indicates that she has not used one herself, and that their efficacy is probably imaginary. Sharp, 190.

26 Forbes, *The Midwife*, 146–7. The oath requires the midwife to report misdemeanours to "me the said Bishop, or my Chancellour."

27 Aveling has also noted this change in emphasis. Aveling, *Midwives*, 7.

28 This would be a surgeon who would bring his instruments to deliveries where destruction of the fetus was required to save the life of the mother. It was with these men that the concept of the male midwife originated.

29 Aveling has found the primary change in the oath one which relates to preserving the exclusivity of the Church of England. Aveling, *Midwives*, 29.7.

30 The same oath was administered in 1635 to a Berkshire midwife. See Appendix C.

regulating a network of mutual assistance and cooperation that upheld the principles to which they had subscribed by oath. In other words, the Church not only
wanted the best possible care for mother and infant, but it readily accepted that
women were still the perceived "experts" in child delivery. Church authorities
remained unconvinced by the claims of male practitioners (male midwives) such
as the Chamberlens who had been proselytising for several generations in an
attempt to gain control over the training and licensing of midwives.[31]

It is instructive to compare the Tudor oath, administered to Eleanor Pead in
1567, to the 1713 oath sworn by Mary Cooke, a widow formerly of Leire in
Leicestershire (Appendix C). For the most part, it is almost identical to the oath
administered in the same archdiocesan jurisdiction to Eleanor Pead almost 150
years earlier.[32] The requirements regarding the baptism of the infant, however, are
gone. Instead the final statement reads:

Moreover if I shall know any woman exercising the Office of a Midwife or doeing anything
contrary to the tenor of this mine Oath I will notifie and disclose the same to the Lord
Archbishop of Canterbury for the time being or to his Vicar Generall or Chancellor or the
ordinary of the place, soe far as I can conveniently.

The rather remarkable change in the oath argues for an increased interest on the
part of the Church in the practical rather than the spiritual qualifications of the
midwife over the course of the Tudor-Stuart period. The omission of the baptism
requirement may merely reflect the Church's moderated attitude toward the rite.
Licensed midwives, however, remain central to the child delivery process both in
a consultive and regulatory sense – by assisting one another in difficult deliveries
and by reporting unlicensed midwives.[33]

There is no question that midwives regarded the process of oath-taking as an
extremely serious matter. For example, in 1664, Mary Franck, midwife of St Anne
Blackfriars, refused to cooperate in the unorthodox baptism of an infant without
godparents since "shee Could not admitt ye child to bee baptised after that way it
being contrary to her Oath."[34] Sarah Fish, an elderly gentlewoman of Enfield,
was well aware of the implications of the midwife's oath when her vicar, Joseph
Gasgoine, sought to have her excused from taking the oath in 1697. Noting that
Mistress Fish, the wife of gentleman Robert Fish, did not need to practise midwifery for profit, he wrote in part:

31 The history of the Chamberlen family has been well documented by other historians. See Forbes,
   The Midwife, 152; Towler and Bramall, 77–81; Donnison, 13–15; as well as the source from which
   most of their information has been culled, J. H. Aveling, *The Chamberlens and the Midwifery Forceps*
   (London, J.& A. Churchill, 1882).
32 LPL MS VX 1A/11/80.
33 Similarly, the main thrust of a French midwife's oath of 1754 lies in the stress it places on the
   midwife's responsibility for ensuring not only the spiritual, but physical well-being of mother and
   child. Like her English counterpart, the French midwife promises to obtain expert assistance from
   other experienced midwives should the need arise. Gélis, *Entrer dans la Vie*, 78.
34 Brian Burch, "The Parish of St Anne Blackfriars, London, to 1665," *The Guildhall Miscellany* 3
   (October, 1969): 36.

. . . she is therefore willing to take out a Licence for that purpose but being aged is loth to be hurryed in ye night and in bad weather [for deliveries] to ye prejudice of her health, therefore, dos humbly desire she may be excused being sworn into that office, which she scruples not out of any singularity in her principles (being a very good churchwoman) but having never before taken any oath which if she could be dispensed with, would be a great benefitt to ye Neighbourhood, especially ye poorer sort of people to whom she is very usefull upon many occasions.[35]

Sara Fish was reluctant to take the oath because her conscience would then oblige her to answer every call for assistance, regardless of time or weather. It appears from Surrogate Cooke's entry that midwife Fish was not excused from taking the oath. Archival evidence relating to hundreds of midwifery candidates of the period indicates that these women took the issue of oath-taking before the chancellor seriously, and it should not be assumed that it was a meaningless exercise.

Although not part of the midwife's oath, the visitation articles issued by Edmund Bonner, Bishop of London, in 1554 included two other duties which the midwife was expected to carry out:

Item, Whether any midwife, or any other woman denieth or letteth, so much as lieth in her, that the child being new born shall not be brought to the church, there to be decently, reverently and orderly baptized, and the mother thereof after a convenient time likewise purified, according to the old ancient and godly ceremonies and customs of the catholic church . . . [36]

In the first instance, the article is referring to the midwife's responsibility in encouraging the early baptism of the infant to signify its acceptance into the Christian community. More than a hundred years later, in 1663, the rector and churchwardens of St Paul's Covent Garden testified that Beatrix Pattison, a long-time resident of their parish, had not only acquired the skills of a midwife through some years as a deputy midwife, but that she "doth orderly bringe the children she is concerned with to the church."[37] Similarly, in 1679, the vicar and churchwardens of St Leonard Shoreditch noted that Hanna Mason not only went to church herself, but went "also in the afternoon with children to be baptised." Rector Duckeson and churchwardens of St Clement Danes testified in 1677 that Phillipa Sampson brought her children "to the font to be baptised."[38] Because of the geographical diversity of a London midwife's practice (see Chapter 3), it is unlikely that a midwife attended the baptisms of all the infants she delivered. At those she attended, she not only played a prominent role preparing the infant and

---

35 GL MS 10,116/14. The reference to her unwillingness to take the oath being based on reasons of health and not on religious grounds is a reference to the fact that Quakers would not take oaths. Evidently Mistress Fish was not excused from taking the oath.

36 Edward Cardwell, *Documentary Annals of the Reformed Church of England* (Oxford: University Press, 1844), 165.

37 GL MS 10,116/3.   38 GL MS 10,116/10.

passing it to the various participants, she would hold a place of high esteem as the one responsible for the safe arrival of a new member of the parish community.[39] In the London parish of St Ann Blackfriars in the early seventeenth century, midwives played a particularly central role in baptisms, many of which were not attended by mothers who were confined to their lying-in beds.[40] Baptisms could also swell the midwife's income as various godparents and guests made gifts of money to the midwife. An anonymous London midwife noted that she had received £1 at a christening in 1695, while gifts of 10s. from various guests were not uncommon.[41]

MIDWIVES AND THE CHURCHING RITUAL

In the preceding quotation, Bonner also included the ancient ritual of "churching," a ceremony taken seriously in this period by church and laity alike.[42] The ceremony of churching sprang from the ancient belief that postpartum women were "unclean" and must undergo a special rite of purification to be held at the beginning of the first church service they attended after giving birth.[43] Cressy has persuasively argued, however, that by the last decades of the seventeenth century, churching was more about conformity than pollution with "multiple meanings" for different actors.[44]

Occasionally, a mother's churching was clouded by sadness. Tiny Marmaduke, son of citizen and draper Marmaduke Spyght of St Botolph Aldgate was buried October 28, 1597, the same day that his mother was churched, at a total cost of 4s.8d. for both services.[45] In the early eighteenth century, candidates for churching

39 David Cressy notes the central role of the midwife in the baptismal ceremony. Cressy, *Birth*, 150, 171. For a description of the key role of the midwife in baptisms in eighteenth-century Italy, see Filippini, 158. Filippini sees the midwife's participation in the baptismal ceremony as a vital element in the Church's control of female sexuality.

40 Cressy, *Birth*, 153

41 BL Rawlinson D1141, fol. 29; the famous diarist and London gadfly Samuel Pepys mentions gifts of 10s. each to midwives attending christenings at which he was present. Robert Latham and William Matthews, eds., *The Diary of Samuel Pepys*, vol. 2 (Berkeley and Los Angeles: University of California Press, 1970), 109, 216.

42 For the ancient Hebrew roots of the custom, see Shay D. Cohen, "Menstruants and the Sacred," Sarah B. Pomeroy, ed., *Women's History and Ancient History* (Chapel Hill: University of North Carolina, 1991), 274.

43 For the best discussion of churching, see Cressy, *Birth*, 197–229. See also Wilson, "Ceremony," 78–80, 88–93. Nor was the rite unique to England. Gélis has noted the church's attitude toward new mothers as objects in need of purification, well into the nineteenth century, as well as the custom of taking two rolls or pieces of bread to the churching ceremony to be blessed, one of which could serve, subsequently, to promote fertility among other women. Gélis, 107, 171–2. Natalie Zemon Davis has described how the new fathers in early modern French urban centres took their newborns to be baptised, while the mother stayed at home until her *relevailles* or purification period was over and she could go to be churched. Natalie Zemon Davis, "City Women and Religious Change," *Society and Culture in Early Modern France* (Stanford: Stanford University Press, 1975), 74.

44 Cressy, *Birth*, 200, 228–9.   45 GL MS 9234/7/6.

in the parish of St James Westminster, their heads decently covered or veiled, awaited their ritual purification in two specially constructed seats or small pews built on each side of the chancel communion table.[46] After the ceremony they were restored to full membership in the Church, with all its attendant privileges.[47] In many cases, the religious significance was buried, if not lost amid the flurry of festivities and it became an important female social occasion.[48]

David Cressy has examined a whole complex of factors, involving issues of religion, authority, and gender.[49] Churching was included in the *Book of Common Prayer* (1662), and Cressy was the first to seriously investigate the practice. In a study of Southwark, however, figures on churching were used in an attempt to measure popular religious conformity in the years 1619–25. It was found that almost 92 % of women who had their infants baptised also partook in the churching rite.[50] The majority of these women were churched two to four weeks after they were delivered.

There are mixed views of how churching was perceived by seventeenth-century parishioners. The Southwark study presents evidence of its unpopularity with some segments of the population, especially radical Protestants who felt it smacked of popery.[51] In addition, opposition to the rite arose, in some cases, because of a customary offering as high as ten pence to the clergyman.[52] At the end of the sixteenth century, parishioners of St Botolph Aldgate paid two pence for being churched while nonresidents paid four pence.[53] The fee for churching in St Saviour's, Southwark, early in the seventeenth century, was four pence for residents (one pence if the child died), and ten pence for nonresidents.[54] Cressy has noted the welcome contribution made by churching fees to parish incomes and with that in mind, speculated on the relative roles of clergy and laity in perpetuating (or abandoning) the ritual.[55] Visitation articles for Canterbury for the year 1605 specifically require the parish officials to name or present any married women who have refused to come for their churching, indicating that there was some resistance to the ritual.[56] Judging also by the tone of midwives' testimonials describing their bearers' responsibilities toward clients' churching, women needed encouragement to conform to the Church's teachings on the ceremony. But aside

---

46 VL MS D 1758/234–5, St James Westminster Vestry Minutes for 1710. Evidently, part of the ceremony included the correct positioning of the woman in the church. David Cressy, "Purification, Thanksgiving and the Churching of Women in Post-Reformation England," *Past and Present*, 141 (1993): 143. Cressy has expanded this pioneering article in his recent book *Birth, Marriage and Death*.

47 Donnison, 4, 13.   48 This is very much as Cressy sees it. Cressy, "Purification," 111–14.

49 Cressy, "Purification," 107–8.   50 Boulton, 278.   51 Ibid., 276–7.

52 *Phillimore's Ecclesiastical Law* vol.1(London, 2nd ed., 1895), 645–47. In France, as recently as the nineteenth century, gifts of money collected by the new mother during her lying-in period were used to meet the expenses of the churching ceremony. Gélis, *Childbirth*, 190.

53 GL MSS 9234/7/6, 9234/8/177.   54 Boulton, 277.   55 Cressy "Purification," 126–7.

56 *Visitation Articles, Canterbury, 1605* (London: 1605; reprint ed., Amsterdam: Theatrum Orbis Terrarum, 1975), 19.

from this there is scant evidence from London records which permits generalisation about how women felt about churching.

Historians have been divided in their opinions as to how churching was perceived by postpartum women. One view, focusing on women's perceptions of the ritual, argues that women disliked it but, for the most part, meekly submitted.[57] Gail Paster has suggested that churching's popularity could be a reflection of women's internalized "shame and embarrassment" which resulted from the birthing process.[58] On the other hand, a more positive assessment of churching as part of the rituals surrounding childbirth concluded that women looked forward to the opportunity of giving thanks for their recovery, particularly women intimidated by the idea that death through childbirth carried particular dangers for the soul.[59] Similarly, Cressy believes that the social and celebratory nature of the occasion led to festivities which women welcomed and thoroughly enjoyed.[60]

The language of the testimonials, in the few cases where churching is mentioned, suggests that midwives played an active role in accompanying the new mothers to the ceremony and that this was viewed in a positive light by the Church. Edward Pelling, rector of St Martin Ludgate, commended widow Mary Garret in 1681 because she "doth bring children to the church to be baptiz'd and women to be churched," while in 1679, vicar Ambrose Atich of St Leonard Shoreditch vouched for Hanna Mason's diligence in going to "Divine service with women to be churched."[61] Dr. Littleton, rector of Chelsea, stated in his testimonial certificate of 1690 that parishioner and midwife Elizabeth Forrest not only came to church herself but "doth constantly bring her women whom she delivers to the church to pay their thanks in publick and their children to receive publick baptism."[62] These testimonies demonstrate the continuing concern of the Church for this aspect of a midwife's function, which it saw as a reflection of her sound character and good citizenship in the "godly commonwealth" that was England. Midwives often received generous monetary gifts during baptisms, but apparently were not tangibly rewarded for their zeal in encouraging their clients to be churched, although attendance with a healthy client proclaimed their skill and competence before prospective parish mothers.[63] While absence of compensation possibly contributed to churching's eventual decline, many Stuart midwives

---

57 Patricia Crawford, "The Construction and experience of maternity in seventeenth-century England," Fildes, ed., *Women as Mothers in Preindustrial England*, 25.

58 Paster, 186, 195.

59 Wilson, "Ceremony," 89; Dorothy P. Ludlow, " 'Arise and be Doing' English Preaching Women, 1640–1660," (Ph. D. dissertation, Indiana University, 1978), 42.

60 Cressy, *Birth*, 199. 61 GL MS 10,116/10,11.

62 GL MS 10,116/13. Perhaps by the late seventeenth century, the purpose of churching was seen in its more modern aspect as a service of thanksgiving. In the prayer book, it is entitled "The Thanksgiving of Women after Childbirth Commonly called the Churching of Women." Donnison, 205, n.54.

63 Cressy, "Purification," 114.

were obviously not simply interested in the pecuniary aspects of their vocation.[64] Even so, the festivities that accompanied many churchings were enjoyable social occasions for participating midwives.[65]

In summary, although a firm date for the inception of licensing of London midwives has never been established, it is certain that the process was in place by the early sixteenth century and that it was originally intended to address a number of concerns including (among others), the ability of midwives to carry out their work competently and to ensure that the soul of the newborn was not placed in jeopardy. By the middle of the seventeenth century, more emphasis was placed on the role of the midwife in ensuring conformity to licensing regulations. In addition, experienced midwives were to cooperate in the instruction of fledgling midwives and in the management of difficult deliveries. The close of the century saw the Church encouraging midwives to participate in (and thus help to enforce) baptisms and churchings, but the main purpose of licensing was to ensure that practising midwives met certain standards with regard to practical knowledge and hands-on experience.

There was, therefore, no single purpose for ecclesiastical licensing. It was the expression of multiple concerns whose relative emphases varied over time. An examination of testimonial certificates and episcopal registers will shed light on how the licensing process functioned for seventeenth-century midwives.

ACQUIRING A LICENCE

The first task facing the aspiring licensee in midwifery was the procurement of testimonial certificates (Appendix D). These were generally endorsed by parish clergy or ward officials, and in some cases, neighbours, medical practitioners, and female clients.[66] The testimonials were presented to the archbishop's or bishop's chancellor (or his representative) who administered an oath of office to the midwife. Six women, including clients, who had personal knowledge of the candidate's ability also attended and were sworn before the chancellor who duly noted the same (in Latin) on the testimonial certificate.[67] This requirement in itself was a distinct departure from the requirements imposed on candidates seeking a licence to practise surgery and physick. The latter two groups were required

---

64 For examples of gifts to midwives at christenings, see John Loftis, ed., *The Memoirs of Ann, Lady Halkett and Ann Lady Fanshawe* (Oxford: Clarendon Press, 1979), 62; *Reports of the Royal Commission on Historical Manuscripts Rutland MSS.*, vol. 4, 466, 522, 540.; Frances P. Verney and M. M. Verney, *The Verney Memoirs* (London: Longmans Green and Co., 1925), vol. 2, 21.

65 Cressy, *Birth*, 202–3.

66 For the clergy's statement, see Richard Burn, *The Ecclesiastical Law* vol. 2 (London, 1842), 513.

67 Bloom and James, in dealing with evidence about several sixteenth-century midwives, have stated that "four or more other women, experienced in midwifery, gave evidence" about the experience and skill of the midwife. They have missed the point that some of the women were, in fact, clients, and not other midwives. I am grateful to the late John Clinard for his assistance in translating these documents in Bloom and James, 11, 84–5.

to present recommendations from practising peers regarding their ability, not from patients.[68] Testimonial certificates presented at the Archbishop of Canterbury's courts usually noted that the successful midwifery candidate was licensed to practise throughout the province of Canterbury. Several, however, were licensed to practise in specific locations such as London, Winchester, Lincoln, Rochester, and Canterbury while two midwives were authorised to work in London and Winchester.[69] Those licensed by the bishop of London could practise anywhere within the diocese of London.

Once the midwife was successful in her application, she was issued a licence. It was this document that she was expected to exhibit at parish visitations. An example of a midwife's licence has been preserved in the Lambeth Palace archives. Written in a fine hand on a small piece of parchment (approximately 7 inches × 6 inches) it was originally issued to Eyton Broughton of Lambeth, Surrey, by the Bishop of Winchester in 1686 and authorised her to practise in the Diocese of Winchester. It reads in part:

Whereas we understand by good Testimony and Credible Certificate that you the said Eyton Broughton . . . are apt, and able, cunning and expert to use and exercise the office, business and function of a midwife. Wee therefore as much as in us is, do admitt and give you power to use and exercise the said office, business and function of a midwife in and through our whole Diocese of Winchester aforesaid with the best diligence you may or can in this behalfe to poore and rich indifferently, and also to performe and accomplish all things about the same according to your oath . . . [70]

Eyton subsequently displayed the document at a visitation in 1691. By 1700, she sought and was granted an extension of her licence to the larger jurisdiction of Canterbury.[71]

---

68 This difference is important if midwives were licensed under regulations other than the statute of Henry VIII. The requirements regarding testimonial certification were much more demanding for midwives than for physicians licensed by the church. See, for example, the testimonial for James Cleverley, licensed in physick in 1669 on the recommendation of the rector, two churchwardens, one man whose occupation was unspecified, a "gentleman," and J. Astell M.D. GL MS 10,116/6. For an example of the minimal theoretical knowledge required to become a surgeon licensed out of Surgeon's Hall in 1789, see George C. Peachey, ed., *The Life of William Savory* (London: J. J. Keliher & Co. Ltd., 1903), 17–18. A handful of females were licensed in surgery by the Church in the seventeenth and early eighteenth centuries. Like that of midwives, their testimonial documentation was much more exhaustive than their male counterparts'. The inescapable conclusion is that gender was a factor in setting the prerequisites for supporting documents for ecclesiastical licences. Doreen A. Evenden, "Gender Differences in the Training and Practice of Female and Male Surgeons in Early Modern England," *Medical History* 42 (April, 1998): 194–216.

69 Most of the midwives who were given permission to practise in other geographical areas were women who resided in London; one was married to a gentleman. LPL MS vx 1A/11, 5, 44, 46, 52, 61.

70 LPL MS vx 1A/11, 61. While licences may have varied from place to place, this one was a very modest document.

71 The midwife may have died or been issued a new document to cover the larger area, including Winchester. The original licence, which noted that the extension was granted, remained unclaimed.

The registers of both the Archbishops of Canterbury and the Bishops of London survive intact for the seventeenth century. They contain records of licences granted to a great many, although not all, of the women who were licensed in the respective jurisdictions in the seventeenth century.[72] There had been sporadic licensing of London midwives in the early sixteenth century. However, the consistency and exactness of the format implemented by the clerks who recorded information in the bishop's registers in the early seventeenth century regarding the midwife's testimonial certification (and also the information on the extant testimonials themselves) suggest that while regulations governing the requirements for women seeking a midwifery licence in London may have been written earlier in the sixteenth century, they were not promulgated until the second half of the century.[73] This process required, as stated above, that *sex mulieres*, or six women, appear before the archbishop, the bishop, or their representatives and give testimony under oath of personal knowledge about the expertise of the applicant.[74] Under Henry VIII's statute of 1511, practising surgeons and physicians were to examine and approve aspiring candidates in surgery and medicine for licensing by the archbishop or bishop, but since the legislation made no mention of midwives, no comparable measures were established for deciding how midwives' licences should be awarded.[75] In 1547, an observer urged that "honest women of great gravitie" (who may or may not have been midwives) should testify to the "Bishop," on the midwife's behalf. But who decided that it should be six women, the number which appears with such regularity in the Vicar General's registers as early as 1608, and how did the responsibility for assessing competence move from practising peer to patient?[76] The register of William Laud, Archbishop of Canterbury, recorded the licensing of Anne Greenewelle of Sevenoaks in Kent in 1636, and included the fact that six women testified on her behalf. The entry is unusual

---

72 For example, the Vicar General's records for London have failed to record the names of dozens of women who were licensed between January 1664 and 1669. GLRO MS. DL/C 345 fols. 21–50v. We have evidence from the testimonials themselves about the women who were licensed during these years. In some instances, the registers list the names of the individuals (both clergy and clients) who gave testimonials or sworn evidence for the midwife, but in many cases the clerk has recorded only such minimum details as the midwife's name, parish, and date of licensing. Other variations of the recording formula provide random information about the midwife's marital status, her spouse's name, and perhaps his occupation. The most obvious gap in the recording process was in the civil war years 1641–61, but there are other omissions both major and minor in nature.

73 Bloom and James have included records of midwives licensed in 1528. In one case, the midwife presented a document attesting to her competence, but in several other cases, the midwife called on one or two women for support. Still later, in 1557, a midwife and three clients appeared before the Registrar of the Vicar General, who subsequently granted the licence to practise midwifery in Essex. The foregoing records do not suggest any standardization of requirements or recording procedures. See Bloom and James, 84–5.

74 It is the persistent recurrence of the Latin term itself which is indicative of a set of "official" requirements regarding the licensing process.

75 Guy, 531.

76 Andrew Boorde in Forbes, *The Midwife and the Witch*, 143; Guy, 537. For examples of licensing requirements in 1608 see GLRO MS DL/C 339/30, 32, 49.

in that it also embodies the following statement, apparently taken directly from
the precedent regulations governing the licensing of midwives:

The oath to be administered to these six women who shall be produced and witnessed,
they being such as have been delivered of child by the within named Anne Greenewell,
who are first to take their oaths laying their hands upon the bible or new Testament you
shall swear that through the experience and skill of Anne Greenewelle in the Art or faculty
of midwifie which you & every of you have had seene or sworne you . . .[77]

Although the quality of testimony given by the midwife's clients has been devalued by historians who have assumed that the women testifying under oath had
not necessarily been delivered by the midwife-applicant, the foregoing evidence
from the archbishop's records and other primary sources from later in the century
supports the view that the women in question had been delivered by the midwife.[78] In the Restoration period, women testifying on behalf of the midwife
continued to comply with the requirement that they attend *personally* before the
bishop or his chancellor. There is every reason to believe that when the midwife
and her clients appeared before the ecclesiastical courts and took their oath on the
Bible or testament, they were fully cognizant of the importance of giving truthful
sworn evidence and honouring their vows.[79]

Since the midwife in some cases sought the support of women who had been
recently delivered, it was not an easy task to arrange court attendance for the
oath-taking process of six clients, and, as we shall see below, applicants for a
midwifery licence did not always have their full complement of six female testa-
tors.[80] An indication of the often complex arrangements involved in assembling
the various components (not to mention individuals) can be found in several of
the testimonial certificates.

Elizabeth Syrette's directions to meet "at ye Crost Dagger near Doctors Com-
ons at Eleven @ cloke for John Bonner" were relatively straightforward.[81] But
when Susan Kempton of Cheshunt, Hertfordshire, travelled to London in her
quest for a midwife's licence, her instructions involved contacting "My Lord
Compton Bishop of Lond. living att Fullsom" and "Sir George Bramstone Chan-
celer att Doctors Commons," as well as seeking the assistance of a Mr. Rupert
Brewer "to be found at the prerogative office." Kempton and three clients (two
from St Brigid in London) managed to find their way to the right place and were
sworn before Chancellor Bramston himself on August 16, 1694.[82] In one instance,

77 LPL *Registers of the Archbishop of Canterbury*, William Laud 1633–1645 fol.244 (1636). Thomas
  Forbes had apparently overlooked the archbishops' and bishops' registers when he noted that he
  had not found the text of any licences from the first half of the century. Forbes, *The Midwife and
  the Witch*, 155.
78 Wilson, "Childbirth," 79; Donnison, 6.
79 Keith Thomas has concluded that the importance of oath-taking declined in the seventeenth
  century, and that the sanctity of the oath was no longer respected by many. Thomas, *Religion*, 76–8.
80 Other variations included testimony by senior midwives or male medical practitioners.
81 GL MS 10,116/13. Bonner was probably a notary public.   82 GL MS 10,116/13.

six women appeared to swear to midwife Laywood's competence in delivering their twenty-three children, but the midwife herself (a busy senior midwife) was prevented from attending because of the demands of her practice.[83]

The Cost of a Midwifery Licence

The actual cost of obtaining a midwife's licence was very high, roughly £1–£2.[84] By charging a substantial fee, church officials helped ensure that only dependable and economically viable women were licensed to practise midwifery. Evidence of what midwives paid for licences is found in testimonial certificates presented in the diocese of London, which survive only for the years after the Restoration. As in Norwich, the fee was made up of a number of smaller sums charged for different services and paid to more than one individual. In some cases, it appears that the fee may have been predicated on the number of women who were "sworn" by the church official, but in other cases the number of women giving sworn testimony was apparently unrelated to the fee charged. The earliest evidence of a London fee is found on the outside of the testimonial certificate of Ann Atkinson of High Holborn in the parish of St Andrew Holborn, licensed in 1662. Surrogate Henry Smith swore six women as well as the midwife. Two sums have been recorded – 6s.8d. and 1s.9d., for a total of 8s.5d. It is unlikely, however, that this is the full fee since it has been noted that the midwife had promised to add certification from "Dr. Winter and Dr. Bowden."[85]

In the years 1673–4, the fee at licensing was recorded for six women, but this fee did not take into account, for instance, what the women paid to have testimonial certificates drafted in the first place. As a general observation on the testimonial certificates, it is possible to ascertain from the handwriting that, in many cases, parish clergy drafted testimonial statements, which were signed by churchwardens and other individuals. In other cases, the women had the statements prepared by a professional scribe (at added expense) and then took them to be signed by the various officials as required.[86] When Elizabeth Beranger of St Peter the Poor was licensed in 1674 and paid £1.7s.8d. to the court, she had possibly already paid a substantial sum to Dr. Hugh Chamberlen, who addressed his testimonial statement to his "honored friend Dr. Exton at his chamber in the Commons."[87] Of the remaining five women, one paid the same fee as Beranger,

83 GL MS 10,116/2.
84 This point was made in both Harley's and Wilson's studies of provincial midwives. Harley, "Provincial midwives," 30; Wilson, "Childbirth," 80.
85 GL MS 10,116/2.
86 There is a strong likelihood that parish clergy charged some women for drafting their letter of reference. See Ludlow, 105.
87 GL MS 10,116/8. Chamberlen's statement appears to have been the only documentation which Beranger presented to the court and therefore we are reasonably certain that the amount recorded was the charge for the licensing process at the ecclesiastical court level, exclusive of any charges incurred by the applicant prior to this.

two paid £1.8s.8d., one paid £1.11s.2d., and one, Elizabeth Withers, paid the lowest fee of the six, at 17s.10d., to be sworn along with her six female clients. In one instance, Dr. Exton the Chancellor received 7s.6d. as his portion of the fee, while in another, the fee of £1.7s.8d. was divided between clerk Moses Jones of Doctor's Commons who received £1, and Exton who got 7s.8d.[88]

Four more testimonials from the years 1677–8 bear evidence of fees; on that of Ursula Stokes, the widow of John Stokes of Stepney, surrogate William Oldys recorded tersely: "Reced. 20 [s] @ noe more by order for this lycense, for seal @ other fees." Midwife Stokes' testimonial certificate was signed by her minister, a churchwarden, and an overseer of the poor. It is possible that the parish had secured a reduced fee or that it was paying for the licence of widow Stokes (described as "altogether expert and every way able to follow the calling of a midwife") not only to meet the needs of parish women, but to enable Stokes to be self-sufficient and avoid becoming a parish charge.[89]

Examples of change in the testimonial documents themselves can be found in the year 1695. The usual practice with regard to the women giving sworn testimony in the court was to record their names as a group. In some cases, the names appeared on the bottom or back of the clerical testimonial; occasionally they were written on a separate piece of paper. But when Ann Day of St Alphage was sworn by George Bramston in 1695, the testimonial documents which have been preserved consisted of a statement by her curate, Edward Lilly, and four separate sheets of good quality paper, each with an embossed seal stamped with the sum of six pence as well as the motto "honi soit qui mal y pense."[90] Information about what midwives paid for their licences in the last five years of the century continues to support the view that fees were set with a fair degree of flexibility for a variety of reasons, most of which are beyond the ken of a twentieth-century researcher. Of the four midwives whose fees for licensing were recorded in 1697, one woman paid £1.2d., the second paid £1.15s., and a third £1.19s.[91] The fourth woman,

---

88 GL MS 10,116/8.

89 GL MS 10,116/10. In addition to Stokes, fees were recorded for Isobel Leigh, Anne Hide, and Anne Goal.

90 This is the motto of the knights of the garter, the order to which the chancellor belonged. GL MS 10,116/13. In two cases, the women signed with their own signatures. Two further examples of this type of document survive in the records for the City of London for the years 1698–9, GL MS 10,116/14. Four examples can be found in the Lambeth Palace archives, all from the last five years of the century. LPL VX 1A/11, 54–7. On each page appeared the name of one female client, with her parish, spouse's name, and occupation, and the woman's signature or mark. Practises like this must have resulted in increased cost to midwives seeking a licence, but unfortunately no fee has been recorded for the six or seven examples of this format which survive. With the greatly increased public expenditure, as a result of waging a war against France, a number of duties were introduced in the 1690s. In 1698, a "long term" duty on vellum, parchment, and paper was imposed which may have been introduced temporarily a few years earlier and been reflected in these midwives' testimonial certificates. See P. G. M. Dickson, *The Financial Revolution in England* (London: St Martin's Press, 1967), 46–9.

91 GL MS 10,116/14. The three women were Mary Russell, widow of Tottenham High Cross, Elizabeth Wynn of Hampton parish, and Martha Tidmarsh of St James in the Fields.

Barbara Collop of St James in the Fields, appeared on September 30 and was given until Christmas to pay the total cost of £2.5s. She left a partial payment of five shillings and was to receive her licence when the balance was paid.[92] It should be borne in mind that in this period, when midwives were generally paying sums of £1 to £ 1.8s. for a licence, those costs represented the equivalent of eight to ten days' wages for a London building craftsman, or approximately fourteen to eighteen days' wages for a London labourer.[93]

It is apparent that in a few cases midwives found it difficult to pay for a licence or were unaware of the costs which were involved, since in a number of cases, the court was willing to accept a partial payment with the promise of further payment at a future date. Sara Wilkins of St Martin Ludgate and Rebecca Smith of St Giles in the Fields were both licensed in 1682 under Canterbury's jurisdiction. In both cases, a partial payment of 10 shillings was accepted.[94] In another instance, the licence was not surrendered without payment; on the outside of Elizabeth Pennyell's certificate is written: ". . . Mr. Cooke desired me to keepe this by me till ye party did come for her Lyc: but left no money."[95] There is no indication of why Hannah Mason of St Leonard Shoreditch was exempted from paying for her licence in 1679; only the word *gratis* was written on her testimonial.[96] In Katherine Howell's case, however, Richard Butler (who acted as a surrogate for the chancellor in some cases) had personally assumed the responsibility of paying for Howell's licence when she and her clients were sworn before surrogate William Oldys in 1678. Butler wrote: "I shall be accomptable unto Mr. Newcourt for Mrs. Howell's License." He added a memorandum: "I payd the Seele out of pocket."[97] Perhaps the midwife, a deputy midwife of long standing, or her husband, Peter, was an acquaintance of the court official.

Personal friendships or social ties were probably the reason why Elizabeth Dean, wife of gentleman Richard Dean of St James Weston, was excused from paying for her licence in 1688. In this case, Richard Newcourt (notary public and court surrogate) requested that "this license passe without fees." Thomas Pinfold administered the oath to midwife Deane and four women, and duly noted on the outside of the testimonial that it had been issued "*gratio.*"[98] Not only did the clients of Sarah Ticer of Laughton sign a statement asking that she be "favourably considered, for her estate being smale," but the vicar of Chigwell added his request that she be used "as favourably as possibly you can in reference to the

92 GL MS 10,116/14. Two of the women were from the same parish. Three women had three supporting clients. Collop was probably charged more because she did not have enough cash at the time of her appearance at the court. There is the possibility, moreover, that Collop never did receive her licence since her name does not appear in the Vicar General's register.

93 John Chartres, "Food Consumption and Internal Trade," Beier and Finlay, *London*, 171.

94 LPL VX 1A/11, 21, 22. In Sara's case, it would be unlikely that she could not afford the full payment, married as she was to a citizen and clockmaker. In Rebecca's case, we know that the total fee was £1.4.6.

95 LPL VX 1A11/42.   96 GL MS 10,116/10.   97 GL MS 10,116/10.

98 GL MS 10,116/12.

taking out of her Licence for the office of midwifery for I believe she is a very poore woman."[99] Evidently the intercessions were effective and Ticer's fee was remitted. In 1664, Temperance Pratt of St Botolph Aldgate submitted her testimonial certificate from her clergyman. It was accompanied by another beautifully written "petition" addressed to "Humphrey Lord Bishop of London" which explained that midwife Pratt was born in Stepney and was sent overseas as a child where she grew up and began her practice of midwifery. She wanted to put her practical experience in child delivery to use now:

but your Peticoner knowing she cannot soe freely exercise the same without approbation and licence to which she is ready and willing to yield unto, But by reason of her Travelle and great charge of children (not haveing any provision or maintenance for herself and children but through her owne labour and Industry) is reduced to great poverty and soe not able to raise any monies for obtaining a licence.[100]

Although Pratt pleaded poverty, her petition was the work of a professional who asked that the licence be granted "*in forma pauperis.*" Pratt's personal petition (the validity of which was certified by her minister, churchwardens, a constable, and a Member of Parliament) conveys the sense of control which the Church exercised in the licensing of midwives. It proved successful and Humphrey Henchman, Bishop of London, personally instructed the court official to administer the midwife's oath to Pratt and grant her a licence without charge.

Only one other case of a licence being granted *in forma pauperis* was found among the more than 500 testimonial certificates. Sara Bent was described as a "poor widow" who had lived in St Giles in the Fields for more than sixteen years and was well experienced in midwifery according to her clergyman, churchwardens, and six female clients. She was licensed by the chancellor Richard Chaworth in 1663.[101] It is apparent that these two women who pleaded poverty were competent and experienced midwives, and their licences were not granted solely on grounds of economic need.

Even though our evidence has not revealed a single fixed fee for a midwifery licence, fees in seventeenth-century London compare reasonably well with those charged in Norwich in 1735, where the fee is estimated to have been nearly £2, and in Chester, where a fee of 18s. 8d. was charged.[102] By charging a substantial sum to obtain a licence to practise midwifery, ecclesiastical authorities, in effect, excluded fly-by-night practitioners and ensured that responsible and stable women of good standing in their respective parishes carried on this important service to women of all ranks. In some cases, where a woman of proven ability but modest means applied, the Church moderated the fee or licensed her without charge.

---

99 GL MS 10,116/3. Although Ticer was described as "very poore," her four clients were described as being of the "best ranck and qualitie in the parish of Laughton."
100 GL MS 10,116/3.   101 GL MS 10,116/3.
102 Wilson, "Childbirth," 80, 11; Harley, "Provincial midwives in England: Lancashire and Cheshire, 1660–1760," Marland, ed., *The Art of Midwifery*, 30.

There is no question, however, that the sizeable outlay of money, time, and energy expended in the mechanics of obtaining a licence were deterrents to a number of midwives whose midwifery skills were on a par with those of licensed practitioners.

MIDWIVES AT VISITATIONS

The responsibility of the Church did not end with the issuing of a licence to the midwife nor did the midwife's expenses end with the cost of the licence. Midwives were expected to attend the periodic parochial visitations, which the bishop or his representative carried out in his diocese. At these visitations, all midwives who had been issued licences were required to exhibit them.[103] Midwives were traditionally charged a fee when their licences were inspected at ecclesiastical "visitations."[104] Not only do fees charged at visitations need to be considered as part of the long-term cost of a midwifery licence, they should be regarded as part of the midwife's and the Church's ongoing commitment to licensing as a meaningful recognition of the midwife's skill. An additional task of the ecclesiastical official conducting the visitation was to ascertain whether there were midwives in the parishes carrying on unlicensed practice. Bishop Bonner's articles for the Diocese of London in 1554 state that one of the aims of the visitation was to establish:

Whether there be any woman that doth occupy or exercise the office and room of a midwife, before she be examined and admitted by the bishop, or ordinary of this diocese, or his chancellor or commisary, having sufficient authority, except in time of extreme necessity when the presence of the midwife cannot be had?[105]

Visitations were, in effect, the main avenue whereby the Church attempted to enforce its control of the licensing process. Midwives practising without licences were summoned to appear and ordered to take the necessary steps toward acquiring a licence. In some cases, licences were issued at the visitation. The visitation

---

103 J. S. Purvis, *An Introduction to Ecclesiastical Records* (London: St Anthony's Press, 1953), 47.

104 GL MS 9537/19. In the back of the Bishop's visitation register for London in the year 1669, there is a list of fees. It is apparently what the authorities charged to inspect the licences and register the names of physicians, surgeons, school teachers, church lecturers, and midwives during visitations. In each case, except for lecturers, the fee was £0.1.4. The fee for church lecturer was £0.1.6. Wilson has estimated that the fee to exhibit in Norwich in 1735 was about £0.2.6. Wilson "Childbirth," 81.

105 See Bonner's "Articles of Visitation"(1554), Edward Cardwell, *Documentary Annals*, 164. For other examples of bishop's injunctions to midwives from this early period, W. H. Frere and W. M. Kennedy, *Visitation Articles and Injunctions of the Period of the Reformation*, vol. 2, 1536–58 (London: Longmans Green & Co., 1910), 23, 49, 292, 385; vol. 3, 383. Of the foregoing, one of the most interesting was that of Bishop Hooper (1551–52), which indicated that some midwives had been reluctant to deliver the wives of former Roman Catholic priests who had now married (vol. 2, 292). For more about these unfortunate women, Mary Prior, "Reviled and crucified marriage: the position of Tudor bishops' wives," Mary Prior, ed., *Women in English Society 1500–1800* (London: Methuen, 1985), 118–48.

process illustrates not only the Church's ongoing concern that midwives obtain a licence, but also the difficulties which faced church officials who were in many cases unsuccessful in enforcing the requirement that midwives be licensed.

Visitation records for the diocese of London in the seventeenth century have survived for the years 1636, 1637, 1664, 1669, and 1680. For the Peculiar of the Dean and Chapter of St Paul's, records are extant for the years 1667–70. The visitation of 1636 was a metropolitan visitation under the agency of the Archbishop of Canterbury covering the entire province. As far as we can ascertain, for 1636, only thirteen parishes lying within the wall and four suburban parishes were visited.[106]

At the 1636 visitation, for six of the parishes that were visited, no midwives were listed. St Clement Danes, which lay outside the walls, noted the greatest number of midwives but, of its nine midwives, four failed to appear. The parish of St Martin Ludgate showed the greatest number of intramural midwives, with all five women marked present at the visitation.[107]

The bishop's visitation of 1637 appears to have benefitted from better organisation and reduced scope. The visitation began in Essex on September 5, 1637 and arrived at the City of London three weeks later.[108] The visitation of City parishes began in the parish of St Augustine on September 26th. It moved in a westerly direction to the parish of St Michael Cornhill on September 27th. The next day, the remaining parishes attended the visitation proceedings held in the parish church of Allhallows Barking which lies in the northeast corner of the City. A much greater number of parishes were visited than at the visitation of a year earlier: eighty intramural parishes, ten extramural parishes, and seven suburban parishes are listed in the records. Forty-two, or more than half, of the intramural parishes reported no midwives while four of the extramural parishes, or 40%, reported no midwives.[109] Of the intramural parishes that were visited, St Martin Ludgate again reported the greatest number at six. Of the suburban parishes, St Clement Danes listed its nine midwives once more (the greatest number for any parish outside of the walls).[110]

Almost thirty years later, on October 6, 1664, the first visitation of Humphrey Henchman, Bishop of London, opened its initial London segment in the parish

---

106 We are using the customary division of parishes with 97 parishes within the walls and 13 parishes considered as "extramural." See Tai Liu, 17–21. The seven suburban parishes were St Mary Islington, St James Clerkenwell, St Leonard Shoreditch, St Clement Danes, St Martin in the Fields, St Giles in the Fields, and St Mary Matfellon: GL MS 9537/15 fols. 51–68 passim.
107 GL MS 9537/14/35–8.
108 The suburban parishes such as St Clement Danes were visited before the parishes within the walls.
109 It is difficult to give a total number of midwives who were listed on the visitation records of intramural and extramural parishes at this visitation because for thirty odd parishes, two lists have been preserved which, in some cases, contain different names for the same parish. For example, on one list, St Sepulchre has reported nine midwives and on the other, only seven. If we use the list containing the greatest number of parishes, there were at least 105 midwives listed.
110 GL MS 9537/15 fols. 51v, 59.

church of Christ Church. The visitation appears to have covered most of the parishes, but again, not every parish reported the presence of midwives.[111] The majority of the midwives had been licensed since the Restoration, but Elizabeth Boycot of St Sepulchre displayed a licence from 1636 and another venerable midwife, Mrs. Lyndsey of St Martin Vintry, exhibited her licence dated almost three decades earlier, July 27, 1637.[112]

The visitation of 1669 concentrated on extramural and suburban parishes, according to the existing records. Only three intramural parishes were visited: St Ethelburga, St Stephen Coleman, and Allhallows Barking. A comparison of visitation records with the registers of the bishop and archbishop reveals that, in many cases, midwives who appeared at visitations were not listed in the registers that recorded the names of licensed midwives. For example, the extramural parish of St Andrew Holborn listed fifteen midwives in the visitation of 1669.[113] Of these, we can establish (by using testimonials and bishop's registers) that six women had licences to practise midwifery. Testimonial certificates and registration were found for a seventh midwife who was also shown as a "licensed" midwife in the visitation records.[114] In three other cases, it has also been noted in the visitation records that the women have produced their licences, although there are no surviving testimonials for them, nor are they found in the registers. This leaves five women who were practising as midwives and for whom there is no proof of licensing at all. One of the five, Mrs. Dodson, was probably the Anne Dodd of St Andrew Holborn who was licensed in 1688 by the Archbishop of Canterbury, which suggests that she may have been a deputy midwife in 1669.[115]

At the visitation of 1680, fewer than half of the intramural parishes were covered according to extant records. The number of midwives shown for the parish of St Andrew Holborn had dwindled to six: Of these we know that three were licensed, one (Dodson or Dodd) was eventually licensed, while two new names have been added. One of the two, a Mrs. Hillyard, was probably a deputy of Elizabeth Hillyard of St Botolph Aldersgate who was licensed in 1678 and whose testimonial mentions a female relative living in St Andrew Holborn.[116]

---

111 In most cases, where a midwife has been listed, we know that she exhibited her licence because the date of licensing has been included in the visitation documents.

112 GL MS 9537/17 fol. 74 and unfol. It is difficult to be precise about these records because they seem to have been partially recopied and, once again, in some instances, where two listings of a parish occur, they contain different information.

113 GL MS 9537/19/64.

114 She was Elizabeth Collins GL MS 10,116/2; GLRO DL/C 344/218.

115 LPL VX 1A/11/46. The possibility that she was a deputy is strengthened by the fact that her testimonial certificate establishes a connection with an older, licensed midwife. The visitation records for 1669 illustrate the haphazard nature of recording practices and emphasize the fragile nature of assumptions based on a single source when dealing with seventeenth-century midwives. It is unlikely we will ever uncover all midwives who practised in seventeenth-century London, although a thorough search of all documentation will yield sufficient numbers for a worthwhile examination.

116 GL MS 10,116/10. Once again, inconsistencies in the recording of information abound in most parishes. The extramural parish of St Sepulchre lists seven women: Four have been named as

Why did both licensed and unlicensed midwives attend visitations with, in many cases, no distinction made in visitation documentation? Or why did so many midwives for whom there is no record of licensing appear at visitations? Among the possible explanations is the most obvious one of deficient records: gaps in bishops' registers, and loss of testimonial certificates or even of the licence itself, in addition to inconsistent recording practices. But other factors may be involved. The midwife may have been licensed in another jurisdiction, or been licensed, widowed, and remarried, her new name having no association with her licensing records.[117] Perhaps the small fee for registration at visitation was resented by some licensed midwives and acted as a deterrent to attendance.[118] Women who occasionally offered midwifery services out of charity would be unlikely to seek a licence.[119] In one or two instances, the clerk has noted that the women were deputies, but this type of information was seemingly added at the whim of the recording functionary. It may, however, allow for the fact that some women were not yet licensed, although practising as midwives, and the number of London women in this category was certainly far greater than these stray notations indicate.[120]

Whatever the reason for the disparity between the number of women for whom we have definite proof of licensing and the number of women who appeared as midwives at the visitation, there is every reason to believe that the Church endeavoured to ensure that midwives were licensed. Visitations were also relatively ineffectual in encouraging midwives to acquire licences. For example, in 1669, which was a visitation year, fewer licences (16) were issued than in the previous year (19).[121]

The parish of St Dunstan in the West is one of the thirteen parishes which has been selected for detailed study (see Chapter 5). Although the overall quality of its other records is good, when visitation records and licensing records are com-

  midwives, although we have elsewhere found proof of licensing for only one. The names of two midwives, Joan Wooden (licensed in 1663), and Katherine Desser (licensed in 1673), appear in the visitation records without any indication of their function whatsoever. Finally, the clerk noted that Mrs. Shaw had displayed her licence but we have found no evidence of a licence having been issued to her.

117 For the difficulty of tracing the careers of widows (not to mention widowed midwives), see Barbara Todd, "The Remarrying Widow," Prior, ed., *Women in English Society*, 57–8.

118 Harley, "Provincial midwives," 30. Harley also notes that some unlicensed midwives in the provinces claimed only occasional deliveries out of charity in order to be excused from penalty when summoned to visitation.

119 Harley, "Historians as Demonologists," 12. Harley has also included Catholics and Quakers with this group of unlicensed midwives, but there is no evidence to indicate that the latter two groups would attend visitations. Since excommunication was the penalty for noncompliance, the Church would be powerless to enforce licensing among these women.

120 Nor was London unique in these recording inconsistencies; Harley's study of provincial midwives has similarly noted gaps in the numbers of recognised practising midwives and those appearing at visitations. Harley, "Provincial Midwives," 37.

121 GL MS 10,116/5,6. For a reference to the way ecclesiastical courts reacted to nonlicensed midwifery practice, G.V. Bennett, *The Tory Crisis in Church and State 1688–1730* (Oxford: Clarendon, 1975), 7.

pared, discrepancies emerge, and parish midwives become almost invisible when viewed from the perspective of visitations alone. Clearly, with a large volume of business to transact, of which verifying midwifery licences was only a small part, the episcopal visitation of several days could not hope to be thorough. The visitation provided a crude form of screening (and a historical source of some value), but the ecclesiastical control of midwifery certainly depended far more upon the regular process of licensing upon request by the presentation of testimonial certification and by the reporting of unlicensed practitioners by midwives themselves.[122]

The records of visitations for the Peculiar of the Dean and Chapter of St Paul's Cathedral describe a process which is different from that adopted by either the Archbishop of Canterbury or the Bishop of London; they support our view that the Church was concerned that women who practised midwifery fulfill certain requirements, but that the various processes by which the Church attempted to enforce its requirements met with mixed success. In the Peculiar, visitations were held monthly, or in some cases bimonthly, during the years 1667–74.[123] During this period, the names of thirty-one women who were engaged in unlicensed midwifery practice, on one level or another, appeared in the visitation records.[124] Of these thirty-one women, fifteen eventually obtained licences, but in a variety of ways.[125] The Deanery and Chapter officials were apparently attempting to ensure that unlicensed midwives within their limited jurisdiction would be compelled to obtain licences. They were not calling before it already licensed midwives.[126]

Fines and Penalties

As noted earlier, the time and expense involved in acquiring a licence were major obstacles for many women. Since the acquisition of a licence had no bearing on the quality of a midwife's performance, the Church was compelled to adopt other measures to enforce its requirement for licensing. Hence, the penalty of excommunication was imposed on midwives who failed to comply. Extant records reveal how ecclesiastical officials of the Deanery and Chapter of St Pauls regularly employed excommunication (or the threat of it) to deal with recalci-

---

122 See chapter 2, for an example of self-regulation by the midwives themselves.
123 In some respects, these visitations resembled the *comperta courts* of Norwich described by Wilson, "Childbirth," 74.
124 GL MSS 25,533/1,2.
125 For a detailed account of these fifteen licencees, see D. Evenden-Nagy, "Seventeenth-century London midwives: their training, licensing and social profile," Ph.d. thesis, McMaster University, 1991.
126 We know of at least three licensed midwives in the parish of St Giles Cripplegate whose names do not appear in these records. Emmet Sare was licensed on May 14, 1662, Elizabeth Ponsam was licensed in February 1664, and Elizabeth Ayre on June 6, 1664. GL MS 25,598.

trant midwives. Midwives who practised without a licence in the jurisdiction of the Bishop of London were similarly liable to the penalty of excommunication. It was a penalty whose efficacy varied with the degree of religious commitment which individual midwives experienced. It was, moreover, totally ineffectual as a means of ensuring compliance in cases where a midwife was not a communicant of the Church of England. Aside from the fact that midwives themselves were under oath to report unlicensed midwives and would, therefore, be less likely to work and cooperate with excommunicated and, hence, unlicensed midwives, the penalty of excommunication had no relevance to the midwife's skill. In the overall scheme of licensing, it was a deterrent to unlicensed practice that enhanced, in turn, the prestige and pride of the midwife in her profession.

In 1665, R. Boreman, the rector of St Giles in the Fields, wrote to Sir Richard Chaworth, the Bishop of London's chancellor, on behalf of two of his parishioners who had been excommunicated for failing to appear in court to answer the charge of practising midwifery without a licence. Boreman asked that the excommunication be lifted for Mary Shelton and Sibil Lee, and that they be granted licences on the grounds that they were experienced and reliable women who depended on their earnings from midwifery for their livelihood and, in Shelton's case, that of her seven children. Both Shelton and Lee were reinstated in the Church and, after submitting testimonial support of former clients, received their licences in February 1665.[127] In 1675, clergyman Benjamin Younge of Enfield wrote to Chancellor Thomas Exton, asking him to lift the excommunication of Dennys Younge who, he said, had submitted to her clergyman's instruction and now wished to be licensed. Exton agreed, even though it was midwife Younge's second offence.[128]

The relative impotence of ecclesiastical authorities in imposing their will upon intransigent midwives who refused to apply for a midwifery licence was demonstrated by the report of an incident some fifty years after it occurred in 1634. A midwife apparently successfully challenged the Church when it tried to enforce its position on licensing; the court's decision was that "the Church could not punish a midwife for unlicensed practice."[129] Although no details about the case have been provided, the midwife, Mrs. Benskin, might have been the midwife Benskin whose name appears on the visitation record of St Ethelburga parish in

127 GL MS 10,116/4.
128 GL MS 10,116/9. See Forbes, *The Midwife and the Witch*, 151, for the full text of the letter. The midwife might have been related to clergyman Younge, who mentioned a second midwife who was excommunicated for practising without a licence. The latter was probably Eleanor Maws of Enfield, whose testimonial certificate from Benjamin Younge bore the same date as his letter concerning Dennys.
129 Wilson, "Childbirth," 41. Although he gives virtually no details about this case, Wilson speculates that the Court of Audience in which it was held may have been that of Canterbury, one of the jurisdictions open to London midwives for licensing. This encourages our supposition that it was London midwife Benskin.

1669.[130] In the intervening years, Mrs. Benskin possibly acquired a licence or she may have continued in unlicensed practice. Benskin's victory apparently had some short-term effect on London midwives' compliance with the licensing process. The Vicar General's registers for the decade 1630–9 (see Table 1.1: Recorded Midwifery Licences: London Diocese 1630–42) suggest a drop in the number of midwives who were licensed in the diocese of London in 1634 and subsequent years up to the civil war period.

Later in the century, in 1662, Anne Spencer, a widow of Holy Cross, Westgate, launched an appeal after a series of events had led to her arrest for producing a false midwifery licence. The eventual outcome of her appeal is unknown, but excommunication had been previously imposed on the "contumaceous" midwife for her refusal to obtain a legitimate midwifery licence.[131] The midwife's troubles with church authorities did not go unnoticed by her sister midwives. In the years commencing January 1661 and 1662, twenty-two and twenty-four midwives, respectively, were licensed in the diocese of London; in the year commencing January 1663, seventy-four women were licensed in midwifery according to surviving records.[132] Both the Benskin and Spencer incidents illustrate measures by which Church officials attempted to ensure compliance with midwifery licensing. Nevertheless, they were measures rewarded by little or no success at the individual level, aside from how their example might have affected their peers.

Midwives themselves played an increasingly important role in the eyes of Church authorities in ensuring that unlicensed midwives were reported to ecclesiastical officials. At the bottom of Margaret Hopkins' testimonial of March 1670 is a note urging church officials to send Christopher Cleeter, the process server, to a midwife living at Mr. Martin's in Tottenham High Cross and compel her to "take out a licence for to doe the office of a midwife." Mrs. Hopkins paid 1s. 6p. to defray the cost of Cleeter's visit to the unidentified midwife.[133] The Church also delegated to the midwives the responsibility for maintaining close and harmonious relationships in order to make available, not only to one another but to their clients, the years of accumulated practical knowledge which they possessed.

Although the origins of ecclesiastical licensing of midwives are hazy, and in the early years linked to the midwife's ability to baptise an infant in grave peril, the Church encouraged the licensing of midwifery practice throughout the seven-

---

130 GL MS 9537/18/65v. Benskin would be an elderly practising midwife by that date. We have uncovered no record of her licensing, but because of the unevenness of recording practices, cannot exclude the possibility that she was licensed at some point.

131 The following information is taken from the records of the Court of Arches at Lambeth Palace Library: Process Books D1960 Spencer v Somner, 1665 Case No. 8596. I am indebted to Miss Melanie Barber of Lambeth Palace Library for bringing this case to my attention, and to Tim Wales for his help in translating the court records.

132 GL MS 10,116/1–3. Unfortunately, no testimonials from the jurisdiction of Canterbury have survived for the 1660s. We have used only testimonial evidence for this comparison because the Bishop of London's registers were spotty for the decade under consideration.

133 GL MS 10,116/7. Cleeter later noted that he had "served" a Sarah Wolingeenne in July 1670 who may or may not have been the midwife in question.

Table 1.1. *Recorded Midwifery Licences: London Diocese 1630–42*

Year	No. of midwives	Year	No. of midwives
1630	4	1636	0
1631	10	1637	4
1632	6	1638	5
1633	6	1639	8
1634	4	1640	4
1635	0	1641/2	0

Source: GLRO MSS 343, 344.

teenth century because of its concern with the midwife's ability and competence in carrying out her work. Even so, the issue is not whether licensed midwifery was actually of a higher quality than unlicensed practice; in all probability there was little difference in most cases.[134] In some instances, the difference between licensed and unlicensed practitioners was presumably that of religion, not skill, since excommunication was an ineffectual penalty for those outside the Church of England. When complications arose, however, the unlicensed midwife who needed assistance might be less likely to call upon other midwives who she feared may report her, thereby depriving her client of critical resources and expertise. The perception of Church officials, clients, and midwives themselves, was, that by taking their oath and giving sworn evidence of satisfactory practice, midwives were providing a better service than unlicensed practitioners.

Licensing undoubtedly meant different things to different midwives at various times throughout the century. In some cases, it was seen as a beneficent and supportive requirement – especially at times such as that of the Chamberlens' attempted takeover – while for others of limited economic resources or dissenting beliefs, it could be viewed with resentment; still others, as busy practitioners, would find it a bothersome waste of time which was irrelevant to the quality of their performance in real life situations. It is important to know about the way ecclesiastical licensing of midwives functioned in seventeenth-century London, but it must also be borne in mind that, in what was essentially a self-regulated system of professional training, the inability of the Church to enforce licensing successfully had little actual effect on the way in which the midwives practised their art.

134 This view is supported by the research of David Harley. Harley, "Historians as Demonologists," 9–10.

2

Pre-Licensed Experience

Licensed as they were by ecclesiastical authorities, midwives were expected to meet prescribed moral and spiritual standards, but there is abundant evidence that training, experience, and competence were also important to those responsible for issuing midwifery licences. Women who sought a licence to practice midwifery in seventeenth-century London had undergone years of practical training, generally under the supervision of a more experienced midwife. In some cases, two or more experienced midwives provided guidance and encouragement to younger midwives seeking to acquire the skills that were necessary for a successful career in midwifery. Parish and ecclesiastical officials, as well as peers and neighbours, set great store by lengthy involvement in the childbed experience. It was an experience, which the midwife shared not only with competent senior midwives, but also with other women who would eventually apply for midwifery licences themselves. Testimonial evidence from the 1660s to the end of the century reveals that representatives of the "official" branches of medicine, as well as the community as a whole, accepted the viability and adequacy of the "unofficial" (but ecclesiastically licensed) system in which seventeenth-century London midwives trained and worked.[1]

LENGTH OF EXPERIENCE

Over 500 testimonials, which London midwives presented to Church officials between the years of 1661 and 1700, have been preserved in London archives. These documents provide a mine of information about midwives, which is analysed below.[2] The results support the view that midwives usually had long expe-

1 By way of comparison, in Paris, midwives in the seventeenth century generally apprenticed to senior midwives, or, after 1630, were associated with the Hotel Dieu, which trained a small number of the most competent fledgling midwives. Even at the Hotel Dieu, however, the instruction was practical rather than theoretical. Petrelli, 279–80.
2 David Harley has described testimonials as "the best source of information on midwives." Harley, "Provincial midwives," 29–30.

rience in midwifery practice before obtaining a licence to practice their art in the vibrant metropolis of London. Testimonials which clergy, clients, and others gave under oath to support the midwife's application for licensing in the years 1600–41 have not survived. In addition, during the civil war period, the licensing process ground to a halt and no testimonials were generated for almost two decades. Instead, the briefer and more dispassionate observations of the clerks who kept the registers of the Vicar General of the Diocese of London and the Archbishop of Canterbury provide information about licensed London midwives. Because of this difference in documentation, relatively few details regarding the length of time which the early Stuart midwife had trained or practised her calling before applying for a licence have survived. Nevertheless, the evidence that is extant tends to support continuity in training over the century as a whole.

We know that when Dorothy Chambers of St Sepulchre's parish received her licence to practise midwifery in November 1608, she already had 13 years' experience in child delivery.[3] In 1611, Anne Ramsay, a widow living in St Olave Hart Street, stated in her application that she had 20 years' experience in midwifery. The readiness of the Vicar General's Office to accept this claim suggests the practice whereby extensive experience preceded licensing was routine. While Elizabeth Keyfar of St Botolph Aldgate and Julian Sutton of St Leonard's Foster Lane both had 10 years' experience in their calling when they were licensed in 1611, Isabel Doubleday of St Dunstan in the West attested to 30 years of midwifery experience the same year.[4] The following year, three midwives were licensed whose practical experience totalled an impressive 50 years.[5] Midwives could be licensed after far shorter, albeit presumably still adequate, periods of service. Several years later, Elizabeth Gilbank of St Martin Ludgate and Sibil Douglas of St Andrew Holborn were licensed with three and two years' "hands on" experience respectively.[6] To date, no record of ecclesiastical licensing has been found for the civil war years 1641–60, either in bishop's registers or by way of testimonial evidence. The absence of an ecclesiastical licensing system during the period 1641–60, however, did not mean that the system of apprenticeship and training practised by London midwives also collapsed. What it does mean is that

---

3 GLRO MS DL/C/339/49. For part of the period, she was probably a deputy midwife with a more experienced mentor.
4 GLRO MS DL/C/340/3v, 5v, 11v.
5 Avis Mallett, 20 years, Barbara Porter, 20 years and Alice Palmer, 10 years. GLRO MS DL/C/340/21v, 22v, 44.
6 GLRO MS DL/C/341/47, 64. Subsequent entries for the period up to 1640 do not record length of experience and there is no way of ascertaining whether this is due to faulty recording practices or other factors. See, for example, GLRO MS DL/C/ 343/143, 165 for the year 1633. The inclusion of information on length of practice prior to licensing was haphazard and seemingly at the whim of the recording clerk. The recording of very short periods demonstrates that entries were not biased in favour of long service; the average length of unlicensed practice where information is available exceeded a decade. There is no way of determining precisely how many years of experience were acceptable to licensing authorities.

we are less able to recover fully the names and practices of those women who had served their apprenticeships in the pre-1641 period, and who entered the system as fully qualified midwives in the 1640s and 1650s.

A collective analysis of all testimonials for seventeenth-century London from the jurisdictions of the Archbishop of Canterbury (61 testimonials), the Vicar General of London (439 testimonials), and the Chapter and Deanery of St Paul's (20 testimonials) reveals certain trends regarding information about the length of time midwives trained before being licensed in midwifery. Early in the Restoration period, midwives' testimonials more frequently contained details about the duration of their practical experience than they did toward the end of the century. Aside from the actual number of years, descriptive terms such as "many years," "long practised," and "divers years" were often used. Since these terms are an expression of the contemporary importance which was placed on the adequacy of a midwife's training, testimonials employing such descriptions have been included in an analysis of the length of time during which midwives gained experience before applying for a licence. Moreover, this emphasis on a lengthy period of experience implies the mature age at which many midwives applied for licensing and the inherent qualities which maturity engenders. Qualities such as "judgement, practical wisdom and self-mastery," not only commanded deference and respect in early modern England, but gave added authority to midwives as a group.[7]

In the years 1661–72, 97 testimonials out of a total of 205 made mention of the length of time the midwife had practised midwifery.[8] Some of this previous experience was under supervision, and some, especially that of "deputy" midwives who had been called to substitute when a mentor was unable to attend, would necessarily be unsupervised, but there is no way of differentiating between supervised and unsupervised experience. Nevertheless, 47% of the testimonials considered the length of time that the midwife had been involved with the midwifery process relevant to the midwife's competence. In 1672–81, of a total of 138 testimonials, 21, or 15%, mention midwifery experience. (See Table 2.1: Length of Experience ([From Testimonials].) The years 1682–91 yielded 101 testimonials with only 10, or 10%, containing information about duration of "training" or experience. Finally, in the years 1692–1700, only 6 testimonials out of 77, or 8%, contained information about the length of time the midwife had worked in her field before applying for her licence.

Although it would be possible to conclude that the length of time which midwives "trained" or gained practical experience became increasingly irrelevant and/or increasingly shorter as the century wore on, it must be borne in mind that no licences had been issued for almost two decades before 1661. A backlog of midwives who had accumulated many years of experience awaited the re-

---

7 Keith Thomas, *Age and Authority in Early Modern England* (London: The British Academy, 1976), 5.
8 For purposes of comparison, the thirty-nine years covered by this analysis have been divided into four shorter periods: 1661–71, 1672–81, 1682–91, and 1692–1700.

Table 2.1. *Length of Experience (from Testimonials)*

	1661–1671	1672–1681	1682–1691	1692–1700
Descriptive term	41	7	4	4
2–5 years	14	5	1	0
6–10 years	15	7	4	1
11–20 years	21	2	0	0
20–30 years	6	0	1	1
30+ years	2	0	0	0
Total	97	21	10	6
Total test.	205	138	101	77

Sources: GL MSS 10/116, 598/2; LPL MS VX1A/11.

establishment of the licensing process in 1661. This can be seen more clearly if we consider the figures for the years 1661–62 separately. In this period, 36 out of 46 testimonials, or 78%, stress the length of time the midwife had practised. Under the circumstances it would be acceptable, even desirable, to cite lengthy periods of unlicensed practice when licensing was first reintroduced. It is true that many midwives customarily acted as deputy midwives for seven years or longer, but later in the century some midwives might have found it more of a liability than an asset to draw attention to the fact that they had been delivering children unassisted for ten years or more without a licence. Testimonial evidence for long periods of unlicensed service late in the century tends to have been in some ways exceptional. When Susan Kempton, of Hertfordshire, however, applied for a licence to practise midwifery in London in 1694, she presented sworn certificates indicating that she ". . . hath used the imployment of a midwife twenty or thirty years last past with good success. . . ." Kempton lived at a distance from London, although she already had clientele in the capital, and it is also possible that she had earlier secured a licence to practise in Hertfordshire.[9]

The vagaries of various officials who were responsible for issuing the midwife's licence could also influence the recording of details regarding the length of the applicant's experience. For example, cryptic, personal notations, quite separate from the sworn testimony of clergy and clients, appear as additions at the bottom of pages or on the outer fold of testimonials. Rebecca Jeffery's and Margaret Pratten's testimonials, both sworn in January 1662, contain this type of minutiae, which has been added in the handwriting of the bishop's surrogate.[10]

Although the notations reflect a lack of standardization in the recording process,

9 GL MS 10,116/13.
10 GL MS 10,116/2. Rebecca Jeffery's testimonial contains the observation "aged 58 yrs. – practiced 18 years." Margaret Pratten's notes at the bottom "practised for 7 yrs."

they are more interesting as an indication of which type of information the official or his clerk considered important. Testimonials which provide a numeric value for the women's experience (excluding those which use descriptive terms) afford a different perspective. For the years 1661–71, 58 testimonials mention the number of years of experience that the women had, for a total of 716 years. For these 58 women, then, the average length of experience prior to licensing was 12 years. In the second period, 1672–81, the average length of experience was 11 years. By the period 1682–91, the average length had dropped to 7.3 years. That was still, by any standard, a respectable length of time to acquire the necessary skills and competence required of a successful midwife, but the reasons for the change are unclear. In the last period, 1692–1700, only two testimonials contained the number of years of midwifery experience. The average of 17.5 years, however, was skewed because one woman had practised for an unusually long time; the other licensee had 10 years of experience.[11] The very partial evidence for the post-1682 period, therefore, suggests that "training" times were falling, perhaps in response to the rapidly increasing population within the metropolis and increasing demands for midwifery services.[12] Despite this possibility, testimonial evidence supports the conclusion that the inhabitants of seventeenth-century London, both lay and clerical, valued lengthy midwifery experience. This experience encompassed active participation in the childbirth process as well as simple observation.

DEPUTY MIDWIVES

A great many trainee London midwives had definite arrangements, including specific time commitments, for serving in the capacity of deputy midwives under experienced or senior midwives.[13] Ecclesiastical records from the seventeenth century described the senior midwife as an *obstetrix supros*.[14] Ecclesiastical authorities, moreover, recognized the role of the deputy midwife as a legitimate one. A section of a midwife's oath to be administered by the bishop or his chancellor read:

Item you shall not make or assigne under you any Deputy or Deputies to exercise or occupie under you in your absence, but such you shall perfectly know to be of right,

11 GL MS 10,116/13; LPL VX 1A/11, 52. The women were Susan Kempton of Cheshunt and Elizabeth Vesey of St Edmond Lumber Street.

12 London's rapid growth in the first half of the century was surpassed in the second half. Roger Finlay and Beatrice Shearer, "Population growth and suburban expansion," Beier and Finlay, eds., *London*, 54. By way of comparison, in Nuremberg there were periodic shortages of midwives in the early modern period. This elicited a variety of responses, but not reductions in the length of time midwives were required to train. See Wiesner, "Early Modern Midwifery," 95–8.

13 There is very limited evidence that indicates London midwives paid a premium to their mentors. In 1696, Mary Griffen paid £5 for three years' training to a licensed and venerable midwife of Deale. Donnison, 8. See also the case of Mary Read, below, 159.

14 GL MS 10,116/3. The testimonial of Katherine Day. The term *obstetrix supros* indicates a midwife who was above or superior to other midwives.

honest and discreet behaviour, also apt, able and having sufficient knowledge and experience to exercise the said room and office.[15]

Demonstration of the status of deputy was sufficient to excuse a midwife summoned before a visitation for unlicensed practice.

Although England had no female guilds, London midwives had developed a system of training very much like the guild apprenticeship system in which artisans, craftsmen, and tradesmen received their training.[16] In a few cases, as in other apprenticeships, seven years was the specified length of time that the midwife served in the capacity of deputy. For other women, the number of years could be less than seven or, as records have shown, it could be considerably more. Early in the eighteenth century, three years' service as deputy midwife could, on occasion, be accepted as adequate.[17]

Although male midwife Percival Willughby had few words of commendation for contemporary midwives, he was moved to acknowledge: "The young midwives at London bee trained seven yeares first under the old midwives, before they bee allowed to practice for themselves."[18] Willughby was an admirer of William Harvey who earlier in the century had criticized "younger," and by implication, less experienced midwives.[19] Willughby takes up this theme and also makes the distinction between "young midwives" and "older sort of midwives."[20] This is a critical distinction that shows an appreciation for the skills of the midwife who has the maturity and experience conferred by a lengthy working association or apprenticeship.

The London system appears in general to have been similar to the training practices employed for midwives in other areas of early modern Europe. In Italy, a lengthy apprenticeship to a "teacher midwife" was the primary qualification for the typical midwife.[21] Spanish midwives also gained their expertise under the tutelage of experienced midwives. In seventeenth-century Zagora, for example,

---

15 T. R. Forbes, *The Midwife and the Witch*, 147, quoting from a book of oaths published in the mid-seventeenth century. See Appendix B.
16 Barbara Hanawalt has pointed out the difficulty which European women faced with regard to guild membership in male guilds in the pre-industrial period. Moreover, women were discouraged from organizing their own guilds. Hanawalt, "Introduction," *Women and Work*, xiii. For information on female apprenticeship in male-dominated guilds in the eighteenth century, see Bridget Hill, *Women, Work and Sexual Politics in Eighteenth-Century England* (Oxford: Basil Blackwell, 1989), 85–102. It is difficult to locate information of a general nature on the apprenticeship system in seventeenth-century London, and Stella Kramer has pointed out the complexity of the topic: Stella Kramer, *The English Craft Gilds and the Government* (London: 1905. Reprint ed., New York: AMS, 1968); Margaret Davies focusses on the seven-year term requirement: Margaret Davies, *The Enforcement of English Apprenticeship 1563–1642* (Cambridge: Harvard University Press, 1956). See also Joan Lane, "Provincial Medical Apprentices and Masters in Early Modern England," *Eighteenth-Century Life* 12 (November 1988): 353–71; O. Jocelyn Dunlop and Richard Denman, *English Apprenticeship and Child Labour* (London: T. Fisher Unwin, 1912). The latter has a useful section on working women as well as information about child labour and apprenticeship.
17 GL MS 10,116/15, testimonials for Margaret Churchwell and Mary Wallis, 1702.
18 Willughby, 73. 19 Aveling, *Midwives*, 37. 20 Willughby, 208. 21 Filippini, 154.

the apprenticeship was for four years.[22] In Nuremberg, where a well-defined system of midwifery apprenticeship was in place in the early modern period, there was also a four-year apprenticeship for German midwives.[23] Mary Lindemann has described an apprentice-like system involving "warming women" in eighteenth-century Braunschweig in which the women served for varying lengths of time, some as long as fourteen years, before becoming fully accredited midwives.[24] Similarly, a "lengthy" apprenticeship to an experienced midwife played a key role in the licensing of eighteenth-century Dutch midwives.[25] Midwives in seventeenth-century Paris apprenticed for three or four years to an accredited midwife or, in a few cases each year, trained at the renowned Hotel Dieu in Paris.[26] Although the length of time varied, what is clearly apparent is that early modern midwives in many European countries recognized the importance of working with other, more experienced midwives in some form of apprenticeship to gain the expertise and confidence which was vital to their important task.

Because of the quality of evidence in the years 1661–1700, it is apparent that many midwives served as deputy midwives under qualified and licensed midwives for varying lengths of time, thereby ensuring that they received both instruction and supervision as they acquired the skills of a midwife. There are, however, indications that this system was already in place early in the century. When Isobel Toller of St Martin in the Fields received her licence to practice midwifery on July 10, 1610, it was noted, along with the customary names of six female clients, that she had served as a deputy to Mary Darley, *obstetrix,* and wife of Matthew Darley.[27] The following year, Joan Joanes of St Botolph without Aldgate, wife of Edward Joanes, painter-stainer, applied for a licence after serving her time as a *deputata.*[28] The accounts for the Overseers of the Poor of St Dunstan in the West

22 Ortiz, 97, 99.
23 A description of the system is found in Wiesner, "Early Modern Midwifery," 98–9.
24 Mary Lindemann, "Professionals? Sisters? Rivals? Midwives in Braunschweig, 1750–1800," Marland, ed., *The Art of Midwifery,* 182.
25 Marland, "The *'burgerlijke'* midwife," 193. The unlicensed Dutch midwife, Vrouw Schrader, worked with other, more experienced midwives to gain expertise at the beginning of her long career, even though she had evidently gained some knowledge of operative obstetrics from her first husband, who was a barber-surgeon. Schama, 526. In turn, Schrader described one of her associates as "pupil" and she herself was called in by other less experienced midwives to assist in difficult deliveries. Marland, " 'Mother and Child'," 19.
26 For the training of French midwives in the sixteenth and seventeenth centuries in a system described as resembling medieval apprenticeships, see Petrelli, 277–9. Petrelli describes a four-year apprenticeship, while eighteenth-century Parisian midwives served a three-year apprenticeship. Gelbart, 133. For eighteenth-century French midwifery training, Michael Ramsay, *Professional and Popular Medicine in France 1770–1830* (Cambridge: Cambridge University Press, 1988), 23, 53.
27 GLRO DL/C/339/132v.
28 GLRO DL/C/339/11/4. "Mistress Fleeke" was probably the senior midwife. The term *deputata* indicates a deputy midwife. See also Sara Garrot and Catherine Mannersley, GLRO DL/C 343/ 257, 193. The term "deputy" is used as late as 1702 on the testimonial of Mary Wallis, deputy to Hannah Winchester for "the usual time." GL MS 10,116/15.

recorded payments in 1638 made to "the midwife and her deputie" for the delivery of Elizabeth Gillam.[29]

Ann Giardina Hess has shown that provincial Quaker midwives were similarly trained by their association with older, more experienced midwives.[30] In London, like their Church of England counterparts, Quaker midwives worked with deputies who eventually were able to assume full responsibility for deliveries. Anne Poore was an active Quaker midwife in the closing years of the seventeenth century and the early decades of the following century. Martha Chamberlain was described as her "deputy" in 1718, but by 1719, Martha was carrying out the occasional delivery on her own, as well as assisting the busy senior midwife.[31] There is no evidence of licensing for Poore or Chamberlain, presumably both of the Quaker persuasion, but, surprisingly, Quaker midwives, in some instances, turned to senior midwives of the established Church either as mentors or assistants at London labours. Senior midwife Elizabeth Fisher was in attendance when Quakeress Mary Howell delivered Hannah Blackman in 1689, while Mary Russell of St Martin in the Fields, licensed in 1664, attended labours with Quaker midwives Anne Albrighton in 1687 and Anne Heariford in 1700.[32]

On the other hand, Sibill Morgan, who received her licence from the Church and was, presumably, a member of the Church of England in good standing, was probably the busy Quaker midwife Ann Heariford's deputy before obtaining her licence.[33] London midwives, both conformist and nonconformist, clearly sought to acquire skills and expertise in their chosen profession and did not permit differences in religion to prevent them from seeking the best training, as well as the most skilled assistance, if the occasion warranted it.

The infrequent acknowledgement of the midwife's professional capacity is a major obstacle in the research of the seventeenth-century midwife. Later in the century, when archival resources permit cross-checking between testimonials and registers, the names of midwives (without occupational designation) have often been found among the women named on the testimonials.

The problem is acute when a widow's name appears with the names of female clients. It is reasonable, however, to speculate that in 1608, when Thomas Pole, notary public, accepted the sworn testimony of Alice Vaughan, widow, regarding the competence of Susanna Williams of Stepney, Mistress Vaughan was acting in the capacity of mentor rather than a recently widowed client. Similarly, in the following year, Hannah Walker of St Mary Mounthaw may have been the deputy of Alice Rikman, widow, of St Leonard Foster Lane.[34] Moving to the period after

---

29 GL MS 2999/1 unfol.   30 Giardina Hess, "Midwifery Practice," 69.

31 PRO RG/6/1628, birth notes 22,40,78,79,91,99,101,169.

32 PRO RG/6/1626/45,31,111,122. Licensed midwives Ward and Wiggens also attended a delivery in 1689 with Quaker midwife Alice Boulton, RG/6/1626/ 48.

33 PRO RG/6/1626/65.

34 GLRO DL/C/339/30, 75. There is evidence later in the century that midwives generally called upon women who had been recently delivered by them to support their applications for licensing; this strengthens the likelihood that at least some of the widows whose names are found on

the re-institution of ecclesiastical licensing, when the testimony of Anne Boggs of St Giles in the Fields was sworn before chancellor Thomas Exton in June 1671, the document stated that she:

... did article and covenant with Alice Herbert of the same parish, an ancient and skilful midwife to become her deputy, which tyme of her Deputyshypp is now ended and determined as may appear.[35]

The great importance attached to training and working under a senior midwife is apparent in the documents supplied by Margaret Cooke of Chelsea when applying for her licence in 1664. Because her senior associate, Mary Leverett, also of Chelsea and a practising midwife for "33 years or thereabouts" had lost the use of her limbs, she could not appear personally to swear to Cooke's abilities. Instead, Sam Wilkinson, rector of Chelsea, took pains to convey Leverett's testimony to the appropriate authorities.[36] Sibil Lee of St Giles in the Fields made her own statement on behalf of her deputy Mabella Hobson of the same parish in 1664: "I Sibilala [sic] Lee testifie that Maibell Hobsess is by mee derected and is a nabell midwife laying many women for me."[37]

A revealing glimpse of the supportive network surrounding midwives-in-training is afforded by analyzing testimonial information as it relates to deputy midwives and their mentors. These documents reveal the complexity of the relationships that existed between midwives of different ages and stages of experience. In some cases, candidates for licensing could claim an association with one, two, or three senior midwives as well as younger, deputy midwives. (See Appendix F.) When Elizabeth Fletcher of St Giles in the Fields applied for her licence in 1664, she had been Mrs. Boshier's deputy for three to four years, and Mrs. Elder's deputy for three years. In addition, she had presided at successful deliveries in the presence of Mary Dowke, another licensed midwife.[38] Three licensed midwives signed the testimonial of Adrey Lucas of St Andrew Holborn in 1667: Ann Adams, Alice Herbert, and Esther Kilbury. Herbert and Kilbury, both of St Giles in the Fields, frequently worked together and their signatures appear on an impressive number of midwives' testimonial certificates.[39] Later in the century, Joan Sinclair of St Martin in the Fields presented credentials signed by midwives Elizabeth Bink, Martha Budd, and Elizabeth Tracee who made the following statement on Sinclair's behalf:

Sir, this woman the wife of George Sinklare was my Deputy her full Terme and p'form'd it very carefully and faithfully and is very diligent and able witness my hand [40]

testimonials were not clients, but midwives. For example, GL MS 10,116/10, certificates of Ann Bell, 1677.

35 GL MS 10,116/3.   36 GL MS 10,116/3.

37 GL MS 10,116/3. Mistress Lee was saying that her deputy was "an able" midwife. Mabella's testimonial also bore the signature of Anne Lamb, the daughter of a midwife, who would receive her own license to practise midwifery in 1678.

38 GL MS 10,116/4.   39 GL MS 10,116/5.   40 GL MS 10,116/11, testimonial from 1684.

The testimonial which William Cave, vicar of Isleworth, supplied for Elizabeth Clark in 1697, noted that she "hath for several years past exercised the office as a Deputy midwife to several persons residing within our parish to their great content and satisfaction."[41]

In addition to the support and instruction of senior, more experienced midwives, midwives applying for licences also included the names of other fledgling or deputy midwives who had been present when they had successfully brought their clients to bed. When Elizabeth Dowke was licensed in 1661, she had already practised midwifery for 20 years; her deputy, Frances Stannard, had 10 years' experience and applied for her own licence later that year.[42] In the same year, Margaret Hall of St Martin in the Fields included sworn testimony by her deputy Mary Jackman. Jackman was subsequently licensed in 1669.[43] There are other examples of women whose names were included among the clients of women applying for licences and who were not identified as deputies but who subsequently obtained licences themselves: Margaret Williscott of St Botolph Bishopsgate supported Sara Griffin of the same parish in 1663, and received her own midwifery licence in 1666; Anne Lamb of St Martin in the Fields testified for Mabel Hobson (St Giles in the Fields) in 1663 and was herself licensed fifteen years later; Joan Wheeler of Stepney was licensed in 1666, three years after her name appeared on the testimonial of Eleanor Rickes, also of Stepney.[44] Later in the century, we find that Hanna Mason, who was licensed in 1679, had been present at successful deliveries attended by Anne Watson, licensed in 1676. Both were of Stepney and Hanna, in her turn, deputized Ann Johnson of Stepney who was licensed in 1692.[45]

Aside from sources related to the licensing process, records such as court depositions support the picture of an extensive "apprenticeship" system of midwifery training. In 1637, Elizabeth Wyatt told the court that she had served five of the seven years agreed on with Mrs. Brown.[46] The latter was probably Anne Brown of St Sepulchre, licensed in 1637. Toward the end of the century, the parents of Mary Read paid an unnamed midwife the substantial sum of £20 to instruct their daughter, who then served as her deputy for a time. Unfortunately, their attempt to provide Mary with a measure of independence was thwarted by the continued interference of an abusive spouse.[47]

MATRILINEAL MIDWIFERY LINKS

Among the most impressive demonstrations of the way in which traditional knowledge and skill in midwifery was passed down from generation to generation within a system of unofficial apprenticeship is the evidence of matrilineal links

41 GL MS 10,116/14.   42 GL MS 10,116/1.   43 GL MS 10,116/1, 6.
44 GL MS 10,116/3,4,10.   45 GL MS 10,116/9, 10, 13.   46 Cressy, *Birth*, 66.
47 GLRO, Consistory Court Records, Dep. Book DL/C/244, Read con Read, October 23, 1695. I am indebted to Jennifer Melville for this reference.

between two, and in some cases, three generations of midwives.[48] The superbly qualified Elizabeth Love of St James Clerkenwell, licensed in 1663, "was for many years bred and brought up with her mother and grandmother both ancient and expert midwives."[49] When Margaret Corney of St Peter Paul's Wharf was licensed in November 1661, her rector, John Wilkins, acknowledged "her mother of knowne experience and ability in her profession of midwifery as by sufficient testimony of many persons she hath delivered will be made good."[50]

Mary Edwards, licensed midwife, signed the testimonial of her daughter Mary Cook of St Mary Matfellon in 1669; Helen Orme, licensed midwife of St James Clerkenwell, also signed her daughter's testimonial certifying that Hester Penney was "able and skillful in the art of midwifery."[51] According to the beautifully written document in Lady Margaret Coventry's own hand and sealed with her seal, Anne Clark of St Peter the Poor, with twelve years' experience in midwifery, was the daughter of a midwife who had practiced "above fortie years from whom she derived her skill."[52]

In some cases, a midwife who received her training at the hands of her mother carried on the family tradition in midwifery in the same parish. In 1678, Anne Lamb, St Martin in the Fields, requested that she be granted a licence to "exercise the office, business and function of a midwife in the place of her mother now deceased. . . ."[53] Anne's mother was Mrs. Wright (alias Ramton) an "ancient" midwife who had been licensed in 1611.[54] Anne's clients, who may have been brought into the world by Anne's mother, faced childbirth with the confidence and trust engendered by decades of experience. Both the daughter and grand-daughter of midwife Susanna Kent, St Dunstan in the East, were midwives although the daughter, Susanna Read, practised in the country.[55] The renowned eighteenth-century midwife and author of a midwifery treatise, Sarah Stone,

48 In France, senior midwives or *matrones jurées* in some cases instructed their daughters in midwifery. Petrelli, 277. For the role of mothers in the transmission of popular medical knowledge, see also Evenden Nagy, *Popular Medicine*, 60, 62 8,81.
49 GL MS 10,116/2.
50 GL MS 10,116/1. The signatures of two midwives appear on Mistress Corney's testimonial, that of Elizabeth Hales, "aged 83," and Mary Soedin, "aged 80." There is no indication of which one was Margaret's mother.
51 Hester was licensed in 1669, and her mother had already sponsored at least one other young midwife, Phoebe Forster of St Sepulchre Newgate, who was granted a licence in the early sixties.
52 Signed and sealed December 12, 1673. GL MS 10,116/8. Margaret Coventry was the daughter of the Earl of Thanet and the granddaughter of Lady Anne Clifford; she married George, third baron of Coventry in 1653. The midwife whose application she supported may have delivered one or two of Lady Coventry's five children at the family's London residence in Lincolns Inn Fields. J. B. Burke, *A Genealogical History of the Dormant, Abeyant, Forfeited and Extinct Peerages of the British Empire* (London: Harrison, 1883), 142–3; D. J. H. Clifford, ed., *The Diaries of Lady Ann Clifford*, (Phoenix Mill: Sutton Publishing, 1990), 130, 151.
53 GL MS 10,116/10.   54 GLRO MS DL/C/340 (fol. no. illegible).
55 LPL VH 95/1136. Barbara Hanawalt has commented on the commonality of women's work experience in this period in Europe and the fact that their primary mentor was usually their mother or another female. Hanawalt, "Introduction," *Women and Work*, viii. For a twentieth-century example of a third-generation American midwife whose early training was influenced by her mother, see Logan, *Motherwit*.

described how she had "been instructed in midwifery by my mother and deputy to her full six years." She noted that her most valuable qualification was her instruction at the hands of her mother and disclosed that her own daughter was now a midwife.[56] Lacking the opportunities for formal education, women were afforded their best opportunities for learning through a close association with their mothers. Very few documented examples of these intimate, instructive relationships survive, but in the case of midwifery, indications are that the tradition was widespread throughout Europe and that in London itself, the practice extended into the eighteenth century.[57]

Paths to Midwifery Training

There are other examples in the testimonials which indicate that midwives were involved with the childbed process, often for many years, as deputies, assistants, or perhaps as observers who at a future date decided to pursue seriously a career in midwifery.[58] Even such rich sources as the testimonials, however, fail to supply answers to the questions surrounding why a woman chose to pursue the arduous, albeit rewarding career of midwifery. In 1663, two women were present at five successful deliveries by a Chelsea midwife that were neither licensed midwives nor clients.[59] Traces of childbed assistants can also be found in parish records: In 1638, two women received 12 pence for assisting in the delivery of Goodwife Ayres while the same parish records acknowledged the assistance rendered by another unidentified parish woman to the midwife and her deputy.[60] Physician William Sermon's midwifery treatise (1671) suggested that, ideally, four women should be in attendance to assist the midwife with a number of tasks, which might include cutting the umbilical cord.[61]

---

56 Sarah Stone, *A Complete Practice of Midwifery* (London: 1737), xv, 148; Grundy, "Sarah Stone," 129. See Elizabeth Whipp and Sarah Sydey, chapter 4. Matriarchal midwifery instruction was not limited to London practitioners; Ruth Rogerson of Norwich had trained under her mother and grandmother. Harley, "Provincial midwives," 28. In Italy, midwifery skills were most frequently passed within a "network of female relations," which included mothers and daughters. Filippini, 154.

57 For an example outside of London, see Harley, "The scope of legal medicine," 47. I am grateful to Peter Earle for an eighteenth-century example of a widow, Sarah Goble of Dowgate Hill, who practised midwifery and was instructing her widowed daughter, Mary Browne, in the art of midwifery. GL MS 9065A/11/302,304.

58 GL MS 10,116/3,7 and MS 25,598/2; LPL MS VX 1A/11, 40, 58. See Chapter 3 for a description of female attendance and participation in childbirth. Jacques Gélis has described virtually the same scene for childbed in early modern France. Gélis, *History of Childbirth*, especially 99–101. See also Natalie Zemon Davis, "City Women and Religious Change," Natalie Zemon Davis, *Society and Culture in early Modern France* (Stanford: Stanford University Press, 1975), 76.

59 GL MS 10,116/3. Margaret Pelling's study of Norwich practitioners mentions women "standing instead of a midwife" in bastardy cases who may have been deputy midwives, or other women helpers and observers. Margaret Pelling, "Occupational Diversity: Barber-surgeons and the Trades of Norwich, 1550–1640." *Bulletin of the History of Medicine* 56 (1982): 408.

60 Records of the Overseers of the Poor of St Dunstan in the West, GL MS 2999/1 unfol.

61 Sermon, 19. Contemporary Sermon assigns a much more active role to the female attendants than Adrian Wilson, who sees their role as largely symbolic in his study of the ceremony of childbirth. Wilson, "Ceremony," 73. See also Chapter 3.

Not to be forgotten are women like Isobel Wilcher who, by 1664, had attended three deliveries by Margaret Cook. These women supported the midwives by their presence without ever becoming midwives themselves.[62] Although not a midwife by profession, Elizabeth Walker, wife of London clergyman A. W. Walker, was knowledgeable in "physick and chyrugery." She would go to women in childbed day or night, taking with her "what might be useful" to assist the midwife in her work.[63] Mrs. Walker perfectly exemplified the literate, well-educated woman whose years of attendance at deliveries afforded yet another source of experience and knowledge to midwives.[64]

SENIOR MIDWIVES

Extant testimonials for midwifery licences from the years 1661–1700 have been analyzed to determine how many women successfully applying for licences in this period claimed an association with experienced midwives, including their own mothers, who had been midwives. (See Table 2.2: Associate midwives, 1661–1700.)

In the years 1661–71, 36% of the testimonials indicate a relationship with at least one other experienced midwife. In the years 1672–81, 24% of the testimonials mention a senior midwife. By the third period, 18% reveal such a connection and, by 1692–1700, 14% of the testimonials convey information about another midwife with whom the licensee has been associated. Thus, whereas slightly less than 26% of all extant testimonials for the period 1661–1700 include an indication of the length of earlier practice/training, slightly more than 26% provide evidence of the role of one or more senior midwives in this training.

The appearance of a gradual but steady decline in the influence of senior midwives toward the end of the century is probably misleading. In general, there is a problem of under-reporting as well as one of detection. Because midwives were frequently not given their professional designation on the testimonials, their names are frequently indistinguishable from those of female clients who were providing sworn testimony on the midwife's behalf.[65] As has already been pointed out, careless recording and loss of records have undoubtedly allowed more than a few midwives to remain undetected. We know, for example, that Sara Sydey of

---

62 GL MS 10,116/3. The presence of these women is particularly apparent in the Quaker birth notes. PRO RG/6/1626–8.

63 Anthony Walker, *The Holy Life of Mrs. Elizabeth Walker* (London, 1690), 180. Early in the century, Lady Margaret Hoby took an active part in the delivery of women of all ranks. Dorothy Meads, ed., *Diary of Lady Hoby* (Boston and New York: Houghton Mifflin Co., 1930), 63, 117, 195, 216.

64 Clergyman Ralph Josselin's wife, Mary, was attended in childbed by other women in addition to the midwife. She in turn participated in the deliveries of friends and neighbours. Alan MacFarlane, ed., *Diary of Ralph Josselin 1616–83* (London: Oxford University Press, 1976), 12, 111, 165, 399, 415, 465.

65 Licences issued after 1700 have not been thoroughly investigated, but a cursory check has revealed at least another ten senior midwives in the first decade of the eighteenth century.

Table 2.2. *Associate Midwives, 1661–1700*

	1661–1671	1672–1681	1682–1691	1692–1700
Worked with:				
1 midwife	43	27	16	11
2 midwives	20	4	2	
3 midwives	4			
mother	7	3		

Sources: GL MSS 10/116, 25,598/2; LPL MS VX1A/11.

the parish of St Ethelburga, licensed in the early years of the Restoration, was the daughter of a prominent midwife of the same parish who was licensed in 1622. Sara does not mention her mother's profession in her own testimonial, although she had no doubt received much of her knowledge and training at her mother's hands.[66] Frances Austen, whose licensing records have not been recovered, gave sworn testimony for Rebecca Searles in 1663, and there is no hint of her occupation. Fortunately, when she supported Anne Alkin's application in 1670, her signed statement added the designation "midwife" after her name.[67] For these reasons, we would argue that the number of midwives who had an apprenticeship with senior midwives before obtaining a licence to practise on their own was higher than our figures have demonstrated, although it is not possible to assert that all London midwives developed within this system. It is noteworthy that the ecclesiastical licensing system encouraged the reporting of this type of training, without making such evidence mandatory. In the same way that only a substantial minority of the testimonials reported on the length of training, we will never know to what extent the role of senior midwives was under-reported.

A picture has emerged, particularly during the 1660s, of highly competent midwives who took an active part in the training of young midwives. (See Appendix F.) The most visible of these women was Alice Herbert of St Giles in the Fields. Alice was responsible for at least seven younger midwives at various times between the years 1661–76. Her protégées included Anne Adams, St Martin in the Fields, licensed in 1661; Gertrude Wigly, St Giles in the Fields, 1662; Audrey Lucas, St Andrew Holborn, 1667; Margaret Venable, St Mary Islington, 1667; Elizabeth Martin, St Giles in the Fields, 1669; Anne Boggs, St Giles in the Fields, 1671; and Anne Dobson, also of St Giles in the Fields, in 1676.[68] Three of the foregoing – Lucas, Venable, and Martin – were also supervised by Esther Kilbury, who worked closely with Herbert for a few years and then moved on to take personal responsibility for at least two other trainee midwives. When Herbert supplied a separate statement for Gertrude Wigly to include with her testimonial certificates in 1662, she wrote:

66 GL MS 10,116/3.   67 GL MS 10,116/3, 7.   68 GL MS 10,116/1, 2, 5, 6, 7, 9.

These are to certifie that the bearer above named hath served me in my imployment and she being my deputie in severall yeares officiate in my absences. She my deputy in being for the space of three years hath faiethfullie performed whatso[e]vear belonged to her in and upon any occasions so fare as eaver it could heave by any whose soeaver I had employment for her. Witness my hand Alyce Herbeart midwife thes 22 yers.[69]

Once again it should be borne in mind that these trainers of midwives brought to their task skills and knowledge acquired through decades of practical experience. Although excluded from access to formal education, the expertise of these women extended far beyond the boundaries of academic learning. It was an expertise acquired within the intimate circle of midwives and female friends which surrounded the childbed. Alice Herbert had more than twenty years' experience to bring to the task of training Anne Adams in 1661. The venerable midwife Susan Swanley of Shadwell in Stepney, who had begun her work as a midwife in the 1630s, had supervised Herbert's associate Kilbury, in her turn.[70] The early years of the Restoration, in particular, saw a group of senior midwives with long careers in the practice of midwifery who were actively involved in the training of younger midwives: Elizabeth Boycott of St Sepulchre licensed in 1636; Eleanor Gillam, St Olave Silver Street, 1637; Elizabeth Hales, St Nicholas Cole Abbey, 1636; Joan Rowley, St Clement Danes, 1632; Helen Orme, St Vedast Foster Lane, 1636; Elizabeth Somner, St Dunstan in the West, 1639; and Mary Melsom, St Thomas the Apostle, 1626.[71]

By the last decade of the century, there are still examples of midwives of long experience who have an association with younger midwives. Eleanor Dickenson of St Martin in the Fields was licensed in 1669. By the time she sponsored Anne Alcroft's and Elizabeth Coleman's applications for midwifery licences, she had over twenty years of experience in midwifery herself.[72] Licensed in 1690, Bridgid Blackborrow of St Botolph Aldgate and Susan Briscoe (whose parish has not been recorded) claimed the testimonial support of Elizabeth Harris and Anne Vere who had 17 and 13 years' experience, respectively. Anne Vere of St Botolph Aldersgate had 20 years' experience by the time Margaret Morse claimed her as mentor in 1697.[73]

69 GL MS 10,116/2. It appears that Wigly served an apprenticeship of unspecified length before becoming Herbert's deputy, competent to act in Herbert's absence.
70 GL MS 10,116/6, 3. Swanley had also supervised Christian Broadgate and Elizabeth Rickes, both of Stepney.
71 GL MS 10,116/1, 2, 3.   72 GL MS 10,116/13, LPL VX 1A/11.
73 GL MS 10,116/13, 14. See Appendix I for a list of midwives, including senior midwives. There do not seem, however, to have been as many senior midwives with long experience in the last three decades as there were in the 1660s. Here again, the evidence may be, in part, deceptive. It seems likely that either the church authorities in general expected a higher standard when issuing licences in the first decade of reintroduction, or else that the candidates were not as certain of what was required and went beyond the authorities' expectations. In consequence, many testimonials are fuller. There exists, moreover, the likelihood that testimonials tended to include testimony primarily from senior midwives who had themselves already been licensed. Many fully experienced midwives of the 1642–60 period may, therefore, have been under-reported as senior midwives in the early 1660s, leaving the impression that training was predominantly in the hands of the more matronly pre-1641 generation.

Thus, the training of London midwives possessed similarities to the system followed by the male-dominated London guilds. Unlike a craft apprentice, an apprentice midwife would, unless related to her mentor, not live with her.[74] Since none of the London midwives about whom we have information had been unmarried, such a residency requirement would have been unrealistic. Many, but by no means all, trainee midwives resided in the same parish as their senior midwife. As we will see, trainee midwives had a more diverse age structure than the traditional young male apprentices.

Since a number of midwives were literate, some recourse may have been had to the gynaecological treatises of the day. Without question, however, the core of the training was "hands on" experience in child delivery. In those cases when senior midwives had several apprentices at one time (for example, Alice Herbert), it is likely that more than one trainee would be present at deliveries. Perhaps novices would have observed several deliveries before being called upon to take a more active role. As several of the above testimonials make clear, more experienced deputies performed deliveries in the absence of their mentors.

MIDWIVES' REFEREES

In assessing the competence of midwives trained in this system, we are not limited simply to internal appraisals. Endorsement of competence and skill came from the "official" branches of medicine.[75] Here the most active supporter of midwives seeking midwifery licences was Hugh Chamberlen of the acclaimed Chamberlen family, inventors and custodians of the (secret) midwifery forceps.[76] Chamberlen, appointed to the position of physician in ordinary to Charles the Second in 1663, carried on his family's traditional interest in the practice of midwifery.[77] Although twentieth-century biases might influence our perspective regarding the value of Chamberlen's testimonials, it must be borne in mind that aspiring male midwives had no recourse to normal deliveries and an association with a traditional midwife was one of the only avenues available for procuring instruction in child delivery. His first recorded endorsement of a midwife appears on the testimonial of Sarah Benet in 1674.[78] Chamberlen has added a statement below that of the curate,

---

74 Apparently in Nuremberg, where married women were discouraged from entering midwifery apprenticeships, midwifery apprentices resided with their mistresses. Wiesner, 98–9.
75 For examples from the provinces, see David Harley, "The scope of legal medicine in Lancashire and Cheshire, 1660–1760," in Michael Clark and Catherine Crawford, eds., *Legal Medicine in History* (Cambridge: Cambridge University Press, 1994), 47.
76 For comment on the possible connection between Chamberlen and the politically active London midwife, Elizabeth Cellier, see Helen King, "The politick midwife: models of midwifery in the work of Elizabeth Cellier," *The Art of Midwifery*, 120–1.
77 Aveling in Snell Smith, 78.
78 Snell Smith seems to suggest that Chamberlen was acting in some sort of "official" capacity as an examiner for the ecclesiastical authorities. Snell Smith, 79. Too few testimonials bear his statement to support this view. Possibly he knew them personally, and adopted his (unwarranted) stance of superior expertise in a manner reminiscent of his father, Peter Chamberlen, who attempted to organize and monopolise the profession of midwifery half a century earlier.

rector, and churchwardens of St Dunstan in the West indicating that he had "examined" Mrs. Benet and found her qualified to practise midwifery.[79] In 1686, he made the following statement on behalf of Mary Lambert of Evesham, Surrey, who was subsequently licensed to practise midwifery in London under the jurisdiction of the Archbishop of Canterbury:

Having at the request of Mary Lambert ye bearer hereof examined her skill in that profession I do hereby certify that I find her sufficiently Qualified both in knowledge and practice for to follow ye said profession.[80]

The following year Chamberlen noted that he had also "examined" Mrs. Mary Bunce and found her "fitt to be admitted to the practice of midwifery."[81] Jane Cooke of St Dunstan in the West presented testimonials in 1684 to which Chamberlen had appended a separate paragraph attesting to her ability as a midwife.[82] Chamberlen's most fulsome statement appears on the testimonial of Elizabeth Deane, wife of Richard Deane, gentleman, of St James Weston in 1688:

These are to certify whom it may concern that upon the desire of the bearer hereof Mrs. Elizabeth Deane of St James I have upon a strict examination found her fitt to follow the practice of midwifery she having also served four or five or more years as Deputy to able midwives.[83]

Chamberlen's statement was an endorsement of Deane's competence and skill, and also of the traditional system whereby midwives served as deputies under highly experienced senior midwives. Aside from that, her "examination" (as well as that of the other midwives whom he "examined") could prove instructive to male midwives, who were generally excluded from the lying-in chamber.

Even more compelling than Chamberlen's statement on Deane's behalf, however, was the statement signed by four of Deane's clients:

These are to certify that the bearer hereof Elizabeth the wife of Richard Deane of the parish of St James Weston, Gent. have layd us safe and well in Childbirth and delivered us by God's help and wee are all of us very much obliged to her care, skill, as a good midwife.[84]

An unusual expression of Chamberlen's interest in a midwife is found in the certificate of Elizabeth Beranger of the parish of St Peter the Poor in 1674. In it, he urged the chancellor, Dr. Thomas Exton, to license Beranger. He points out that in a previous communication he had forgotten to mention that Beranger was not only a staunch adherent of the Church of England, but that she had a certificate from the Hotel Dieu of Paris, "famous all the world over for the Instruction of midwives." Beranger received her licence on the strength of Cham-

79 LPL MS VX 1A/11/6.   80 LPL MS VX 1A/11/41.   81 LPL MS VX 1A/11/45.
82 GL MS 10,116/11.   83 GL MS 10,116/12.   84 Ibid.

berlen's testimony without the benefit of testimony by clients or clergy.[85] Although Chamberlen's court connections might give him added credibility when supplying testimonials, the Chamberlen family had a long history of entrepreneurial designs on midwifery and an association with a skilled midwife like Beranger would have provided a marvellous opportunity for self-styled man-midwife Chamberlen to hone his skills.

When Sarah Trip of Isleworth, Middlesex, presented her statement of competence to the licensing authorities in 1661, she obtained the signatures of "medical doctor" R. Hodges, surgeon John Gisby of Brentford, apothecary Frances Phillips, also of Brentford, and midwife Mary Elin, of Richmond. All four attested to the fact that Sara had ". . . longtime performed the office of midwife in these parts with good success and with great approbation from all those who have made use of her."[86] John Knapp, "Dr. medicina," and G. Constable, bachelor of medicine, signed the testimonial of Alice Thwaites of Stepney, the wife of Thomas Thwaites, "one of his majesties lifeguards" who subsequently was licensed to practice midwifery in February 1663.[87] Katherine Pinchon of St Martin Vintry enclosed a separate statement from N. Paget, a member of the "London College of Medicine," which read: "These may certify that I judge Mrs. Katherin Pinchion to be a sufficient midwife, July 20, 1663."[88] Two medical doctors, Joseph Hinton and Edmond Cooper (who also claimed to be an honourary member of the "Medical College of London") spoke to the abilities of Elizabeth Mercer of St Mary Savoy in 1666.[89] Signatures of apothecaries, surgeons, and physicians appear on other testimonials of women applying for licences in the years 1669, 1681, and 1697.[90]

Although recent publications, such as that edited by Hilary Marland, have begun to revise traditional perceptions, historians have generally sympathised with the views of medical authors with vested interests such as Percival Willughby, that midwives were, as a group, poorly trained and ill prepared for their calling. Some representatives of the medical profession were, for whatever motives, clearly prepared to give sworn testimony to the ability and competence of midwives.[91] It should be borne in mind, however, that other factors such as social status may have had a bearing on the fact that these particular women obtained some accreditation from the "professionals." Elizabeth Deane, Mary Bunce, and Mary

85 GL MS 10,116/8. Donnison notes that in the eighteenth century there was a head midwife at the Hotel Dieu who was independent of the medical staff and who called in a surgeon only when she thought instruments were necessary. Donnison, 27.
86 GL MS 10,116/3.   87 GL MS 10,116/3.   88 GL MS 10,116/3.
89 GL MS 10,116/4. Hinton was possibly related to Sir John Hinton, physician-in-ordinary to the King.
90 GL MS 10,116/3, 14. In the case of Katherine Coal, the "medicos" claimed an acquaintanceship of nine years. GL MS 10,116/11. I suspect, as was the case with Chamberlen, that some of these practitioners were aspiring to the practise of midwifery, if not already engaged in it.
91 Willughby did have a somewhat higher opinion of London midwives than their provincial counterparts. David Harley, in commenting on the frequent testimonial support of physicians and surgeons for provincial midwives, has suggested it might imply a "close working relationship" between some midwives and medical practitioners. Harley, "Provincial Midwives," 29.

Glasse were married to gentlemen; Alice Thwaites was married to a man who had a connection with the court; Katherine Coal was described as a "gentlewoman"; and Elizabeth Beranger's father was a Proctor of the Arches.[92]

Like the unnamed midwife and gentlewoman who sought instruction from the anatomist Dr. Thomas Wharton in 1673, the midwives may have approached the medical practitioners to acquire theoretical knowledge.[93] It is also possible that these women claimed an association with these men based on mutual social ties and friendships within the circles in which they moved. As such, it reflects the high status of some London midwives. On the outside of Elizabeth Deane's testimonial, court official Richard Newcombe had written: "Let this pass without fees." Since Deane was married to a gentleman and could well afford the expense of obtaining her licence, this can only be taken as an indication that she had friends of influence in high places. Male practitioners may also have cultivated an association with midwives of the upper class for what they could offer by way of an entry into the homes of upper-class clients.

In total, twelve testimonials, or 2% of all surviving testimonials, contain these recommendations from a variety of medical practitioners.[94] It is apparent that the ecclesiastical authorities on occasion accepted the testimony of medical professionals as to the practical skills of applicants for midwifery licences. Of these individuals, Chamberlen was unique in asserting that he had "examined" the women's competence. But the point that should be stressed is that an association with a midwife afforded unrivalled opportunities to male practitioners eager to learn about normal childbirth processes. These opportunities will loom large in the events of the eighteenth century, which saw the eventual displacement of the female midwife from her position of superiority by the male midwife.

COMPETENCE VS. CHARACTER?

To modern eyes the striking feature of these documents [certificates or testimonials] is that the principal, and sometimes the only, mentioned qualification of the midwife was that she was a person of good character. If there was any reference to her professional competence,

---

92 Mary Glasse was supported by an apothecary and a surgeon. GL MS 10,116/3. It is possible that midwives of some social standing were working with male professionals who became the prototype for the male midwife. It is generally acknowledged that the surgeon was the practitioner who worked most closely with the midwife because of his involvement in complicated deliveries when instruments were required for the removal of a dead infant. Of the twelve women above who claimed support from medical practitioners, only three included the support of surgeons. Hugh Chamberlen, however, styled himself a male midwife and would have profited and learned through a working association with upper-class midwives like Deane.

93 Notts. Record Office DDA 67/9.

94 For purposes of this analysis, the testimonial of Elizabeth Francis, who was licensed as a midwife and surgeon, was excluded. She will be dealt with in a later chapter. GL MS 10,116/14. Since the sole reason for seeking the support of a medical professional was to facilitate the acquisition of a licence, this feature would not likely be subject to under-reporting. This differs from the evidence on training with senior midwives, and we can conclude with some degree of confidence that only a very small minority of seventeenth-century midwives were licensed following examination or recommendation by other branches of the medical profession.

it was usually the number of years she had functioned as a midwife, although laymen sometimes testified to her skill. Thus, like her training, the licensing of the midwife was seriously inadequate by modern standards.[95]

The consequence of statements of this nature, by historians living in the twentieth century, is that it is generally (and erroneously) believed that the seventeenth-century ecclesiastical licensing system paid scant regard to the skill and training of midwives, with the obvious corollary that professional standards were low.[96]

We have determined that the licensing authorities were concerned with far more than the applicant's character (see Chapter 1); what evidence do the testimonials contain about the way clergy and laypersons assessed candidates' qualifications? Contemporaries did not make a clear distinction between character and professional competence. For them, the two were obviously and intimately associated.

It is true that a number of clerical testimonials (or in some cases, those of churchwardens) speak only of the character and high principles of the prospective midwife.[97] In the context of licensing in the 1661–1700 period, however, far more testimonials comment on the midwife's skill and competence as well as her character than on her character alone. Indeed, in 1678, when Anne Hide of St Mary Islington applied for her licence, the clergy and churchwardens acknowledged a midwife's priorities: They noted that Anne "frequents her parish Church except at such times as shee is hindred by the business of her profession which is that of a midwife."[98] Similarly, in 1693, the curate John Ewer and the churchwardens of St Mary Mattfellon allowed that Mary Salmon "hath and doth constantly come to her parish church on the Lords days (so often as her office will permit)."[99] Mary Duckett of St Dunstan in the West applied for a licence in 1669. Her testimonial certificate stressed her service as deputy for a licensed midwife (Mrs. Hatton) but did not even mention the fact that she was the wife of a clergyman.[100]

In 1661, of 20 testimonials signed by clergy, 17 attest to the midwife's competence as well as her character, 2 mention only her character, and one speaks only of her skill. In addition to the testimonials of the clergy, one midwife was licensed who apparently presented only sworn testimony from female clients, although there is a possibility that some of her documents may have been lost.[101] Testimo-

---

95 Forbes, *The Midwife and the Witch*, 155.
96 One historian has dismissed both licensed and unlicensed midwives in the seventeenth century, concluding that "their qualifications were rudimentary." In justification of his overtly negative view, Thomas has cited two brief, but damning comments, both taken from seventeenth-century writers with vested interests in changing midwifery practice. Thomas, *Religion*, 15. The two writers were Percival Willughby, male midwife, and Elizabeth Cellier, a midwife who wanted to found and head a school for midwives at a handsome profit for herself. Unfortunately, the view that competence was not a consideration for licensing still prevails. See Cressy, *Birth*, 63–4.
97 The term "character" is used to encompass the candidate's religious attributes as well as other more secular characteristics.
98 GL MS 10,116/10.   99 GL MS 10,116/13.   100 GL MS 10,116/6.
101 GL MS 10,116/1. For these observations, only full statements by women with a personal knowledge of the midwife's work and not merely the usual listing of several women's names as sworn witnesses have been considered.

nials from representative years of 1672–7 still show that competence was not neglected in issuing midwifery licences: Of 22 testimonials signed by clergy, 7 refer to both skill and competence, 12 to character, and one to competence only. In the years 1690–95, of 23 clerical testimonials, 6 refer to the woman's competence as well as her character, 1 refers solely to her competence, and 16 to her character alone.[102]

As a general observation, conformity to the tenets of the Church of England appears to have been an increasing preoccupation of clergy, as well as of the laity, who testified on the midwives' behalf in the last decade of the century. For example, female clients usually commented only on their knowledge of the midwife's skill, but in 1696, four women swore to Ann Pedro's experience in midwifery and, in a separate statement at the bottom of the page, it was noted "All the persons above testified of Mrs. Pedro's conformity."[103] One possible explanation for the increased emphasis on a midwife's conformity could be heightened clerical apprehensions following the passage of the Toleration Act in 1689. When Lucy Wetherby of St Giles in the Fields presented her accreditation from her minister and churchwarden in 1690, it was in the form of a communion certificate. It stated that Wetherby had taken the sacrament on April 13, 1690 and was signed by John Sharpe, D.D., and Nathaniel Chandler, churchwarden.[104] Thomas Tenison (the future Archbishop of Canterbury) was particularly conscientious in mentioning the candidates' participation in the rite of sacrament.[105]

Although most of the testimonial documentation includes a statement of one sort or another by parish clergy, by no means all of the applicants supplied clerical testimony. Again, there is the possibility that loss of documents is a factor. However, it does not appear that the licensing authorities absolutely *required* an authoritative statement on faith or character before issuing a midwifery licence.

There are other indications at the parish level of the Church's concern that midwifery licences be issued on the basis of a woman's experience and skill in her chosen field. Rectors and vicars, as well as church wardens, frequently relayed information about the midwife's experience, particularly as it related to her association with another, more experienced midwife. The minister of the parish of Stepney, Spitalfields, presented the statement of Temperance Pratt, widow and midwife, that Ursula Stokes of the same parish was "altogether expert and

---

102 GL MS 10,116/13.   103 GL MS 10,116/14.

104 In addition to the certificate, Wetherby presented sworn testimony of four women. GL MS 10,116/13. The same type of communion certificate was presented by Mary Higdon of St Botolph Bishopsgate in 1681. GL MS 10,116/11.

105 GL MS 10,116/12, midwives Rathbone's and Walford's testimonials, and LPL MS VX 1A/11, 35, Mary Wood's testimonial, contain examples of the vellum communion certificate issued by Thomas Tenison who became the Archbishop of Canterbury in 1695. Since only a handful of midwives submitted communion certificates, they could not have been a requirement for licensing. David Harley similarly notes only one instance where a provincial midwife submitted a communion certificate and does not believe that they were a requirement. Harley, "Provincial Midwives," 35.

every way able to follow the calling of a midwife."[106] Thomas Tenison, then rector of St James Weston, took his responsibility seriously when he supplied sworn support for Anne Hopper, one of his parishioners in 1690: "I have made inquiry about Ms. Ann Hopper of my parish." He concluded, on the basis of reports by "grave matrons," that Anne was "well qualified . . . for ye office of a midwife."[107] Before he swore that Elizabeth Syrett was fit for the office of midwife, Thomas Pettiplace, curate of St Giles in the Fields, sought out the opinions of Syrett's neighbours.[108]

In the intimacy of the crowded London parish, a midwife's neighbours were possibly in the best position to give a trustworthy account of midwives' abilities.[109] They would know of her successes as well as her failures. An unidentified London midwife who practised in the late seventeenth and early eighteenth centuries recorded her deliveries of several close neighbours.[110] Dozens of testimonials stress the length of time that the midwife had lived in her parish.[111] Rector John Williams of St Peter Paul's Wharf noted that his parishioner Margaret Corney, licensed in 1661, had lived in the same parish for forty years.[112] The churchwardens of Stepney pointed out that Martha Grymes had lived in their parish "for twenty years or thereabouts."[113] The "good success" of long-time midwife Emmett Sare and her excellent personal qualities were known to "hundreds" in her home parish of St Giles Cripplegate.[114]

Statements such as these were not only proof of the stability of the midwife; they were an indication of the high esteem in which these women were held as they worked and lived under the close scrutiny of neighbours, clients, and other parish residents. In the words of the rector of Rayleigh, not only had Elizabeth Moors lived more than 20 years in her parish, she was "well known to exercise the office of midwife among us."[115] Elizabeth Dowke had lived for forty years in the parish of St Bartholomew the Great with "good credit and reputation among her neighbourhood."[116] Judith Newman of Allhallows the Less, was perceived to have "demeaned herself honestly and in love and charity with her neighbours" throughout her more than thirty years of residence and "many years past" of midwifery practise.[117] A resident of St Giles in the Fields for more than twenty years, Dorothy Rosson "alway behaved herself justly, soberly and honestly among her neighbours," while Emma Cayford, also a twenty-year resident of her parish,

---

106 GL MS 10,116/10.   107 GL MS 10,116/13.   108 GL MS 10,116/13.

109 Margaret Pelling has noted the importance of community approbation in the case of apprentices' masters. Margaret Pelling, "Apprenticeship, Health and Social Cohesion in Early Modern London," *History Workshop Journal* 37 (1994): 47.

110 BL, Oxford, Rawlinson MS D/1141/34, 60.

111 Again, implicit in the idea of long-term parish residency are the concepts of respect and authority, which these women commanded. Thomas, *Age and Authority*. Ancient is used in the sense of having the wisdom of age: SOED.

112 GL MS 10,116/1.   113 GL MS 10,116/1.   114 GL MS 25,598, (1662).

115 GL MS 10,116/3.   116 GL MS 10,116/1.   117 GL MS 10,116/1.

had "always been observed" to have been an "able midwife" as well as a woman of "good life and conversation."[118]

This sense of neighbourhood endorsement emerges time after time and it is obvious that the parish clergy and churchwardens were acting as the semi-official voices of their parochial communities when they provided their testimonials. In 1663, both the rector and curate of St Clement Danes swore that Clare Baxter was

. . . of honest life and conversation and an expert and skilful midwife who hath brought to bed and delivered many women with much commendation amongst her neighbours.[119]

Parish officials of St Bride's noted in 1663 that they "have a report" from the neighbours of Margaret Stevens regarding her ability and character, while almost thirty years later the vicar and churchwardens of St Dunstan in the West also cited the evidence of neighbours regarding Sara Mainwaring's suitability for the office of midwife.[120]

Rector Barton and churchwarden Poole of St Margaret New Fish Street testified on behalf of neighbourhood women when Anne St John applied for her licence:

[Anne] Hath manifested both her skill and care in safe delivering some of her neighbours in the parish of child bearing as many women on theyr own experience can testifye and therefore we do conceive her to be fitt that she may be licensed for that office.[121]

The testimonial of Elizabeth Cooper of St Martin in the Fields was a statement by her "neighbours and parishoners," including nine men of the parish, while Elizabeth Hill of St Michael Wood Street was commended for the "good order in her house" and "living peacably and quietly as a good neighbour ought to do."[122] The next-door neighbour of Alice Pinnock of Shadwell vouched for her suitability as a midwife in 1673.[123] Parish clergy and their communities could not help but be concerned about both the technical competence and the moral conduct of the prospective licensee. The parish clergy would not entrust their wives, daughters, and parishioners to an individual, no matter how well trained, who was untrustworthy. It seems clear that licensing was the end product of a system that began with extensive experience and a good reputation within a parish.

As a general rule, aside from clergy and churchwardens, the majority of witnesses giving sworn testimony on behalf of women seeking a midwifery licence were female. There was, however, some evidence that in a society where women gained their legitimacy as they related to a male (be he parent, sibling, or spouse), midwives believed that male witnesses would give their application increased legitimacy. Frances Cloys of St Botolph Aldgate obtained the statement of Val-

118 GL MS 10,116/13, 1.   119 GL MS 10,116/3.   120 GL MS 10,116/3, 13.
121 GL MS 10,116/3.   122 GL MSS 10,116/3, 5.   123 GL MS 10,116/8.

entine Waite, her landlord, as well that of her minister and one churchwarden to support her claim that she had gained competence and experience as a deputy to Jane Ward, a licensed midwife whom she had served for many years.[124] Joseph Peterburow made the following statement on behalf of Alice Bunworth of St Andrew Holborn in 1671:

She lived in my house and was marreyd out of my house & did always behave herself very modestly and faithfully during that time & I believe will doe in any place or imployment whatsoere.[125]

Joan Cockson of St Dunstan in the West obtained brief signed statements from three males including her neighbour of many years, John Jermyn, who commended her sufficiency in the office of midwife.[126]

Aside from the customary cleric and two churchwardens, various other parish officials were called upon to attest to a midwife's competence and character. Margaret Digborrow of St Mary Woolchurch and Temperance Pratt of St Botolph without Algate both obtained the signatures of parish constables.[127] Anne Goodwin of St Andrew Wardrobe, Margaret Johnson of St Clement Danes, and Mary Knott of St Bride's, licensed in 1661 and 1663, claimed support from their parish clerks.[128] Still other women presented documents witnessed by parish overseers of the poor.[129] In addition to parish officials, civic and other government officials occasionally gave their stamp of approval to applicants: Judith Newman of Allhallows the Less and Jane Ward of Allhallows the Great both obtained the signatures of two common councilmen while Margaret Digborrow, Katherine Pinchon, and Mary Duckett presented documents sworn by a single common councilman. Temperance Pratt's testimonial bore the signature of a member of Parliament.[130]

A survey of testimonials to ascertain how many contained the signatures of men who could not be considered parish officials or clergy revealed the following: In the period 1661–71, 60 women out of 205, or 29%, obtained male signatures beyond those of parish officials and clergy.[131] In the years 1672–81, only four testimonials out of 138, or not quite 3%, carried additional male signatures. There was a slight increase in the period 1682–91 to just under 4%, or 4 out of 101 testimonials. By the last period, 2.5%, or only 2 out of 77 testimonial documents, bore men's signatures that could not be associated with clergy and parish officials. Again, one possible explanation for the decreasing number of male signatures could lie in the fact that midwives in the period following the re-establishment of ecclesiastical licensing were uncertain of just how much documentation or certi-

---

124 GL MS 10,116/4.   125 LPL VX 1A/11/2.   126 GL MS 10,116/1.
127 GL MS 10,116/2, 3.
128 GL MS 10,116/1, 3. Later in the century, Mistresses Fendell, Whitehorne, and Fowler enlisted the support of their parish clerks. GL MS 10,116/10, 12.
129 GL MSS 10,116/6 (Martyn) and 10,116/ 10 (North).   130 GL MS 10,116/1, 2, 6, 3.
131 For purposes of this survey, two signatures were arbitrarily allowed for churchwardens, even if they were not designated as such.

fication they needed and were ensuring that they had enough support. For example, Jane Johnson's testimonial (1661) contained fourteen men's names and Charity Langton's (1663) contained nine.[132] Hence, it would appear that in some cases, the women obtained the signatures of vestry members as well as signatures of other men of standing in the parish. This, however, was a short-lived development. Those who testified on behalf of candidates were overwhelmingly drawn from the applicant's parish clergy, parish officials, fellow midwives, and former clients.

In conclusion, midwives seeking licences to practise midwifery in London secured sworn evidence which not only showed them to be of good character and upright conduct, but also demonstrated that they had frequently undergone lengthy training by way of practical experience under the supervision of highly skilled midwives whose expertise had been acquired through decades of midwifery practice.[133] Fledgling midwives worked closely with senior and deputy midwives while they were acquiring the experience, which was necessary for licensing. Members of the medical establishment acknowledged the competence of a number of midwives and, by extension, the adequacy of the unofficial system of apprenticeship that the women underwent. Neighbours, civic and parish officials, including clergy, testified under oath that midwives seeking licences were women in every way qualified to carry out the work of child delivery successfully. Issues of training, competence, character, and faith were addressed by testimony from all four groups. Although the ecclesiastical licensing process was not concerned with supervision of licensed midwives, it did ensure that certain standards of competence and good conduct were met before a midwifery licence was issued. It also encouraged the supervision of inexperienced midwives or deputies by experienced midwives and the interchange of knowledge and assistance among midwives when difficult deliveries were encountered. The substantial outlay of cash which was required to obtain a midwifery licence was, in itself, a form of insurance against the temptation to dabble in midwifery on a whim or merely to avoid the pangs of poverty. The majority of the women who emerge from these pages were career professionals who dedicated years to their training and then went on to practise for decades.

The tracts of Elizabeth Cellier have been cited repeatedly as evidence from the midwives themselves that a new system of training was needed.[134] When the terms of Cellier's grand scheme for a training school for midwives are examined, how-

132 GL MS 10,116/1, 3. Anne Boggs, licensed in 1671, who had eleven male signatures, seems to be the last midwife to have a large number of male signatures on her testimonial. GL MS 10,116/7. See Appendix D.
133 To compare requirements and training for Dutch midwives in the eighteenth century, see Marland, " 'Stately and dignified,' " 296.
134 See also King, "The politick midwife," 115–30. For a perspective on Cellier, which is at odds with this study, see Kirstin Evenden, "The 'Popish Midwife': Printed Representations of Elizabeth Cellier and Midwifery Practice in Late Seventeenth-century London," *Racar*, XX (1–2, 1993): 43–58. The problem with the foregoing interpretation is discussed in the Conclusion.

ever, it becomes apparent that the major beneficiary would have been Mrs. Cellier herself, and that her criticisms of ecclesiastical licensing were rooted in her Roman Catholicism which excluded her from the contemporary avenue for obtaining a midwifery licence.[135] Given the state of medical knowledge which prevailed, it is clear that the traditional system, whereby midwives of long experience worked alongside new midwives, was superior to any instruction which the physicians or surgeons could offer, despite the sweeping accusations and allegations of critics among the doctors.[136]

The overwhelming majority of births was normal and did not require the intervention of medical practitioners whose services were restricted to medical emergencies. The male professionals gave no details of any proposed curriculum whereby the "ignorant midwives" of their diatribes could be taught the principles of midwifery. In 1634, when Peter Chamberlen attempted to monopolize midwifery in London, offering "instruction" in return for being the only practitioner authorised to answer a midwife's summons in cases of "dangerous and unnaturall travile," the midwives firmly pointed out his ignorance of the mechanics of normal childbirth.[137] As a result, the College of Physicians gave its stamp of approval to the ecclesiastical system of licensing midwives, and the consequence of a hearing into Chamberlen's proposal was that he was ordered to stop harassing the midwives and to acquire a licence himself to practise as a physician.[138] Jane Sharp had published midwifery information for midwives and while acknowledging in the "forward" to *The Midwives Book* that some midwives had no formal knowledge of anatomy, she stressed the preeminence of practical experience over knowledge acquired from books in the actual childbirth situation: "It is not hard words that perform the work, as if none understood the Art that cannot understand Greek." Deferring to the prevailing mind set of the seventeenth century, Sharp allowed the suitability of men for contemplating the "things of deeper Speculation than is required of the female sex," and then continued: "But the Art of Midwifry chiefly concerns us, which even the best learned men will grant."[139]

Much has been made of male midwife Willughby's knowledge of the technique of podalic version, implying that this granted him an expertise which female midwives lacked. Midwives, however, would certainly have been aware of the problems involved in abnormal presentations, which estimates have placed at four

---

135 Aveling, 66, 74.   136 See Shorter, *A History*, 47.   137 GL MS 9531/12–13.

138 For an interesting example of the gulf between midwives and male professionals of the early modern period, see the account of events surrounding the death of a member of the French royal family in childbirth in 1627. The renowned French midwife Louise Bourgeois and male practitioners became embroiled in a series of allegations and counter-allegations. Wendy Perkins has seen the incident as a clash between theory and practice with élitist and gender overtones. See Wendy Perkins, "Midwives versus Doctors: The case of Louise Bourgeois," *The Seventeenth Century* 3 (1988): 135–57. See also Thomas G. Benedek, "The Changing Relationship between Midwives and Physicians during the Renaissance," *Bulletin of the History of Medicine*, 51 (1977): 563–4.

139 Sharp, 1–3.

in every hundred births.[140] In many cases, experienced midwives devised a method of turning the child guided by their own observation and empirical knowledge.[141] Donegan has pointed out that the sexist attitudes of the age so coloured the thinking of male practitioners that they believed that gender rendered even a highly experienced midwife incapable of dealing with the deviations from the normal: If she performed a successful version, it was considered to be merely a stroke of luck.[142] Culpeper, it may be noted, in his popular *A Directorie for Midwives* of 1651 gave no practical instructions about how version could be carried out. He recommended that the midwife attempt to correct the malpresentation manually on the assumption that experienced midwives would understand how this could be accomplished.[143] In addition, midwives could avail themselves of published works, such as that of Guillimeau who described podalic version, and there were other ways that knowledge of such obstetrical techniques could be acquired and disseminated among the network of London midwives. For example, version techniques were taught at the famous Hotel Dieu in Paris and at least one London midwife trained and received her certificate at the renowned French hospital.[144]

Despite Jane Sharp's worry in 1671 that some midwives were deficient in their knowledge of anatomy, a London practitioner in the Stuart period gave evidence before the Royal College of Physicians that he had learned anatomy from a midwife who did dissections.[145] Moreover, it was possible for a midwife to improve her understanding of anatomy by private instruction.[146] It was not un-known, however, for uncharitable male practitioners to practise exclusionary tactics in an effort to keep midwives from invading their territory. Percival Willughby described how a midwife tried to observe an operative procedure that he carried out, but he managed to block her view and keep her in ignorance.[147] Eighteenth-century male midwife William Smellie credited an "illiterate" Irish midwife, Mary Donally, with successfully performing a Caesarean section, al-

---

140 Adrian Wilson, "William Hunter and the Varieties of Man-midwifery," W. F. Bynum and Roy Porter, eds. *William Hunter and the eighteenth century medical world* (Cambridge: Cambridge University Press, 1985), 344. Elsewhere, Wilson has acknowledged that some midwives "might have mastered the technique of podalic version," Wilson, "Participant or Patient?", 137.

141 For version techniques practised by German midwives in the early modern period, see Wiesner, 101. In the Netherlands, Vrouw Schrader was highly successful at performing manoeuvres to turn the fetus *in utero*. Hilary Marland, trans., *"Mother and Child were Saved": The memoirs (1693–1740) of the Frisian midwife Catharina Schrader* (Amsterdam: Rodopi, 1987), 37.

142 Donegan, 40–1.   143 Donegan, 17.

144 She was Elizabeth Beranger, licensed in 1674. GL MS 10,116/8. Jane Donegan notes that there are examples of seventeenth-century midwives in the English colonies in America who carried out podalic version. Donegan, 17.

145 Harold Cooke, *The Decline of the Old Medical Regime in Stuart London* (Ithaca: Cornell University Press, 1986), 33.

146 Notts. Record Office, DDA 67/9, letter of introduction to Dr. Thomas Wharton, by John Smith, April 9, 1673. I am grateful to David Harley for this reference.

147 Eccles, 110. Ironically, Willughby was highly critical of what he considered midwives' deficient knowledge.

though continental midwives had lost to the surgeons their traditional capacity for performing Caesareans by the fifteenth century.[148] For the great majority of deliveries which were, as now, free from complications, London midwives offered services which were vastly superior, because of their extensive training and practice, to those of male practitioners. In the occasional instance where operative intervention was needed, the midwife was obliged to call on the services of a male practitioner who possessed the required instruments of destruction and, in most cases, the child was sacrificed in the course of the procedure. The prominent eighteenth-century midwife Sara Stone railed against the fact that women had to call in surgeons for difficult deliveries which, almost inevitably, ended with the infant's death. London midwives' training was not perceived as deficient except by a few parties motivated by self-interest.

With respect to training and competence, one important conclusion arising from the study of extant evidence is that the licensing system illuminates an apprenticeship system that was based upon self-regulated community standards. The curate and churchwardens of Stepney parish noted in 1674 that although Mary Burnham, a widow with children to support, had served as a deputy for three years (her testimonial bore the mark of Hester Laramitt, midwife), "the midwifes do threaten to prosecute her of being not sworn."[149] Because it was self-regulatory and the midwives were expected to enforce the requirement for licensing, the system did not collapse with the removal of ecclesiastical licensing in the middle of the century. The clerical hierarchy knew that this system existed and approved of it (as did a critic as caustic as Willughby), but it played no direct, perceivable role in controlling it. The Church's role was to regulate – through licences – the end product. It did so largely by accepting the testimonial evidence that was generated by the apprenticeship system and, more generally, from the applicant's parochial community. It must also be borne in mind that deputy midwives were women who, in many instances, had years of experience, but were content to continue in their role of substitute for, or assistant to, a mentor, and thereby left no traces in the documents relating to licensing. The important point is that whether licensed or not, as Willughby conceded, the vast majority of London midwives underwent a lengthy training period under the tutelage of one

---

148 R. W. Johnston, 63. Blumenfeld-Kosinski has argued that the exclusion of continental midwives from performing the operation near the beginning of the fifteenth century was the "first step" in the male takeover of medicine. Renate Blumenfeld-Kosinski, *Not of Women Born* (Ithaca, N.Y.: Cornell University Press, 1990), 91. In Malta, in the eighteenth century, midwives were required by the Roman Catholic Church to have the skill and knowledge to carry out Caesarean sections. C. Savona-Ventura, "The Influence of the Roman Catholic Church on Midwifery Practice in Malta," *Medical History* 39 (1995), 24.

149 I suspect that this was the case with at least some of the women who claimed to be midwives and who have come to light in court depositions, but for whom I have found no evidence of licensing. Peter Earle, Jennifer Melville, and David Cressy have generously passed on the names of midwives whom they have uncovered in these sources and, in at least one instance, the woman was, indeed, a deputy to a licensed midwife.

or more experienced midwives. Since the testimonial and licensing system was not intended to reveal the full nature and characteristics of the training of midwives, what we find in this documentation is important but fragmentary evidence: a window into a larger world.

3

Mothers and Midwives[1]

Previous studies of early modern midwifery have paid scant attention both to the identities of midwives' clients and to clients' perceptions of the women who were so intimately involved with their personal well-being and that of their infants.[2] Valuable insights into the work and world of midwives can be gained, however, by directing our attention away from the London midwives themselves and focussing upon their clientele, a previously undefined constituency.

MIDWIVES AT WORK

Before beginning an examination of midwives' clients themselves, a brief exploration of the wife/client nexus is presented through a reconstruction of the midwife's activities in the lying-in chamber.[3] My reconstruction has been influenced by evidence from wills and inventories, which suggests that a midwife's kit would include such practical items as maps, saddlebags, aprons, medicine bottles, spare nightgowns, and linen (towels and napkins).[4] It is difficult to recreate childbed events without recourse to secondhand or prescriptive information from nonparticipating males, but these are not always reliable guides to actual childbed

1 An earlier version of this chapter appeared as Doreen Evenden, "Mothers and their midwives in seventeenth-century England," Hilary Marland, ed., *The Art of Midwifery* (London: Routledge, 1993), 9–26.
2 For comment on the authority and power invested in the midwife at the time of delivery, see Adrian Wilson "Childbirth in seventeenth and eighteenth-century England" (Ph.D. dissertation, University of Sussex, 1983): 127–8, 226; "The ceremony of childbirth and its interpretation," Valerie Fieldes, ed., *Women as Mothers in Industrial England* (London: Routledge, 1990), 71–3. The testimonial evidence used in this study affords a different perspective on the perception of midwives by their clients since it was recorded sometime after the delivery and was thus distanced from the situation which conferred unusual power on the midwife.
3 For a study of this nature, I would argue that the actual mechanics of midwifery are irrelevant. Because of our twentieth-century preoccupation with technical and medical details, however, questions about "what," as well as "who," have prompted me to attempt this discussion.
4 GLRO AM/PI(2)/1681/19, AM/PI(2)/1745/1, AM/PI/(2)1690/17. For an eighteenth-century French midwife's work plan, see Gélis, 158.

experiences.[5] Turning to several treatises which incorporate the insights of female practitioners will, perhaps, afford a glimpse into the darkened space that enclosed the woman in labour and her attendants.[6]

It has been well established that giving birth in the seventeenth century was still "women's business" and once the husband had summoned or ridden for the midwife, he was banished from the actual birth chamber, leaving the hustle and bustle of preparation, delivery, and aftercare to midwife, female relatives, neighbours, and friends.[7]

Upon her arrival, in some cases on horseback, the midwife donned a fresh apron, checked to see that "a little bed, or couch, of moderate height" was ready, and that other supplies of linen, swaddling, etc. were at hand.[8] If the prospective mother lacked the necessary sheets or bedding, the midwife could supply them from her own linen stock.[9] The room would be dark and warm and the woman decently, as well as warmly covered. A midwives' advice manual from 1680, written by a woman who identifies herself as the mother of a midwife and was a midwife herself in all likelihood, suggests that the newly arrived midwife should

5 For example, doctors were advising warmth and darkness for the seventeenth-century birthing chamber while by the eighteenth century, as male midwives grappled with fixing the blame for postpartum deaths, medical treatises urged airy and cool surroundings. Yet most women would have given birth in rooms which reflected their socioeconomic circumstances and personal habits with little or no choice involved. See Adrian Wilson "Ceremony," 73. For eighteenth-century views regarding temperature and ventilation, see John Aitken, *Principles of Midwifery or Puerperal Medicine* (London: 1685), 186; Charles White, *A Treatise on the Management of Pregnant and Lying-in Women* (London: 1773), 330.

6 The treatises in question are discussed in the Introduction: See notes 41, 45, 54. See also Cressy, *Birth*, 53–87 for a different and interesting perspective on childbirth, its rituals, and activities. A deputy or junior midwife was frequently in attendance with her mentor. The maternal grandmother was also often in attendance. Quaker birth notes give the names of women present at the birth of Quaker infants. The number varied from as few as two, to as many as nine, in addition to the midwife. Most commonly, four or five women were present. PRO RG/6/1626–8.

7 According to the midwife's oath (Appendix C) only if an emergency occurred, which the midwives could not manage, were males (surgeons) to be admitted to the secrecy of the birthing chamber. So strong was the association between death and the appearance of a male that one puritan mother thought she was doomed when the male midwife appeared. Houlbrooke, 108. See also Adrian Wilson, "Ceremony," 70–3, "Participant or patient," 133–5; R. V. Schnucker, "The English Puritans and Pregnancy, Delivery and Breast Feeding," *History of Childhood Quarterly* (Spring 1974): 640–1. For France, where there were striking similarities as well as differences, see Gélis, 99–103. For a different interpretation in which the seclusion of the mother is rooted in the shame and embarrassment surrounding the female body, see Gail Kern Paster, *The Body Embarrassed: drama and the disciplines of shame in early modern England* (Ithaca: Cornell University Press, 1993), 185.

8 T. C. [Catherine Turner] et al., 76. The preparation of bed linen – older linen to be used during labour and finer linen for the lying-in period – was an important consideration. The Verney family letters give priority to the preparation of "old bed linens" for the delivery of a family member. Frances P. Verney and M. M. Verney, *The Verney Memoirs* (London: Longmans Green and Co., 1925), vol. 2: 64.

9 The testimonial of Anne Miller mentions the fact that she rode to her patients. GL MS 10,116/16. After examining a number of midwives' inventories and wills, their liberal supplies of linen (sheets, towels, napkins, pillow covers) suggest that they were prepared to loan these necessities to their clients. For similarities and differences in the preparations undertaken by a French midwife, see Perkins, *Midwifery and Medicine*, 57–61.

"See that the Bed be well made for the woman that is to be brought to bed . . . put on her a little smock and waste-coat, and other linen necessary."[10] In 1649, the overseers for the poor of St Olave Jewry approved payment for a pillow, coverlet, waistcoat, and stockings, "necessaries" for a poor woman who was delivered in the home of a parish widow.[11]

The midwife could then check the woman's abdomen to see if the child had "fallen down" and carry out an internal examination, after first anointing her hand with fresh butter or other oils, to establish the amount of cervical dilation.[12] The midwife might position herself close to the woman on a stool or chair that was lower than the bed.[13] If the labour was well underway, she perhaps encouraged the prospective mother to assume a favoured position: kneeling, crouching, sitting (on a stool, chair, or another woman's lap), standing, or, most commonly, lying.[14] Ideally, a "little cricket" or footstool would be at hand since, in some cases, the contractions could have more force by placing the woman with "her feet bowed."[15] If no nourishment had as yet been readied by the other women attendants, and in the event of a "long travail," the midwife would arrange that small quantities of a nourishing "broth, yolk of a poached egg with some bread, a cup of wine or distilled water" be offered.[16]

After placing pillows under the woman's head, in the small of her back and

10 C. R. [Rachel Cotes], *The Compleat Midwives Practice Enlarged* (London: 1680), 27.

11 GL MS 4409/2 unfol. The churchwarden's accounts for this parish contain several references to women who were lodged and delivered at parish expense at widow Bull's, who was not a midwife. My thanks to Linda Hayner for this reference. By 1752, these homely tasks relating to the preparation of linen and bedclothes had been relegated by male midwives to nurses. See William Smellie, *Treatise on the Theory and Practice of Midwifery* (London: 1752), 450.

12 T. C. et al., 80; Sermon, 99.   13 Sermon, 99.

14 Sarah Stone describes her arrival, wet and tired, after riding eight miles on bad roads. She took some time to dry out before going up to the mother. Stone, 51. Evidence from inventories points to a midwife's apron. For a discussion of various positions adopted by women in early modern Europe, see Gélis, 121–33. In France, the horizontal position was the least favoured. In England, a three-legged stool was frequently used in the early seventeenth century. Although the little evidence that we have points toward a greater use of the bed for delivery in the latter part of the seventeenth and the eighteenth centuries, women were not confined to their beds for their labour and, in some cases, delivery. Cressy, *Birth*, 69. H. Spencer, *The History of British Midwifery from 1650 to 1800* (London: John Bale, Sons & Danielsson Ltd. 1927), 164; Aveling, *English Midwives* 31, 37. Sarah Stone also comments on the superiority of the bed over the birthing stool for delivery. Stone, 46. In the eighteenth century, in some rural areas, sitting on the lap of an assistant or delivering in the standing position was still popular. Stone, 55; Charles White, *A Treatise on the Management of Pregnant and Lying-in Women* (London: 1773), 285, 289, 302, 306, 307). White, a male midwife, felt that it was dangerous to deliver women in the sitting or upright position, positions which lessened the control of the male midwife. One commentator observed that midwives in England, France, and Germany were more fortunate in their use of the bed for deliveries than Italian midwives whose use of stools caused them to go home "all aches and pains." Filippini, 156.

15 T. C. et al., 77. A manual by a male author suggests that a piece of wood laid at the foot of the bed could act as a support against which the woman could brace her bent legs. This suggestion is missing from the midwives' manual, possibly because it was impractical or ineffectual, in their view.

16 T. C. et al., 77; C.R., 27.

under her pelvis "that her rump may be elevated," and to assist in the spreading of her knees and thighs, the midwife might begin her work by attempting to stretch the opening through which the infant was to emerge.[17] Various sweet oils or lubricants were applied to the perineal area and the midwife's hands to encourage softening and relaxation of the tissues as they were manipulated and stretched. In the early stages of labour, the midwife would have an opportunity to assess various potential complications such as a bowel impacted by faeces. The preferred treatment for the latter, a common enough affliction in the seventeenth century without the added burden of pregnancy, was purging. A receipt "For one bound in the body, though a woman with childe" contained white wine, Damask Rosewater, twenty Damask prunes, forty "sunstoned" raisins, whole mace, aniseed, and sugar.[18] But for a woman in labour, more heroic measures would be called for.[19] For relief of "colick" or "indigestions of the stomach" which could be as troublesome as labour pains, the midwife might administer oil of sweet almonds with cinnamon water or try a "wind dispelling glyster" or enema. Alternatively, the gas pains could be treated with warm compresses.[20]

Some midwives had their own prescriptions and stocks of ingredients, and traces of equipment for making and storing medicines have been found in inventories of midwives' and their relatives.[21] An unnamed London midwife practising in the first half of the century claimed to have a miraculous "Spanish roote" which, when applied to the birth passage, enlarged it so that "the child is instantly brought forth." Predictably, she would not disclose its name or source to anyone.[22] For midwives who were not prepared to carry their own remedies, the 1680 advice manual written by midwives instructs: "You ought to give orders for things to be had from the Apothecaries with her consent."[23]

If the labour was slow, the midwife might try one of the concoctions such as Lady Thanes's "hors dung water," purported "to cause speedy labour"[24] or Dr. Stephens Water, a polycrest medicine with a myriad of uses including stimulating labour pains.[25] Another popular treatise offered: "To Help a Woman in Labour

---

17 T. C. et al., 78.   18 W. M., *The Queen's Closet Opened* (London: 1655), 159.
19 Sarah Stone describes an interesting case in which a woman who thought she was miscarrying was successfully treated for extreme "costiveness" by Stone's administration of an enema. Stone, 62–4.
20 T. C. et al., 79.
21 Elizabeth Thompson, the Kendal Midwife, lists a number of stock ingredients in the back of her record book as well as a favourite receipt which, in keeping with the practice of the period, was probably used for a variety of obstetrical problems. She numbered two apothecaries' wives among her clientele that may account for the exactness of her measures and the sophistication of the ingredients. See Cumbria Record Office MS WD/Cr. In addition to purging, Gélis has noted that some midwives administered "vomits" to stimulate contractions. Gélis, 137.
22 It was probably spanish liquorice root, described as having a soothing, as well as oily quality. When applied according to the practice of the period, it would have some lubricative effect. Samuel Hartlib, *Ephemenides* (London: 1650). I am grateful to Mark Greengrass for this reference.
23 C.R., 27.
24 Diana Astry, "Diana Astry's Recipe Book," Bette Stitt, ed., *The Publications of the Bedfordshire Historical Record Society* 37 (1957): 155.
25 Ibid., 112. Almost every seventeenth-century compendium of medical treatments contained a version of "Dr. Stephens Water." This particular version was attributed to Culpeper.

. . . Give her a Date-stone that hath a perfect round circle, with half a Nutmeg in a draught of Renish Wine" or the midwife could try "A receit for a woman that cannot be delivered," attributed to Goody Wilsheirs who may have been a midwife. It contained the yolk of a newly laid egg, two pennyworth of saffron, and a little sugar, and was to be followed by a drink of mace ale or burnt claret.[26] Country midwives might resort to still other means such as girdles and charms.[27] If the woman had not voided for some time, the midwife might be obliged to put a "fit instrument in the bladder, and force it to expel the urine."[28]

In a smooth and uncomplicated delivery, the midwife would have little more to do than offer encouragement and support as the pains increased in intensity and frequency. The midwife or friends of the woman might gently massage the abdomen with a downward motion "to thrust down the infant by little and a little" and encourage her to hold her breath with the pains and bear down "as if she were doing the ordinary deeds of nature."[29]

A task which female attendants might undertake was the winding of a "swathe band" a foot wide around the woman's abdomen. This would then be held on each side by a woman who pulled on it with each contraction. Intended to help ease the woman's discomfort, the midwives' treatise warned that unless the women pulled with the same degree of strength, "it does more harm than good."[30] If required, mild restraint could be applied by two women beside the bed, each holding a hand and shoulder of the woman in labour.[31]

Midwives were warned against the more painful "dry birth," which would result if they tore the membranes with their fingernail "in haste to be gone to other women."[32] The correct way to deal with a stubborn membrane was to soften it by setting the woman over warm water containing a "softening liniment." Once the membranes had ruptured, care must be taken to prevent the patient from chilling.[33]

Patience was the key while nature did her work. Not only did the midwife need to be physically strong, "it being required that she should be stirring at all hours and abiding long time together with her patient," but, in the midwives' own words:

She ought, moreover to know that God hath given to all things their beginning, their increasins, their Estate of perfection, and declination: Therefore the said midwife nor any of her assistants must not do anything rashly, for to precipitate or hasten nature.[34]

The midwife would "catch" the baby (possibly using her apron) and place the baby on the mother's abdomen where it could be examined for possible defor-

---

26 F. Philiatros, *Nature Exenterata: or Nature Unbowelled By the most Exquisite Anatomizers of Her* (London: 1655), 233; J. Stevens Cox, ed., *Dorset Folk Remedies of the 17th and 18th Centuries* (Dorchester: The Dorset Natural History and Archaeological Society, 1962), 3.
27 Thomas, *Religion*, 222.   28 *Sermon*, 16.
29 T. C. et al., 78–9. A medieval Hebrew midwifery manuscript also recommends massage and controlled breathing to facilitate the expulsion of the fetus. Ron Barkai, "A Medieval Hebrew Treatise on Obstetrics," *Medical History* 33 (1988): 110.
30 T. C. et al., 78; *Sermon*, 95.   31 *Sermon*, 95.   32 T. C. et al., 81, 83.   33 Ibid., 81.
34 Ibid., 75–6.

mities and to establish its sex.[35] Next came the important task of cutting the umbilical cord or "navell string" with a knife or, preferably, "good sharp scissors." Aware of the possible effect on a male infant's genital development, the midwife was cautioned to carry out the task "leaving the length of four fingers," first tying it with silk thread "as near the belly as maybe."[36]

If the infant was in good condition, it could be "laid aside" after ensuring that its head, face, and stomach were well covered.[37] For an infant that failed to breathe, the midwife might try some extraordinary measure such as burning a "little Coventrey blew threed" and allowing the smoke to enter the child's nostrils.[38] Each midwife would have her own method of stimulating respiration before cleaning the infant with warm water and soft cloths, made, in some cases, from clean old linen which she had brought with her. Assured of the child's well-being, either she or one of the other attendants, often the wet nurse who was already in attendance, would apply oil of sweet almonds or fresh butter to the infant's skin in the belief that this would make its skin firm and close up the pores, thereby protecting it from the air.[39] A dressing made of fine linen and cotton saturated in oil of roses was recommended to protect the newly cut navel cord.[40] Before the child was swaddled, the midwife was advised to gently:

. . . put one hand upon the bone of the forehead and another upon the bone called the coronal bone and softly close up the gap which was made during the time of travail, closing also the suture one against another, exactly.[41]

The same treatise warns against trying to shape the nose and head except in cases where the child is born with the nose "awry." Then the midwife can "gently stroke [it] with a moistened finger but lay no stress upon it." Finally, the midwife would "gently" put her finger under the infant's tongue to see if there was "a string or no." If one were present, she would clip it with the point of sharp scissors.[42] The child could then be swaddled using strips of cloth and warm napkins or "clouts" and before being carefully placed in its cradle near the

---

35 In France, midwives held their aprons to catch the baby, giving rise to the phrase "being born in an apron." Gélis, 129.

36 T. C. et al., 15, 83. Earlier in the treatise, the midwife was warned that cutting the cord too short would affect the length of the "yard" or penis. One advice manual suggests leaving the child on the mother's abdomen and delivering the afterbirth after which both are carried "to the fire," the infant to be attended to, and the afterbirth, presumably, to undergo a closer inspection before its disposal by burying. Sermon, 105–6.

37 T. C. et al., 83. Jane Sharp also emphasises the need to keep the infant in darkness. Cressy, *Childbirth*, 82.

38 W. M., *The Queen's Closet Opened* (London: 1655), 159.   39 T. C. et al., 92.

40 Sermon, 106–7.   41 T. C. et al., 100.

42 Ibid., 100. The women stress the gentleness with which the infant should be handled throughout their discussion. This aspect is missing from the treatise by William Sermon, which drew heavily upon the midwives' publication.

fireplace, be given "a little sack and sugar in a spoon" or a concoction of mithridate, molasses, wine, and cardus water.[43]

Experienced midwives would be well aware of the importance of delivering the afterbirth, and ensuring that, if it did not separate cleanly, no pieces remained in the woman's uterus which could cause postpartum haemorrhage and, in some cases, death. To speed up the process, she might massage the woman's abdomen, give a pinch of sneezing powder or try another popular receipt such as a caudle made from rye: "To bring away the After burden although a day or two after the Delivery."[44] Whatever method was used, the midwife knew that the secundines or afterbirth must be removed with care and without force.[45]

When perineal tears occurred in a first-time mother, the midwife would gently cleanse the area (white wine was often used for this purpose), and then apply an ointment and plaster to the wound to assist healing. More severe tears might require suturing, a task that the midwife might competently carry out, or a surgeon could be called to perform the task.[46] After washing the rest of the woman's "privities" and limbs, she would carefully place a cloth or pad to catch the lochia or postpartum vaginal discharge. In some cases, a tightly rolled linen swathe band, a triangular compress or other arrangements of napkins would be applied to the abdomen to support the womb.[47]

If the mother's waistcoat had become soiled, the "fustian waistcoat and petticoats usually worn during the lying in" would be donned.[48] Avoiding remedies that might inhibit the flow of breast milk, the midwife could apply a warmed linen cloth which had been dipped in a number of recommended solutions.[49] Depending on the woman's economic resources, the lying-in bed might be freshly

43 Ibid., 92. Mithridate was a compound thought to be an antidote for poison, while cardus water was derived from a member of the thistle family, commonly the artichoke.

44 W. M., 159. It is interesting that eighteenth-century physicians decried the custom of serving the new mother a "cawdle," claiming it was one of the reasons they succumbed to childbed fever. Obviously the women saw a positive medicinal benefit, in some cases at least, in it. The same treatise contains other receipts for bringing away the afterbirth, 159, 160.

45 T. C. et al., 84.

46 For an example of a treatment of this type using egg yolks and black soap, which was "spread on fine flax" and combined with linen dipped in a mixture of egg whites and flour, see Philiatros, 334. For other examples of plasters, see J. White, *A Rich Cabinet with Variety of Inventions* (London: 1651), sections F and G. Seventeenth-century manuals directed to midwives discuss the possibility of sutures for severe tears, as do others intended for surgeons. Sermon, 167; James Cooke, *Mellificium Chirurgiae* (London: 1648), 261.

47 T. C. et al., 86, 102; La Vauguion, *A Compleat Body of Chirurgical Operations Containing the Whole Practice of Surgery with Observations and Remarks on each case Amongst which are inserted, the several ways of Delivering Women in Natural and Unnatural Labours* (London: 1707), 210. Eighteenth-century doctors were critical of the practice of binding the abdomen, claiming an application that was too tight could cause childbed fever. Charles White, *A Treatise on the Management of Pregnant and Lying-in Women* (London: 1773), 114.

48 White, 115. Eighteenth-century male midwives were critical of the practice of wearing a waistcoat and petticoats for the lying-in since they believed that overheating was one of the main causes of childbed fever.

49 T. C. et al., 89.

made with "child bed" linen of the finest quality and if two hours had passed since the delivery, the midwife would again offer the new mother a drink of "warm, cherishing, and cordial broths or yolk of poached egg, or cinnamon water."[50] Before taking her departure, the midwife might instruct the new mother regarding her bathing regimen for the lying-in period. For the first eight days, a handful of chervil steeped in boiling water and honey of roses was recommended while for the second eight days, "province roses boiled in water and wine" was preferred.[51]

In the seventeenth century, the new mother could expect a lying-in period of four weeks when she would be free from the demands of domestic and other responsibilities. If the family could not afford the expense of providing the necessary domestic help, the parish would often pay a poor parish woman to attend the new mother during her four-week recovery period. In some cases, the parish paid for the woman's delivery and four weeks' room and board at approved parish homes such as widow Bull's of St Olave Jewry or "nurse" James' and "nurse" Ray's of St Bride's.[52] Midwives, however, avoided carrying out deliveries in their own homes lest they be accused of performing abortions.[53]

If, instead of a normal birth, a malpresentation or an obstructed delivery developed which the midwife could not correct, she would send for other midwives for advice and assistance. Surviving evidence indicates that experienced midwives, especially senior midwives, were able to correct malpresentations by turning the infant *in utero*.[54] In the rare case where all the women's efforts were defeated, a surgeon or male midwife would be called who would, in most cases, be required

---

50 C. R., 27. See the will of Elizabeth Whipp for a reference to fine childbed linen, chapter four. A Cambridgeshire father bequeathed his dead wife's childbed linen to his daughter in 1622, Mary Abbott, *Life Cycles in England 1560–1720* (London: Routledge, 1996), 167.

51 T. C. et al., 95, 98. Nothing in particular was suggested for the last two weeks of the lying-in period.

52 In 1649, the parish of St Olave Jewry used the home of widow Bull for this purpose on a number of occasions, GL MS 44092 (unfol.). Nearly fifty years later, James and Ray were accommodating deliveries, boarding lying-in women, and caring for "nurse" children, perhaps temporarily, until they could be placed at nurse in the country. GL MS 6552/2 (unfol.) 1696–1702 (passim). It is interesting that lying-in women in parish workhouses in the early eighteenth century were similarly afforded rest and nursing care during their lying-in period. See VL D 1758/450 St James Westminster Vestry Minutes.

53 T. C. et al., 126.

54 Evidence survives which suggests that thirteenth-century Hebrew midwives had access to information about malpresentations and the method for correcting them. Barkai: 104. The midwives' handbook, published by four midwives in 1656, includes pictures of malpresentations, as well as instructions of how to correct them. T. C. et al., 118–28. Sarah Stone, the early eighteenth-century midwife who learned her art from her mother, an outstanding seventeenth-century midwife, describes how she corrected abnormal presentations. See, for example, Stone, 33–4, 42–3. Evidence from the continent also supports the view that midwives were competent in correcting abnormal presentations. See Marland, "The *'burgerlijke'* midwife," 194; Filippini, 156. Even Edmund Chapman, London surgeon and man-midwife, writing in the prescriptive vein in the early eighteenth century, admitted, "many women midwives may know how to turn a child." Edmund Chapman, *A Treatise on the Improvement of Midwifery chiefly with regard to the Operation* (London: 1735), vi.

to use his surgical instruments to remove the infant, usually by dismemberment or craniotomy, in an effort to save the mother's life.[55]

THE CLIENTS

Hundreds of midwives' testimonial certificates provide the best surviving evidence of the ecclesiastical licensing process in seventeenth-century London and information about the midwives' clientele. In addition, the records of an anonymous London midwife who went about her work of child delivery from 1694 to 1723 supplement the more impersonal church records, which also include bishops' and archbishops' registers. A careful examination of these records has permitted insights into the work of London midwives with regard to what we have called "repeat business," the geographical distribution of their practices, the social standing of their clients, and the client and midwife referral system. Finally, we will hear from the childbearing women themselves what they thought about their midwives.

In assessing the relationship which existed in seventeenth-century London between midwives and clients, among the most illuminating themes to emerge are those of the extent of repeat business and the nature and prevalence of personal referral from satisfied clients to prospective mothers. One might assume that midwifery services in a large cosmopolitan population centre such as London would follow a different pattern from that of the more intimate rural parish. In fact, the evidence points to the existence of long-term and intricate relationships between many London midwives and their clients, similar to what might be found in rural England.[56]

The evidence for repeat business is derived from both testimonial certificates provided by satisfied clients and the anonymous midwife's account book. Testimonial documentation in some cases specified the number of children the midwife had already delivered for the referee. In 1662, testimonials for all twenty-four successful candidates recorded the number of children they had delivered for each of the women testifying on their behalf. The account book provides information on the number of deliveries per client, thus giving a reasonable indication of the relationships that existed in late Stuart London between a midwife and her

---

55 In the case of complicated deliveries requiring surgical intervention, specific instructions of how to position the woman and assist the surgeon, or in some cases, where a surgeon is unavailable, the way in which the midwife should deal with haemorrhage caused by the placenta obstructing the opening and other obstetrical emergencies, is explained in some detail in *The Compleat Midwifes Practice*, the handbook published by four midwives in 1656, 112–18. For a description of the various instruments and techniques employed by male midwives, see Wilson, *Man-midwifery*. In the seventeenth century, the surgeon's or male midwife's instruments would not have included obstetrical forceps that were a closely guarded secret of the notorious Chamberlen family.

56 For a rural midwife's practice, see the transcript of a Kendal midwife's diary, covering the years 1665–75, Cumbria Record Office MS WD/Cr. The diary records Elizabeth Thompson's practice in an area where there were one or (at most) two practising midwives. It demonstrates, not surprisingly, very extensive repeat business.

clients. It demonstrates that the midwife routinely carried out her work to the satisfaction of many of her clients who continued to use her services throughout their childbearing years.

Information about the number of deliveries that a prospective licensee had carried out for clients testifying on her behalf is valuable as an indication of the clientele's level of satisfaction with a midwife. The six women delivered by Debora Bromfield of St Andrew Holborn had borne a total of thirty-two children when they supported her application for a midwifery licence in 1663.[57] Elizabeth Philips of St Clement Danes had been delivered of five children by Bromfield; Susan Brownell of the parish of St Andrew Holborn of three children; Susan White of St Martin Iron Monger Lane of four children; Mary Huntley of St Salvator Southwark of seven children; and Elizabeth Boggs of St Benet Paul's Wharf had used Bromfield's services on thirteen occasions. The high degree of confidence which women placed in the skill of their midwives was exemplified by women such as Boggs or by Bridgette Richards, of St Mildred Poultry, who was brought to bed thirteen times by Elizabeth Davis of St Katherine Cree Church or again by Martha Marshall, of St Martin in the Fields, who was successfully delivered by midwife Elizabeth Laywood twelve times.[58] In 1662, twenty-four midwives presented the sworn testimony of 142 clients; of these, eighty-six clients were delivered more than once by the same midwife, and more than 60 percent of the deliveries by this group of wives could be termed "repeat business." For the number of women delivered more than once by the same midwife, see Table 3.1: Frequency of Contact with Clients 1662 (Testimonials).

The testimonial evidence sheds light on the extent of repeat business at only a single point in the ongoing relationship between a midwife and a client: the time of an application for licensing. It could be expected that the reliance of many of these women upon a particular midwife would continue, and thus the actual extent of repeat business would exceed the figures provided here. A general pattern is discernible, confirmed by the account book of the, as yet, unidentified midwife which covers the years 1694 to 1723. During that period, this active midwife attended over 376 clients, more than one-third of whom she delivered several times. In addition to the 243 clients that Mistress X delivered on a single occasion, 433 deliveries involved clients who had previously utilized the midwife's services. That is, out of a total of 676 deliveries, 64 percent involved a client who had used the midwife on more than one occasion. The midwife delivered eight sets of twins (counted as one delivery), and in all but one of these cases the mothers were delivered of other children by Mistress X. At least twenty-two of the clients who used the midwife's services only once did so in the last five years of her recorded practice. This would have decreased the opportunity for repeat business. (See Table 3.2: Frequency of Contact between Mistress X and Her Clients 1694–1723, account book.)

57 GL MS 10,116/3.   58 GL MS 10,116/2.

Table 3.1. *Frequency of Contact with Clients 1662 (Testimonials)*

Number of deliveries (same client)	Frequency (%)
1	56 (39%)
2	35 (23%)
3	17 (12%)
4	11 (08%)
5	13 (09%)
6	5 (04%)
7	4 (03%)
12	1 (.7%)
13	2 (01%)

Note: Percentages are approximate, having been rounded off in most cases. There is no indication of whether or not any of the foregoing included multiple deliveries; our calculations have assumed the delivery of a single child.
Source: GL MS 10,116/2.

The majority of Mistress X's clients expressed a high level of confidence in her skills by summoning her repeatedly when they were brought to bed and they freely recommended her services to other family members. Mrs. Page, who used her services three times, no doubt played a role in the referral and subsequent delivery of her sister by the midwife.[59] Mrs. Duple of Blackfriars was delivered by Mistress X six times between 1703 and 1714; her sister became a client in 1704 and 1706. One of our midwife's most fecund clients, Mrs. Dangerfield of Whitechapel, first used her services in July 1699. By March 1712, she had called upon the midwife nine times. Dangerfield's trust in and reliance on her midwife's skills undoubtedly influenced her own sister who became a client of Mistress X in 1713. Mrs. Osten, an apothecary's wife, and her sister both placed their confidence in our midwife's abilities. All told, at least six clients referred their sisters to the midwife. Madam Blackabe, an affluent client who had been brought to bed of two sons and two daughters, referred a kinswoman who paid the midwife handsomely at £4.6.0. for her services.[60]

The women of the socially prominent and wealthy Barnardiston family showed a similar satisfaction with the midwife's abilities. Six Barnardiston women used her services on a regular basis. Madam Barnardiston from Leytonstone was deliv-

59 Bodleian Library, Oxford, Rawlinson MS D1141/31, 32, 40, 56.   60 Ibid., fol. 15.

Table 3.2. *Frequency of Contact between Mistress X and Her Clients 1694–1723 (Account Book)*

Number of deliveries per client	Frequency (%)
1	243 (65%)[a]
2	48 (13%)
3	38 (11%)
4	22 (06%)
5	10 (03%)
6	7 (02%)
7	1 (02%)
8	2 (.5%)
9	3 (.8%)
10	0 (00%)
11	1 (.2%)
12	1 (.2%)

[a]Or 192 (58%) excluding the last 5 years of Mistress X's practice.

Note: In most cases, the percentages have been rounded. The delivery of twins was counted as one contact.

Source: Bodleian Library, Oxford, Rawlinson MS D 1141, used with the kind permission of the Bodleian Library, Oxford.

ered three times; Madam Barnardiston from "The Fig Tree" twice; Madam Barnardiston living in "Cornewell" sought assistance in childbed four times and Madam Barnardiston of Budge Row used the midwife's assistance on two occasions.[61] The midwife also delivered Barnardiston women living on Granoch Street and Watlen Street. In total, fourteen small Barnardistons were brought into the world by the "family midwife."[62]

Since several of the anonymous midwife's clients were themselves the daughters

61 In 1726, teaman Richard Beach was located at the "Figg Tree" in Newgate Street and, in 1755, grocer George Snowball occupied the "Figg Tree" on Salisbury Street in the Strand. Sir Ambrose Heal, *The Signboards of Old London Shops* (London: B.T. Batsford, Ltd., 1947), 164, 87. A member of the Barnardiston family of merchants may have been the owner and occupant of one of these two businesses in 1715, the year Madam Barnardiston was delivered.

62 There are frequent references to the family midwife, Mrs. Mitchell, in the letters of the prominent puritan family of the Barringtons, Hatfield, Broad Oak in Essex. Arthur Searle, ed.,*Barrington Family Letters 1628–1632* (London: Offices of the Royal Historical Society, University College, 1983), 58, 123, 141. She may have been Joan Mitchell, licensed in 1610, or Isobel Mitchell, licensed in 1611.

of women who had been brought to bed by the midwife, there is every possibility that Mistress X was attending women whom she had brought into the world, a remarkable tribute to the level of confidence and personal rapport she enjoyed. For example, Mrs. Tabram of Butcher's Hall Lane was delivered by the midwife four times from 1697; 20 years later, our midwife delivered "Ms. Tabram's daughter" who was living in Chapter House Lane.[63] The popular midwife brought to bed altogether at least nine daughters of former clients. Two clients, Mrs. Maret and Mrs. Benet, summoned Mistress X when their serving women gave birth. Other London "family midwives" who practised in the seventeenth century included Lucy Lodge of St Leonard Shoreditch, licensed in 1663 and supported in her application for a licence by three female members of the Samwaye family, in addition to eleven other women. Judith Tyler of Hendon, Middlesex, who was licensed in 1664, claimed four clients with the surname "Nicoll."[64]

Although the occasional midwife, such as Alice Davis of St Paul Shadwell, might be described as "the midwife of the parish," London midwives did not restrict their practices to the parish in which they lived.[65] This is an important distinction, which undermines the assumption that midwives carried out too few deliveries to gain the experience necessary for competence. But archival evidence shows, for example, that Bridgid Jake of St Leonard Shoreditch, who presented her testimonials for licensing in 1610, was one of the relatively few seventeenth-century midwives whose six supporting clients all resided in her home parish.[66] Even this, of course, did not mean that Jake's practice then or in the future was restricted to her own parish. On the other hand, the abundant evidence that midwives seeking licences normally provided references from satisfied clients beyond the boundaries of their own parish demonstrates that even at that point in their professional career, London midwives practised over a large geographical area. Rose Cumber, licensed in the same year as Jake, presented sworn testimony from women who resided in St Swithin and St Andrew Holborn although she herself resided in St Bridgid's Fleet Street.[67] Elizabeth Martin of St Giles Cripplegate called on only one client from her home parish in 1626 when she applied for her licence. Women from St Antholin, St Dunstan in the West, St Martin in the Fields, and St Michael Pater Noster added their testimonies.[68] In 1629, Alice Carnell of St Dunstan in the West was licensed after presenting evidence from clients, none of whom resided in her parish.[69]

Licensing of midwives broke down in the civil war period but after it was reinstated in 1661, midwives' clients were distributed much as they had been earlier in the century. Most testimonials indicated that midwives drew their clients from both their own parish and from other parishes. Some midwives found more

---

63 The daughters of Mrs. Abel and Mrs. Chapman, both clients, were also delivered by Mistress X.
64 GL MS 10,116/3.   65 GL MS 10,116/9.   66 GLRO DLC/339/1/102.
67 GLRO DLC/339/1/133.   68 GLRO DLC/339/13/172.
69 GLRO DLC/339/14/68v.

clients close to home, in adjoining parishes, while others extended their practices far beyond parochial boundaries. In 1664, Ursula Nellham of All Hallows the Great provided testimonial support from women residing in St Dunstan in the West and the easterly parishes of St James Duke's Palace and St Botolph Aldgate, as well as from women of her own City parish which lay along the Thames.[70] In some cases, the prospective client could only be located by using a map. It may have been necessary for the midwife to hire a coach and, if travelling to a delivery at night and outside the city walls, pay the watchman to open the gate.[71]

The account book of our unidentified London midwife, Mistress X, demonstrates a similar mobility and geographical diversity of practice. Although addresses were not recorded in every case, clients from at least thirty parishes within the city walls claimed her services. But these formed only a part of her practice: in the years covered by her records, the busy and popular midwife travelled far beyond the confines of the city walls. To the east, she journeyed to Leytonstone, Spitalfields, and Whitechapel where she attended, among others, Mrs. Dangerfield in her numerous confinements; to the north, to the area of Finsbury Fields and the northern reaches of the vast ward of Cripplegate Without; to the west, she delivered women in the Strand, the Haymarket, and Drury Lane. Among her clients on the south bank was the prosperous Mrs. Sims, who was brought to bed five times by the peripatetic midwife. Mistress X's practice encompassed not only the City, but also almost all of suburban London north of the River Thames, as well as Southwark.

Her sprawling practice is all the more remarkable in view of the backward state of intra-metropolitan communications. At the same time as the anonymous midwife was travelling ill-lit streets to the numerous night-time confinements which she recorded, one visitor commented that the city was "a great vast wilderness" in which few were familiar with even a quarter of its streets.[72] In the last year of recorded practice, most of Mistress X's deliveries were in the east end of London or its eastern suburbs, close to where the midwife resided. The shrinking catchment area was probably a result of ill health or old age.[73] It is uncertain how representative Mistress X was, but it is clear that very few, if any, licensed

---

70 GL MS 10,116/3. Testimonial evidence touched on only a fraction of a midwife's practice, but it is still a useful indication of the geographical range of individual midwifery practices.

71 GL MS 6552/3 February 10, 1710. See also note 9, above. Midwife Anne Miller rode to deliveries. GL MS 10,116/16.

72 Jeremy Boulton, *Neighbourhood and Society: A London Suburb in the Seventeenth Century* (Cambridge: Cambridge University Press, 1987), 231. There are few indications in London sources of how midwives travelled to their deliveries. No doubt, in many cases, transportation (either by horse or carriage) or a guide would be provided by clients' families but, in others, she would travel alone on foot or on horseback to the site of the lying-in.

73 This pattern of an aging midwife restricting her practice to deliveries closer to home was also demonstrated by Vrouw Schrader, the eighteenth-century Frisian midwife. See Hilary Marland, M. J. van Lieberg, and G. K. Kloosterman, *"Mother and Child were Saved": The memoirs (1693–1740) of the Frisian midwife Catharina Schrader* (Amsterdam: Rodopi, 1987), 11.

midwives (of whom almost 1,200 have been uncovered) restricted their practices to a single parish.

There is no evidence that midwives advertised their skills by means of printed advertisements.[74] Word-of-mouth recommendation by satisfied clients living close to one another apparently played a key role in establishing pockets of women who used the midwife's services, and may explain some of the cases which lay at the geographical periphery of the practice of Mistress X. Mrs. Rowden of Drury Lane employed her in March and less than six weeks later, a client from nearby Tower Street called on her. On October 29, 1707, Mrs. Nicolls of St Martin's Street was delivered; a few days later, on November 7, Mrs. Hampton of the same street called the midwife to her delivery; a month later, Mrs. Wood, also of St Martin's Street, was delivered of an infant daughter by Mistress X. Mrs. Field and Mrs. Hobkins, both of Aldgate Street, were delivered within three days of each other. Also delivered within three days of one another were Mrs. Duple's sister (referred by Mrs. Duple) and her neighbor, the shoemaker's wife in Swan Yard.[75]

Unconstrained by the "ethical" considerations restricting twentieth-century practitioners, our anonymous midwife delivered a substantial number of family members. She attended her daughter, Elenor Campion, five times and had the satisfaction of bringing four grandsons and one granddaughter into the world.[76] In September 1695, she delivered a niece and was handsomely reimbursed for the delivery at £1.10s. In addition, "sister Parker" made her a present of 7s.6d. and she received an additional £1 at her niece's christening.[77] Four of the midwife's cousins were clients: "Cusen Brown" was delivered of a daughter shortly after midnight on February 17, 1705; Mrs. Jackson sought her cousin's assistance with four deliveries between July 24, 1708 and Easter Day 1716; cousin Fowler was delivered three times beginning in 1706 and, unlike cousins Jackson and Brown who did not pay the midwife, gave between 15s. and £1 for each of the deliveries; similarly, cousin Dosen paid £1 for her delivery in 1707.[78] Since cousins Fowler

74 Patricia Crawford, "Printed Advertisements for Women Medical Practitioners in London, 1670–1710," *The Society for the Social History of Medicine* Bulletin 35 (1984): 266–9. Even in the early eighteenth century, advertising was restricted to special cases such as the anonymous woman purporting to be a midwife who advertised her "cure" for an illness which could develop into a malignant "Womb." William B. Ewald, *The Newsmen of Queen Anne* (Oxford: Blackwell, 1956), 108.

75 Although the evidence needs to be developed, I suspect that these referrals, which resulted in deliveries within a few days of one another, are also an indication that at least some women limited their contact with the midwife to the actual date of delivery.

76 Bodleian Library Rawl., MS D 1141/69, 8, 13, 26, 14. The midwife noted a charge of ten shillings for the birth of her first grandchild (a male). In addition, the happy father gave her a present of a pound. She received no fee for the other four grandchildren. For Quaker midwives who delivered their own grandchildren, see Giardina Hess, "Midwifery Practice," 50, 60.

77 Ibid., fol. 28v.

78 Ibid. fols. 58, 1, 11, 63, 66, 70. The midwife delivered at least one more cousin, whose surname is illegible, on July 31, 1707.

and Dosen obviously chose to use the midwife for reasons other than those of economy, it is likely that they believed that they would receive skillful service from their relative, a reflection on her competence that extended beyond considerations of kinship.

Testimonial evidence suggests that female clients, on occasion, sought a midwife on the basis of recommendations by women whose husbands were employed in the same craft or trade as that of the prospective father. For example, when Mary Taylor of St Olave Silver Street sought her licence in 1661, of the six clients who supported her application, two were butchers' wives (one from Christ Church parish and one from St Sepulchre) and two were shoemakers' wives, both from different parishes, indicating a link through their spouses' occupations.[79] The following year, Winnifred Allen of St Andrew Wardrobe enlisted the wives of three tailors from two different parishes when she applied for a licence, and Elizabeth Davis of St Katherine Cree Church supplied the names of three women (one of whom had used her services six times) all of whom were married to men employed in the relatively exclusive goldsmith trades. Similarly, among the seven clients sworn for Elizabeth Ayre of St Giles Cripplegate in 1664, Lucy Buffington was the wife of goldsmith John Buffington of the midwife's parish, and Elizabeth Swift was the wife of Abraham Swift, a goldsmith of St Alban Wood Street. Three of the remaining clients attesting to Ayre's expertise were wives of brewers.[80] In the case of Eleanor Stanfro of St Leonard Shoreditch, where a large number of weavers made their home, parochial and occupational links converged: four of the six testimonial clients from her home parish were married to weavers.[81] The wives of seamen also apparently referred their midwives to other women whose husbands were similarly engaged. All six of Elizabeth Willis's clients, all three of Mary Salmon's, and all four of Sarah Griffin's were married to seafaring men.[82]

Out of the fifty-three testimonials that gave occupational designations for clients' husbands in 1663, thirteen, or almost 25 percent, demonstrated similar occupations for two or more spouses. Similarly, in the years 1696–1700, out of the forty testimonials which declared occupations, twelve testimonials, or 30 percent, gave the same occupation for at least two of the women's husbands. Although Mistress X seldom recorded occupational information for spouses, among the few instances where she has done so, we have two examples which confirm testimonial evidence of occupational links between clients of individual midwives: In 1704, the midwife "laid" two shoemakers' wives within five weeks of one another; similarly, in 1715, two tailors' wives were delivered less than five weeks apart, one of whom lived in the Minories and the other at considerable distance to the west in the Strand.

The existence of other networks between women and their clients can be

79 GL MS 10,116/1.   80 GL MS 10,116/2. All of Davis's clients were from different parishes.
81 GL MS 10,116/3.   82 GL MS 10,116/1, 2, 3, 13.

traced in the testimonials. Mary DesOrmeaux, wife of Daniel, a jeweller of St Giles in the Fields, was a member of the "French" church in the Savoy (home of the Huguenot congregation) when she applied for a midwifery licence in 1680. All five women who gave sworn testimony on her behalf were French immigrants: Catherine Faure, Marguerite Gorget, and Marguerite Fournie were residents of St Giles in the Fields, while Mere Lamare and Marie Colas were from the parish of St Martin in the Fields. Catherine Bont of Stepney had been a member of the Dutch church in London for 3 years when she applied for a midwifery licence in 1688. Catherine was the wife of Jonas Merese, but she retained her own name after her marriage, as was the custom amongst Dutch women. Similarly, two of her clients, from Stepney and St Leonard Shoreditch, were Dutch women who gave their maiden names when they testified under oath.[83] It is apparent, and understandably so, that, whenever possible, female immigrants turned to midwives of their own nationality, who spoke the same language and shared the same cultural heritage, to assist them when they were brought to bed. Indeed, the refusal to allow midwives of their own Protestant faith to attend them was one of the precipitating factors in the flight of Huguenot women from France in the 1680s.[84]

More surprising is recently uncovered evidence that ecclesiastically licensed midwives numbered Quaker women amongst their clients: apparently for these women the demands of childbearing overrode, at least temporarily, religious concerns.[85] At least thirty-three London midwives who received ecclesiastical licences in the seventeenth century and the first decades of the eighteenth century delivered the infants of Quaker mothers. Twenty-four women had endorsed Alice Blackman's testimonial in 1706, adding "Sir I am very sorry you dou not make us midwifes all a Like [Blackman]." Eleven years later, the popular Anglican midwife delivered the newly widowed wife of a Stepney Quaker.[86] In some cases, the conforming midwives claimed a single Quaker client, but Elizabeth Clarke, licensed in 1673, for example, presided at the deliveries of ten Quaker mothers. (See Table 3.3: Licensed Midwives who Delivered Quaker Mothers.) Moreover, several of the mothers called on their conformist midwife more than once. Mary Ann White delivered Dorothy Wyatt, the Quaker wife of London citizen and draper Zedekiah Wyatt, three times in four years.[87] This argues against their employment in an emergency situation when other women who were coreligionists were unavailable. Even more surprising, although Quaker midwives in some areas were prohibited from seeking assistance from women "of the world," London Quaker midwives apparently were not adverse to employing the services

83 GL MS 10,116/11, 12. Samuel Biscope was the minister of the Dutch congregation in London and he signed the testimonial certificate.

84 A. P. Hands and Irene Scouloudi, *French Protestant Refugees Relieved Through the Threadneedle Street Church, London 1681–1687* (London: Huguenot Society of London, 1971), 49–51: 9.

85 I am grateful to Ann Giardina Hess for directing me to the sources which enabled me to establish this connection.

86 GL MS 10,116/16; PRO RG 6 1627/227.   87 PRO RG 6 1626/280, RG 6/1627/50, 123.

Table 3.3. *Licensed Midwives Who Delivered Quaker Mothers*

Licensed Midwife	Quaker Deliveries	Years
Bennett, Mary	1	1689
Blackman, Alice	1	1717
Broughton, Eyton	1	1710
Budden, Susan	1	1707
Cardiffe, Joanne	1	1711
Carter, Mary	1	1713
Chesmore, Ursula	4	1698–1704
Churchwell, Margaret	1	1702
Clarke, Elizabeth[a]	10	1676–1719
Cope, Mrs.	1	1698
Dixon, Mary	1	1701
Dodson, Anne	1	1719
Dunsley, Mary	1	1713
Hill, Anne	1	1707, 1718
Johns, Elizabeth	2	1704, 1705
Kist, Anne	2	1719
Leefs, Mary	1	1720
Lestocart, Elizabeth	5	1717
Martin, Elizabeth	15	1698–1703
Mitchell, Mary	1	1710
Moore, Elizabeth	3	1698–1700
Pell, Elizabeth	1	1711
Reynolds, Sarah	1	1710
Saunders, Anne	1	1702
Saunders, Mary	1	1707
Sherwood, Elizabeth	1	1704
Silverthorn, Susan	1	1714
Simmonds, Mary	3	1707–17
Thodee, Anne	2	1706
Warren, Elizabeth	1	1719
White, Mary Anne	4	1705–11
Whyte, Elizabeth	2	1683, 1686
Woodford, Sarah	2	1703, 1720

[a]Two Elizabeth Clark(e)s were licensed: one in 1673, the other in 1697 and we have no way of separating their practices.

Note: In addition to the above, at least six other licensed midwives were shown as being present at Quaker deliveries: one was the Quaker midwife's deputy while four others were midwives of long standing, possibly there to assist at difficult labours.

Sources: Quaker Birth Notes: PRO RG 6 1626, 1627, 1628; GL MS 10,116.

of non-Quakers as deputies.[88] Quaker Ann Heariford was one of the most active London midwives of her faith, particularly in the years 1698–1700 when she delivered more than two dozen Quaker mothers. Although Quaker women accompanied her in some cases, her preferred assistant in 1698 was Sibill Morgan of St Giles Cripplegate, who received her ecclesiastical licence from the Church of England in 1703.[89] It is obvious that not only Anglicans, but Quakers believed that competence and skill were key when choosing the practitioner to whom such an important task was to be entrusted. While "neighbourly obligation or financial incentive" might have played a part in the interchange between Anglican midwives and nonconformist clients and Quaker midwives and "people of the world," it is more likely that the universal and elemental drama shared by women in childbed in some cases created stronger bonds than those imposed by religion (See Appendix G).[90]

The authors of two studies of midwifery and gynaecology in the early modern period both concluded that women turned to male midwives because they believed that male practitioners could offer them better care.[91] If this was the case, women of the upper echelons of seventeenth-century London society could reasonably be expected to be among the first to desert the traditional midwife and seek the services of the male midwife. Our evidence, however, points to a different conclusion. Wives of London gentlemen continued to use the services of midwives into the third decade, at least, of the eighteenth century, as both testimonials and the anonymous midwife's account book demonstrate.

Midwives applying for licences frequently included the name of a gentlewoman among those giving sworn testimony on their behalf. Debora Bromfield of St Andrew Holborn was exceptional, with three of the five clients shown on her 1662 testimonial, delivered of a total of twelve children, married to "gentlemen": Elizabeth Philips of St Clement Danes; Susan Brownell of St Andrew Holborn; and Susan White of St Martin Ironmonger Lane.[92] Since all three women lived in different parishes, some distance apart, the midwife was probably referred by means of a social network among women of the urban gentry. At least six midwives licensed between 1677 and 1700 included the names of two gentle-women among those testifying on their behalf.[93] The curate of Laughton, parish

---

88 Giardina Hess, "Midwifery Practice," 63–4.

89 It would appear that Morgan was her deputy for at least one year. PRO RG 6 1628/53–122 passim; GL MS 10,116/15.

90 Giardina Hess has similarly concluded that concerns about competence and neighbourliness could override religious concerns. Giardina Hess, "Midwifery Practice," 53. As an example outside of London, the Kendal conformist midwife Elizabeth Thompson delivered a Quaker mother. CRO MS WD/Cr Feb. 24, 1670, March 26, 1674.

91 Wilson, "Childbirth," 317–22; Eccles, 124. The weaknesses of this argument, based mainly on the perceptions of male practitioners, have been dealt with at length in Evenden-Nagy "Seventeenth-century London midwives."

92 GL MS 10,116/2.

93 This number includes only those women whose husbands were designated "gent." It does not include the dozens of women whose names and signatures appear on these documents, many of whom were apparently literate and probably reasonably well-to-do.

of midwife Sarah Tricer, noted in 1664 that all four clients named in the testimonial were "of the best ranck and qualitie in the parish of Laughton."[94] Similarly, in 1669, the curate, vicar, and churchwarden of Shadwell, Stepney, testified pointedly that Katherine Botts had been "very successful in the safe delivery of many persons of very great reputation and quality in the said parish."[95]

In rural England, a midwife's practice could be expected to cover a wide spectrum of social and occupational groups. For example, the diary of the Kendal midwife lists clients whose husbands were drawn from over fifty diverse occupations. This included professionals, such as apothecaries, schoolmasters, attorneys, and clergy, and members of the gentry and the aristocracy. Elizabeth Thompson also delivered the children of at least four or five estate owners including a squire, the two children of Sir Thomas Braithwaite and, more unusually, the infants of a tobacco cutter and a fiddler. The clientele of the Frisian midwife Catharina Schrader was also drawn from a wide occupational spectrum which included labourers, farmers, doctors, vicars, merchants, and skippers and members of various trades associated with the sea.[96]

In London also, midwives continued to administer to the needs of women from all classes of society. Of the seventy-five testimonials which have been preserved for the years 1663–64, fifty-three contain information on the status of clients' spouses. Of 249 given spousal occupations, nine clients (4 percent) were designated as "gentleman." (See Table 3.4: Occupation/Status of Midwifery Clients, 1663–64 and 1690–1700.)

An indication of the continuing loyalty of gentry women to their midwives can be found in testimonial evidence at the end of the century. Of seventy-five testimonials presented to the vicar general for the City of London in the years 1690–1700, sixty-five contain occupational and status designations. Of 198 possible designations, fourteen husbands were recorded as members of the gentry. Thus, 7 percent of the women supporting the midwives' applications were from the upper level of society. The testimonials preserved in the Lambeth Palace archives were analysed separately for purposes of comparison. Of the sixty-two testimonials that survive for the years 1669–1700, fifty included occupational information. Out of a possible 174 designations, twenty-three spouses were named as "gentleman" (over 13 percent). This would indicate not only that midwives who sought licences from the jurisdiction of the Archbishop of Canterbury, rather than the jurisdiction of the Bishop of London, drew their clientele from a more affluent sector of society, but that this elevated group continued to use the services of the traditional midwife.

If the occupational designations for 1663 and the 1690s from the records of the Bishop of London and the Archbishop of Canterbury are combined and averaged, we find that around 10 percent of the designated clients giving testimonial evi-

---

94 GL MS 10,116/3.   95 GL MS 10,116/6.
96 CRO MS.WD/Cr; Marland et al., *"Mother and Child were Saved,"* 13.

Table 3.4. *Occupation/Status of Midwifery Clients, 1663–4 and 1690–1700*

	1663–64	1690–1700
Building	14	21
Clothing	54	48
Decorating/furnishing	7	2
Distribution/transport	54	33
Labouring	4	4
Land/farm workers	21	15
Leather	10	12
Merchants	5	3
Metalwork	14	7
Miscellaneous production	8	4
Miscellaneous services	8	10
Officials	1 (+2)[a]	0
Professions	9	4
Victualling	31	21
Gentlemen	9	14
Total	249	198

[a]Two spouses served as churchwardens in addition to their occupations.

Note: The foregoing classifications were adapted from A. L. Beier "Engine of Manufacture: the trades of London," in A.L. Beier and Roger Finlay, *London 1500–1700: The Making of the Metropolis,* London and New York: Longman, p. 164.

Source: GL MS 10,116/3/, 13, 14.

dence for midwives applying for licences to practice in the City of London and its environs were drawn from the gentry. Using Gregory King's estimates for the year 1688, we might assume that the gentry made up a little more than 2 percent of the population of England and Wales. Our figures, therefore, support the view that educated and affluent members of London society continued to turn to midwives to deliver their offspring throughout the seventeenth century.[97]

In seeking referees, midwives quite possibly looked to respectable members of society, and the evidence from the testimonials is not necessarily representative of their practices as a whole. The practice of Mistress X, however, reflects the range of clientele listed in testimonials – indeed, her accounts suggest higher levels of employment by the well-to-do. Her account book makes a clear distinction

97 Gregory King cited in D.C. Coleman, *The Economy of England 1450–1750* (Oxford: Oxford University Press, 1977), 6. King's figures are for all of England and Wales, while we are dealing with London, where the population would contain proportionately fewer gentry and more tradesmen, craftsmen, shopkeepers, and artisans.

regarding the status of clients: women from the lower and middle class are designated "Ms" or "Mistress," while women of the upper ranks of society are given the more respectful form of address, "madam." We are therefore able to identify a sizeable segment of her midwifery practice which was largely made up of women whose husbands were men of affluence and prestige. Although there is a very close connection between the size of the fee charged by the midwife and social designation, there are indications that the courtesy title of "madam" was extended, in some cases, for reasons more social than economic. Madam Andrews of St Bartholomew Lane, for example, paid less for her deliveries, at £1.14.0. and £1.16.0. than many a mistress among the midwife's clients.

Our anonymous midwife identified no fewer than twenty of her clients as "madam" and, in addition, delivered a lady. Lady Clarke paid £6 in 1720 when she was delivered of a daughter. These twenty-one women, several of whom were extremely fertile, accounted for roughly 9 percent of the busy midwife's practice, and provide some support for the argument that midwives were not deserted in favour of male practitioners by women of substance at the turn of the century. On one of the last folios of the casebook, the names of Lady Shaw, Lady Clarke, Arthur Barnardiston (a wealthy merchant), Samuel Barnardiston, John Barnardiston, and Lady Barnardiston appear, indicating the elite status of a section of Mistress X's clientele.[98]

At the other end of the social scale, we find evidence that midwives remained faithful to their oath, which required that they not discriminate between rich and poor women who were in need of their services. Susan Kempton's testimonial (signed by her vicar) stated that "she is not only helpfull to the rich and those that can pay her but also to the poore."[99] Individual parishes frequently assumed responsibility for paying for the delivery of poor women of the parish and also of vagrant women who could not be removed from the parish before they gave birth. Fees paid to the midwife by the parish ranged from the modest sum of 2s.6d. paid by the parish of St Gregory by St Paul's in 1677 for delivering a "poore woman that fell in labour" in the parish, to the 5s. paid in 1655 and the 10s. paid in 1684 and 1686 by the wealthy parish of St Mary Aldermanbury.[100] Mistress X delivered a female felon held "in the stocks" at the marketplace in 1712 and was not paid for her services.[101]

98 See Anon., *The Directory Containing an Alphabetical List of the names and Places of Abode of the Directors of Companies, Persons in Public Business, Merchants etc.* (London: 1736). The midwife usually referred to Lady Clarke as "Madam Clarke" and always referred to Lady Shaw as "Madam Shaw." At least one other client was the wife of a well-to-do member of London financial circles – Mrs. Bodicete – whom the midwife delivered on four occasions. See *The Directory*, 8. Some sixty years earlier, Thomas Barnardiston had been one of the City's parochial and civic leaders.

99 GL MS 10, 116/13.

100 GL MSS 1337/1/16, 3556/2 (unfol.), 3556/3 fols. 33v, 47 (churchwardens' accounts). The midwife delivered "Mr. Todds maide" in 1684 and was paid by the parish. Mr. Todd would not be liable for the expense of delivering an unmarried maidservant who was probably dismissed as soon as she became the mother of a bastard, according to the accepted practice of the period.

101 There is no indication in the midwife's records whether or not the woman was temporarily released from the stocks in an unspecified London marketplace in order to give birth.

If an obstetrical "disaster" occurred which required more than the manual removal of a dead foetus, midwives were obliged to call for the help of a surgeon who owned and was permitted to use the requisite instruments such as hooks, knives, and crochets.[102] Since surgeons were called upon when an operative procedure became necessary, it has been suggested that they were the group from which male midwives would logically evolve.[103] There is, however, evidence that the wives of surgeons themselves continued, throughout the seventeenth century, to turn to midwives when they were brought to bed and not to their husbands' colleagues.

By the year 1662, Rebecca Jeffery of St Botolph Aldgate had delivered Susan Noxton, wife of surgeon Peter Noxton of the same parish, five times. The following year, midwife Elizabeth Dunstall of St Anne and St Agnes included the names of two surgeons' wives among the satisfied clients who supported her application for licensing. This pattern persisted throughout the century, with no evidence of change. In 1689, Catherine Goswell of St Andrew Holborn claimed among her clientele Sarah Pettit, wife of Gersham Pettit, citizen and barber-surgeon of St Katherine next to the Tower. Not only did Mistress Pettit live at a considerable distance from the midwife, but there is a possibility that her husband was the resident medical attendant for St Katherine's, a hospital for almswomen, a position that afforded practical experience in treating ailing women. Even so, the Pettits chose the services of a midwife when Mistress Pettit was brought to bed.[104] As late as 1698, testimonial evidence shows that the wives of surgeons continued to rely on the traditional skills of a competent midwife rather than those of the surgeon. The account book of the anonymous London midwife, although containing scant reference to husbands' occupations, records that in August 1712, a Mistress Mos, who was a surgeon's wife, was delivered of a son.

According to Irvine Loudon, before 1730, "the surgeon-man-midwife had, . . . little or none of the extensive experience of normal midwifery which is the basis of good obstetric practice."[105] Apparently very few surgeons were married to

---

102 See Eccles, 109–18 for a discussion of the role of surgeons in the birth process, which usually encompassed the death of the child, the mother, or both. In 1688, midwife Elizabeth Cellier attacked the medical profession for their lack of practical experience in delivering children in a scathing, albeit humourous, pamphlet *To Dr. . . . An Answer to his Queries concerning the Colledg of Midwives* (London: 1688).

103 Adrian Wilson has developed this argument. See Wilson "Childbirth," 311, 318–20. Our evidence supports Wilson's view that it was an evolution which took part mainly in the eighteenth century. See also Wilson, *Man-midwifery*.

104 Frances Sowden of St Martin Outwich and Mary Garland of St Bridgid obtained testimonial support from wives of variously a surgeon and two barber-surgeons in 1689. GL MS 116/2, 3, 5, 12. In light of recent research on London barber-surgeons' records, there is the possibility that these men were barbers and not surgeons. D. Evenden, "Gender Differences," 195–8. Quaker midwife Margaret Robards delivered a surgeon's wife in 1707, PRO RG 6 1628/262.

105 Irvine Loudon, *Medical Care and the General Practitioner 1750–1850* (Oxford: Clarendon Press, 1986), 86. Although Loudon dates the beginning of the male takeover of midwifery at around 1730, he is sketchy about details of how the surgeons acquired their midwifery training. He suggests that treatises published by Smellie (1752) and Denman (1786) were instructive, as were Smellie's

midwives who could have instructed them in obstetrical techniques.[106] Seventeenth-century surgeons (and their wives), aware of the shortcomings in menmidwives' knowledge and experience of normal birth processes, ensured that when their own children were born, an experienced midwife was at hand.

Finally, we may consider the role of clients in the licensing process and the significance of the testimonials as evidence of women's personal involvement and concern for the maintenance of adequate midwifery services. As the century wore on, women's signatures, as well as their names, appeared with greater regularity and in more substantial numbers on testimonial documents presented to the courts of the Bishop of London. In the years 1661–62, out of forty-six testimonials, only one contained a statement signed by the women themselves. In it, six women, from five different parishes, appended their signatures to a statement attesting to the bearer's "sufficient experience and ability to perform and exercise the office of a midwife."[107] In the years 1663–64, women's voices are heard, unmediated, in five testimonials. The lengthiest list of names appeared on the documents of Isabel Ellis of St Martin in the Fields: twenty-four women were willing to vouch for the "long experience," and competence of midwife Ellis. In the case of Anne Gill of High Barnet, also licensed in 1664, all six women signed with their own distinctive marks. The testimonial of Mary Dowdall of Chipping Barnet contained the following statement about the woman who had been employed as a midwife "these many years past":

wherein she hath had the blessing to be a meanes for the safe delivery of others whose names are here subscribed and many others whome we knowe witness our hands the 23 Day of May 1664.[108]

Similarly, the four women who signed in their own "hands" Sarah Tricer's certificate (and who were described as "gentlewomen" by the curate of Laughton), noted:

. . . inhabitants of Laughton doo certifie that we have good tryall of the good skill and Gods blessings upon the endeavour of Sarah Tricer in the office of midwife; and have

courses in London, which began in 1744. Smellie's private courses, however, were not a requirement for the practice of midwifery. Loudon, *Medical Care*, 85–94. In the late 1740s, when John D' Urban, having already completed an apprenticeship in surgery, wished to become knowledgeable in midwifery, he undertook a separate course of training in London (possibly the one offered by Smellie). After successfully completing an M.D. degree at Edinburgh in 1753, he became physician and man-midwife at the Middlesex Hospital: British Library, Additional MS 24,123 fol. 82 As late as 1788, surgeons who had completed their apprenticeship were obliged to seek out private courses in midwifery. That was the year William Savory paid five guineas to a male midwife in London for two courses in midwifery, given at the doctor's own residence and his "labour house" near St Saviour's. George C. Peachey, *The Life of William Savory* (London: J. J. Keliher & Co. Ltd., 1903), 12. The first professor of midwifery in England was appointed in 1828 at London's University College. Loudon, *Medical Care*, 92.

106 Bloom and James list one example of a barber-surgeon married to a midwife early in the century, while Harley names two provincial midwives who were wives of surgeons. Bloom and James, 20; Harley "Provincial midwives," 29.

107 GL MS 10,116/1.   108 GL MS 10,116/3.

heard of the like good success to many more . . . we doe conceive her to be skilfull, discrete & honest . . . [109]

The 1668 testimonial of Mary Parsons of St Mary Matfellon contains the customary sworn testimony of six clients. Eleven other women added their names: one signed with a mark, but the other ten names appear as signatures, presumably executed by the women themselves. In addition to the four women who gave sworn testimony in June 1670, twenty other women signed a "petition" on behalf of Elizabeth Paulson of St Botolph Aldgate stating that they had "good experience of the great care and ability . . . in the safe delivery of women in childbearing."[110] Two years later, fifteen women set their marks to the certificate of Mary Burton of Rosemary Lane in the parish of Whitechapel, confirming her suitability for the office of midwife.[111] The testimonial of Joan Elsey of Enfield, submitted in 1689, contained the names of ten women who had been delivered by her and who had done very well "under her hands."[112]

The last five years of the century, in particular, demonstrate an increasing involvement by female clients in the formulation of testimonial certificates. Susan Warden of New Brentford and Elizabeth Thorowgood of Chipping Ongar presented statements containing the signatures of ten and seventeen women respectively in the years 1697 and 1698.

The testimonial submitted in 1696 by Margery King of Chipping Ongar, Essex, was signed by twelve women and bore witness to her:

. . . good skill, experience and success in wifery . . . hath safely delivered severall women in child bed with good success, and more particularly some of us whose hands have subscribed to this testimoniall.[113]

The women also commented on her "sober" life, thereby preempting one of the customary concerns of the clergy who in this instance were not represented in the testimonial.[114]

In addition to statements by groups of women, there are examples of individual women's voices. Ann Bell of St Martin in the Fields secured sworn testimony from four women who appeared in the consistory court on October 13, 1677. She also obtained the following statements (all in different handwriting) from three other women:

For I will assure you that I was safe delivered by ye help of mistris bell the midwfe of a son september ye 10 my name is Filadelfa Rogers liveing next dore to ye doge and duck in Pickadily.

109 Ibid.   110 GL MS 10,116/7.
111 Ibid. In addition, four women gave testimony under oath, one of who was included in the fifteen signees.
112 GL MS 10,116/12.   113 GL MS 10,116/14.
114 In the eighteenth century, provincial testimonials saw medical men replacing clergy as signatories according to Harley, but in London, there is no evidence of this trend. Harley, "Provincial midwives," 31.

Sir my name is market Grimes I was safely delivered by *ye hands* of Mrs Bell a midwife than [that] is with her now that can justifie ye same.

Ser i was safely deliverd by *ye hands* of Mrs bell the midwife the second of this present month my name is Susan Jackson [115]

Midwife Bell's clients emphasised not only the safeness of their deliveries, but their midwife's capable hands. In the previous decade, midwife Sell's testimonial certificate, written by a literate, upper-class woman, noted that no woman had ever "failed under her hand."[116] In the last decades of the century, mothers still preferred the warm and compassionate touch of their midwives' hands of flesh and blood to the cold instruments of the male midwives so aptly described by the eighteenth-century midwife, Elizabeth Nihell:

... where is the kingdom, where is the nation, where is the town, where in short, is the person that would prefer iron and steel to a hand of flesh, tender, soft, duly supple, dextrous and trusting to its own feelings for what it is about; ... .[117]

Women were becoming more actively involved in the testimonial process of the Bishop of London's ecclesiastical courts. They were drafting petitions (either personally or with the assistance of a clerk), signing their own names (whether by mark or full signature), and continuing to appear before representatives of the vicar general to deliver evidence under oath regarding the midwives' competence. One possible explanation for this trend could be that women were experiencing difficulty in obtaining the midwifery services that they needed in a city whose burgeoning population was placing increased demands on midwives.[118] Women decided perhaps to take matters into their own hands and licensing authorities acquiesced to their petitions by waiving, in some cases, the customary requirement of supportive clerical testimony.[119] The evidence clearly demonstrates the Church's perception of clients as being a (perhaps the) central feature of the testimonial system.

The clientele of seventeenth-century London midwives were drawn from a broad spectrum of society. They lived not only in their midwife's parish but, in many cases, well beyond its confines. Many of them turned time and time again to the midwife who had already proven her competence and care in previous

---

115 GL MS 10,116/10 (my emphasis). Ms. Grimes is referring to Bell's deputy.

116 GL MS 10,116/4.

117 Elizabeth Nihell, *A Treatise on the Art of Midwifery* (London: 1760), 36. The powerful imagery evoked by the term "soft hands" can be traced to ancient times according to Helen King, "As if None Understood," 185.

118 For a discussion of urban population growth, which continued to the end of the seventeenth century, see Roger Finlay and Beatrice Shearer, "Population growth and suburban expansion," Beier and Finlay, eds., *London 1500–1700*, 37–57. The number of midwives who were licensed by the vicar general showed a marked decline in the 1680s, with some recovery in the 1690s.

119 Although I have not found any regulation which specifies that clerical testimony was a requirement for licensing, the evidence arising from the practice of the period indicates that it was standard practice.

deliveries. The gentry, as well as the poorest parish residents, continued to call on midwives throughout the century. Clients voiced their satisfaction with the services provided by these women both by maintaining a network of referral among relatives, neighbours, and wives of their husbands' co-workers, and by becoming more individually (and personally) involved in the testimonial process. In all of these ways, clients not only expressed their concern for, and satisfaction with, their midwives, but gave their implicit stamp of approval to the traditional system in which midwives worked.[120]

120 No examples of client dissatisfaction were found in the ecclesiastical records.

4

A Social and Economic Profile of London Midwives

Elizabeth Whipp was the only midwife listed in the visitation records of 1637 for her parish of St Ethelburgha.[1] Midwife Whipp, widowed in 1628, was granted the administration of her husband's estate.[2] As one of the city's most prominent midwives, Elizabeth Whipp, along with Hester Shaw of All Hallows Barking, presented a petition to Parliament in 1633 against the attempt of Peter Chamberlen III to organise and incorporate London midwives under his direction. The midwives objected strenuously to Chamberlen's efforts, pointing out that he had little or no experience in normal deliveries, having garnered his knowledge of childbirth in "desperate occasions" when he used his surgical instruments with "extraordinary violence." The midwives' counter-petition was accepted by the bishop's enquiry held at Lambeth Palace in 1634, and Chamberlen's efforts were quashed, at least for the time being.[3] Whipp and Shaw, from parishes at opposite sides of the City, collaborated on this project, working together in the unofficial network which existed among members of their profession.

Details of certain aspects of Whipp's life have survived and afford fascinating insights into this midwife's circumstances. Elizabeth Whipp bore eight daughters and one son between 1601 and 1617, at least two of whom died in infancy.[4] The economically viable widow Whipp was assessed a substantial 13s. for repairs to her parish church in 1635.[5] Although Whipp's annual rent of £7 was average for this wealthy parish, it was higher than the rents paid by both of her sons-in-law.[6] By the time of her death in 1645, she was survived by a son, George Whipp, two married daughters, Sara Sydey and Ann Shepheard, an unmarried daughter, thirty-

---

1 GL MS 9537/15/65v. 2 GLRO DL/C 342/52(blurred, may be 54).
3 Aveling, *The Chamberlens*, 40–8.
4 Bruce Bannerman, ed., *The Registers of St Mary Aldermanbury* vol. 62, part 2 (London: Harleian Society Publications, 1932), 92–6.
5 Her assessment of thirteen shillings was not exceptional: Of the 121 assessments, 50 were lower, 10 were the same as Whipp's (including that of her son-in-law, Waldegrave Sydey) and 60 were higher: GL MS 4241/1/341.
6 T. C. Dale, "Citizens of London 1641–1643," Unpublished typescript (1936), 55. Sydey, not yet fully established, was shown at £6, and George Shep(he)ard at £4 and £6, although one of these was for property, which Shepheard rented to four tenants and was not for his own use.

seven-year-old Hester Whipp, and six grandchildren. The latter included the three children of her daughter, Mrs. Jones, who had predeceased her mother.[7] Elizabeth Whipp's oldest daughter, Ann, was married to Dr. George Shepheard, who was listed among the "ablest" inhabitants of Bishopsgate ward in 1640.[8] Mrs. Whipp's second daughter, Sara, married Waldegrave Sydey, a prominent citizen and merchant tailor.

The care with which she listed her bequests has permitted some rare glimpses into Mistress Whipp's material world, including a look into her well-stocked linen cupboard. Her "fine Holland sheets" were obviously items of pride while the "fyne childbed sheete," which she left to each of her married daughters, reflected not only a concern with personal "niceties" but also her professional pride.[9] Whipp's three married children each received five dozen napkins, flaxen and "coarse" tablecloths, towels, and everyday sheets – our midwife had lived very nicely indeed. A peep into Whipp's clothing cupboard reveals a woman with considerable flair whose tastes ran to the sumptuous, if not flamboyant. In her damask gown and red petticoat with "two gold laces" (left to Ann Shepheard) and her watered taffeta gown with its crimson satin petticoat with "small silver laces" (left to Sara Sydey), she was a colourful presence. A Mrs. Clark was the recipient of a small bequest from Whipp, and it is possible that she was Elizabeth Clarke, licensed in 1673 as a midwife in St Ethelburga, who may have had an association as deputy to the older midwife.[10] Eventually, Whipp's grandson and Clarke's niece would marry.

Whipp's cash bequests to family and friends, set out in a lengthy and detailed will, totalled more than £520, a figure indicative of substantial personal wealth. In addition to linens and personal belongings, which she left to each of her children, there was £10 to each family, specifically designated for the purchase of mourning gowns for the women (at £6) and new cloaks for the men (£4). The rest of her estate was to go to her daughter, Hester, who was also her executrix. At the time of her death, Elizabeth Whipp was living, along with her servant, Mary, in the home of her daughter Sara and son-in-law Waldegrave Sydey.[11] There is no question that Elizabeth Whipp was a London midwife who made her presence felt in a personal, political, and professional sense.

The next midwife whose licence was recorded for the parish of St Ethelburga was Sara Sydey, the daughter of Elizabeth Whipp. At the time of her licensing in February 1663, Sara had already been practising as a midwife "skilfully and carefully" for thirty-four years, as attested by the rector and churchwardens of St

---

7 The source of this, and most of the ensuing information about her, is Elizabeth Whipp's original will, probated February 17, 1646: GL MS 9052/13.

8 *Principal Inhabitants*, 3. St Ethelburga was in Bishopsgate ward.

9 Evidently these sheets were of the best quality and used during the postpartum period when the new mother could expect numerous friends and "gossips" to visit, in which case they could be regarded as part of the "ceremony" of lying in. Wilson, "Ceremony," passim. See also Chapter 3.

10 GL MS 10,116/8.   11 We believe this is so because of bequests to three of Sydeys' servants.

Ethelburga.[12] Beginning her practice in 1629, Sara was able to draw on the experience and wisdom of her mother who was still practising as a midwife and who was almost certainly her teacher and mentor. Sara's name also appears on records of the visitation for her parish in September 1669.[13]

There is abundant evidence of the wealth and prominence of the Sydey family. Citizen and merchant tailor Waldegrave Sydey played an active part in parish affairs, serving as a questman in 1646–47, a churchwarden in 1649–50 and auditor for the parish accounts in 1655, the year of his death.[14] The Sydey residence on Helmut Court was comfortable and of moderate size with six hearths.[15] Indications of Sydey affluence were the high assessments against Mrs. Sydey in 1666 and 1668 for royal aid: the 1666 tax at 14 shillings was the second highest assessment in the parish.[16] In addition to the family home in St Ethelburga, Waldegrave Sydey owned property on Ratcliffe Row in the suburbs of St Leonard Shoreditch, which included a building, "yard, gardens and orchard."[17] Sydey also owned lands and buildings in Bury St Mary, Suffolk, all of which became his wife's property at his death. Aside from a bequest of £600 to their son Waldegrave, Sara acquired a lifetime interest in her husband's entire estate for which she was also executrix.

Sara Sydey's will, dated April 30, 1670, is a lengthy and complex document consisting of "seven sheets of paper," to use Sara's own description.[18] It is a fascinating document because of the continuity which it establishes with family members already familiar to us through their relationship with Elizabeth Whipp. We find that Elizabeth's unmarried daughter Hester (who inherited the bulk of her mother's estate) was now married to Robert Langridge, whom Sara named as overseer and advisor to the executors of her will. Two of Sara's orphaned cousins, Elizabeth and James Jones, were among the beneficiaries of her estate. Elizabeth was now Elizabeth [Jones] Forshaw, the wife of Thomas Forshaw of St Benet Fink. Elizabeth was licensed in 1684 to practise midwifery, thus becoming a third generation midwife in this prominent London family.[19] Sara appointed her cousin

---

12 GL MS 10,116/3. Sara Sydey was incorrectly catalogued in the Guildhall list of midwives licensed in 1663 as "Hanna Hyde." The hiatus in ecclesiastical licensing during the 1640s and 1650s was probably a factor in the length of the period during which St Ethelburga failed to record the licensing of a midwife.

13 GL MS 9537/18/65v.

14 GL MS 4241/1. See insert between fols. 423–424 and fols. 425–440, passim. The office of churchwarden was the most important parish office. For a description of his responsibilities, Alice McCampbell, "The London Parish and the London Precinct 1640–1660," *Guildhall Studies in London History* 2 (October 1976): 115. For a discussion of churchwardens' accounts, see Tate, 83–107.

15 CLRO 25.9/34; 25.9/5.   16 CLRO Assess. Boxes 66.3, 71.13.

17 PRO prob. 11/222/318: will of Waldegrave Sydey probated December 19, 1655.

18 PRO prob. 11/343/136: will of Sara Sydey probated May 2, 1673.

19 LP VX 1A/11, 25. Elizabeth Whipp's will left legacies to the three Jones orphans with the provision that John Jones live with Dr. Shep(he)ard, who was to administer his funds, and James and Elizabeth were to live with Waldegrave Sydey, who was to receive and administer their legacies. Thus, Sara would have been, in effect, Elizabeth's mother. This would have strengthened

Rowland Worsapp, the son of Elizabeth Whipp's "sister Worshipp," as one of her executors and left him money for a memorial ring. Sara's only brother George was now dead and Sara left an annuity to her widowed sister-in-law, Martha Whipp, to be paid from rents of an agricultural property in Geldham, Essex. Sara's only son, Waldegrave junior, died in 1667; he noted in his will that he and his mother were joint owners of the Essex property, and that it would eventually pass to his son, Waldegrave.[20]

At the time of her death in 1673, Sara left the bulk of her estate to her two grandsons: John, the younger, was to receive £800 at age 21 with the residue to go to grandson Waldegrave. The sophisticated concepts regarding property bequests in her will attest to Sara's keen grasp of financial matters and her competence in administering a complex and valuable estate. Sara Sydey, midwife Sydey's great-granddaughter, was baptised in the parish church of St Ethelburga in 1676.[21]

St Martin Outwich was the home parish of Mary Sherwood, the wife of citizen and grocer Ralph Sherwood, who was licensed in 1676.[22] Her testimonial was signed by Rector Richard Kidder, the future Bishop of Bath and Wells. Of the four women who gave sworn testimony, two of them were associated with midwifery. Elizabeth Forshaw, the niece of Sara Sydey of St Ethelburga, would be licensed herself in 1684. At the time of Sherwood's licensing, Forshaw was possibly gaining experience, perhaps as a deputy midwife. The name of Sara Sydey (widow of Waldegrave junior) also appears on the testimonial, in all likelihood in the capacity of an assistant midwife. Ralph Sherwood, the midwife's husband, was a wealthy and prominent citizen and grocer of London. Midwife Sherwood had borne at least four daughters and a son. The son, John, was born in 1674, but lived less than two years. A daughter, Margaret, also died before the age of two. The family's links with the gentry were evident in 1679 when a gentlewoman was buried from their house. Other indications of wealth and social prominence were the high fees paid by Sherwood for the burial of their children in 1678 in the chapel of the parish church.[23]

Sherwood was a parish questman in 1680, and in the following year was chosen as churchwarden for his parish. In 1690, the Sherwood household was comprised of Ralph, his wife, one daughter, a grandchild, two maids, and a journeyman. By

even more the matrilineal aspect linking the three generations. There is also the strong possibility that Sara Sydey's daughter-in-law, who was also named Sara Sydey, was a midwife since her name appeared as a deponent on the testimonial of Elizabeth Forshaw in 1676, with the designation "widow." We know she had been widowed for nine years and would therefore not likely be supporting Forshaw's application as a client.

20 PRO prob. 11/ 323/11: will of Waldegrave Sydey Jr.
21 *The Registers of the Church of St Ethelburga The Virgin within Bishopsgate* (London: Press of the Church of Saint Ethelburga, Bishopsgate, 1915) unfol.
22 GL MS 10,116/9; CLRO DL/C/345/155. According to Calamy, Kidder was ejected as vicar of Stanground, Hunts. in 1662 but was reinstated after proof of conformity. A. G. Matthews, *Calamy Revised* (Oxford: Clarendon Press, 1988), 307.
23 GL MS 11394/1 unfol.

1695, Ralph Sherwood had attained the important City position of common councilman. Upon the death of her husband, whose will was probated in January 1703, Mary Sherwood became the principal heiress of Sherwood's extensive property holdings, including their residence on Threadneedle Street in St Martin Outwich, the adjoining residence leased to a gentleman, a vintner's shops, cellars, and warehouses in St Olave Hart Street and two properties on Ivy Lane in St Faith the Virgin parish. Sherwood also made cash bequests totalling almost £900, indicating the magnitude of his personal resources.[24]

Sherwood indicated his previous generous provision for his two widowed daughters, but named them to inherit the various properties after his wife's death. Daughter Mary was the widow of Edward How, a cleric, of Battersea; she was living with her parents at the time of her father's death. One of Mary's three daughters had also married a clergyman, Richard Staverton of Eversley in Hampshire, while a second daughter married doctor of laws Thomas Taylor of Canterbury. Sherwood's other daughter, Rebecca, had been widowed twice. She had one son, John Burman, by her first husband.[25] Her second husband was Dr. Robert Plott, doctor of laws, whose prestigious career encompassed appointments as the first keeper of the Ashmolean Museum, 1683–90, secretary to the earl marshal (1687), registrar of the Court of Chivalry (1687), Mowbray herald extraordinary (1694), registrar (1695), and historiographer royal (1688).[26] Plott had extensive property holdings in Kent, including a manor, timberlands, and marshlands. The extent of Plott's personal wealth was reflected in the cash endowments and material bequests which he left to his wife and family at the time of his death in 1696.[27]

His wife Rebecca, the daughter of our London midwife, received, among other valuables, a pearl necklace and bracelets. Indicative of the quality of the Plott household furnishings were the "curtains vallence and bases of silke imbroidered now upon the bedd in the Chamber over the Parlour at Sutton Barne together with the imbroidered tablecloath belonging to them" which were left to John Burman, Plott's stepson (midwife Sherwood's grandson).

In the event that Rebecca Plott should die without surviving heirs, Plott requested in his will that the proceeds from some of his leases be used to establish a chair of Natural History at Oxford with the professor to be called "Plotts Professor of Naturall History." Plott wished his stepson John Burman to be the first appointee to the professorship if he were "capable and willing." John Burman, however, who entered University College in 1697 and remained there until

24 PRO prob. 11/485/100: the 1705 will of Ralph Sherwood. The marriage tax rolls of 1695 show Sherwood as having an estate of at least the value of £600. CLRO Marriage Tax 56.2.

25 Rebecca's first husband was a gentleman, Henry Burman. The name of physician William Burman, who was probably a relative of Rebecca Sherwood's first husband, appears on a list of chemical physicians in 1665. Henry Thomas, "The society of Chymical Physitians," E. Underwood, ed., *Science, Medicine and History* 2 (Oxford : Oxford University Press, 1953), 63.

26 *DNB*, 1310–2.

27 PRO prob. 11/432/99: the will of Dr. Robert Plott, probated June, 1696.

1715, the last four years as a fellow, left to become the rector of a parish in Newington Kent.

Plott specifically addressed midwife Sherwood in his will, requesting that his "much honoured" mother and father-in-law assist with the guardianship of his two young children and in the administration of his estate which he left to his executrix, his "intirely beloved wife" Rebecca. As the son-in-law of a respected midwife, it is not surprising that Plott discounted any connection between midwifery and witchcraft in England.[28] At the time of his death, Rebecca Plott was carrying their second son who was named Ralph Sherwood Plott after the husband of midwife Mary Sherwood.

Few midwives have left their mark on the records of seventeenth-century London as vividly as the wealthy and articulate Elizabeth Whipp and Sara Sydey, or the respected and well-connected Mary Sherwood. Yet it is rewarding that so much can be recovered about the socioeconomic circumstances as well as the lives and careers of London midwives. To do this, it was necessary to look beyond the records generated by the licensing system which contained relatively few details. For this purpose, sampling was obligatory and the records of midwives of twelve parishes, chosen as representative, were examined. But, wherever possible, this information was supplemented by evidence relating to the larger population of midwives. Themes such as midwives' age at licensing, marital status, children, spousal occupations, literacy, fees, homes, and furnishings were addressed. In addition, reference will be made to immigrant midwives who practised in London.

AGE AT LICENSING

Early in the century, there are fragments of information about midwives' ages at the time of licensing. When Anne Ramsay, widow, of St Olave Hart Street presented her certificates for licensing in August 1611, she was sixty-five years old and had twenty years' experience in midwifery. Later the same year, Audrey Claybrook of St Lawrence Jewry, a fifty-year-old widow, Elizabeth Keyfar, a fifty-four-year-old matron of St Botolph Aldgate with ten years' experience, Isobel Doubleday, St Dunstan in the West, sixty-years-old with thirty years' experience, and Sara Curry, a forty-five-year-old widow from St Mary Matfellon were licensed. In 1612, Alice Warner of Stratford, also widowed, was fifty-six years old when she applied for her licence.[29] Later in the century, Rebecca Jeffrey, of St Botolph Aldgate, was fifty-eight years old at the time of applying for her licence.[30]

If these women are at all representative, licensed London midwives were mature women with long experience in their chosen calling, who began practising

---

28 Harley, "Historians as demonologists," 10.
29 GLRO DL/C 340/3v, 10, 11, 11v, 13v, 30v.   30 GL MS 10,116/2.

midwifery in their thirties and forties. Maturity was also a key concern in other areas of Europe. In Braunschweg, most midwives and their apprentices, or "warming women," were over the age of forty; in rural Italy, a woman's chief recommendation for the occupation of midwife was her advanced age. In seventeenth-century Spain, an aspiring midwife must have attained her thirty-sixth year.[31] Historians have tended to view early modern midwives through a lens clouded by twentieth-century ageism, but it is evident that in the seventeenth century, a midwife's longevity was to be applauded, not denigrated.[32]

MARITAL STATUS

Although provincial midwives could be unmarried, there are strong indications that marriage or widowhood were informal requirements for licensing as a midwife in London.[33] Of twenty-six midwives identified in the Vicar General's Register between December 1607 and June 1611, seventeen were identified as married women and nine as widows.[34] In the first four decades of the century, there is an occasional omission regarding either a husband's first name or the designation *vidua*, but there is no indication that any of the women who applied for licences were unmarried. Similarly, in the period 1661–1700, testimonial records reveal that 346 married women were licensed. The same period saw eighty-five widows receiving licences; ninety testimonials gave no indication of marital status. The percentages for the period 1661–70, therefore, are: married 66%; widowed 16%; unspecified 17%. Although the occasional unmarried midwife has been uncovered in the provinces, London records support the view that licences were granted only to married or previously married women.[35]

31 Lindemann, 182; Filippini, 154; Ortiz, 99. Harley notes examples of young midwives in provincial England. Harley "Provincial midwives," 34. In Nuremberg, "young, light-headed" girls were discouraged from taking up the practice of midwifery in the early modern period. Wiesner, "Early modern midwifery," 99. In sixteenth-century France, older midwives instructed "young girls or daughters" according to Petrelli, 277. The Frisian midwife Catharina Schrader was 38 when she began practising and she delivered her last child at age 88. Marland, "Mother and Child were Saved," 7.

32 See, in particular, the testimonial of Margaret Corney, where the ages of two venerable midwives, both in their eighties, are recorded as an obvious comment on their wisdom, and by extension, Corney's superior training. GL MS 10,116/1.

33 There may have been regulations, as yet uncovered, regarding the requirements for licensing of London midwives, which addressed marital status. David Harley notes several spinsters, one of whom was extremely young, who were practising midwives in Lancashire and Cheshire. See Harley "Provincial midwives," 33, 34. By way of comparison, Nuremberg's midwives were described as older, unmarried women or widows. Wiesner, "Early modern midwifery," 99.

34 GLRO DL/C 339. Because of ensuing gaps in the recording process, we are unable to extend our analysis beyond this period.

35 Percival Willughby mentions his daughter in 1655. She was probably in her early twenties at the time, presumably unmarried, and already practising midwifery on her own as well as in conjunction with her father in Derby; see Willughby, 119. So unusual was the presence of an unmarried woman at a Quaker delivery, when Elizabeth Whyte of St Paul Shadwell (licensed in 1675)

Similarly, in most areas of early modern Europe where studies of midwives have been done, marriage or widowhood was a prerequisite.[36]

MIDWIVES AS MOTHERS AND GRANDMOTHERS

While not a requirement for licensing, many London midwives had conceived and borne children themselves.[37] Testimonial certificates contain scattered references to midwives' children: widow Elizabeth Collins of St Peter Paul's Wharf had four children in 1662, while Mary Buskill of Whitechapel, a widow of eleven years, had three children to support in 1664. Temperance Pratt, widow, of St Botolph Aldgate had "a great charge of children." Widow Shelton of St Giles in the Field had seven children.[38] Joan Maxey of Hammersmith in Fulham had at least one child and was helping to support her two orphaned grandchildren in 1666 when she applied for licensing.

By examining wills, parish registers, and other records, we have been able to find evidence relating to the offspring of approximately half of the midwives from the twelve parishes subjected to detailed examination.[39] As could be expected, we were more successful at identifying the children of midwives in the period 1661–1700 than in the period 1600–41.[40]

The majority of London midwives had completed their own childbearing cycle at the time of licensing, a practice which was common in continental Europe and

delivered Quakeress Elizabeth Johnson of Shadwell, the birth records note that one of the two other women in attendance was Lydia Marshfield "maide." PRO RG 6 1626/16.

36 See Ortiz, 101; Fillipini, 154; Lindemann, 181–2; Wiesner, "The midwives of south Germany," 89. The exception seems to have been Nuremberg where midwifery candidates were older, unmarried women and widows. Wiesner, "Early Modern Midwifery," 99.

37 Midwives in Braunschweig were customarily women who had borne children (although past childbearing age) as were Italian midwives of the sixteenth and seventeenth centuries. See Lindemann, 182; Filippini, 154. Regulations in late seventeenth-century Haarlem in the Netherlands similarly required midwifery candidates to have borne children. Marland "The *'burgerlijke'* midwife," 197.

38 GL MS 10,116/2,4.

39 In the early period, we were able to find evidence about the relationship between twelve or thirteen midwives and their children while in the later period, there is some evidence of the maternal relationships of twenty-seven midwives.

40 Since a number of midwives were identified only by their surname in visitation records (and in some cases in licensing records also), it is difficult to establish with certainty that there was a relationship between a given midwife and children with the same surname whose baptisms and burials were recorded in parish registers. Children were usually identified in parish records by their relationship to their father, but, in many instances (especially in records showing burial costs), even the father's name was not given. Where the midwife had a commonly occurring surname, and her spouse's Christian name was unknown, it becomes almost impossible to identify offspring. Assumptions are equally precarious when the spouse's name is known but the records give only the child's name, unless the surname is an unusual one. Compounding the difficulties is the fact that parish records frequently failed to distinguish between infants, children, and adults who often shared the same Christian name as well as surname. For identifying mature children of midwives, wills proved the most valuable single source.

encouraged in advice manuals such as Jacques Guillimeau's treatise on childbirth, published early in the seventeenth century.[41] There were, however, exceptions. Joyce Meagon, St Dunstan in the West, combined careers as mother and midwife: by the time she was licensed in 1616, she had already borne two sons, one of whom had died in 1613. She subsequently bore two, possibly three daughters (in 1616, 1619?, and 1621), one of whom died in 1620.[42] For some women, the timetable was altered by economic circumstances: Elizabeth Whitehorne of St Mary Aldermanbury was a young widow with three children, the youngest of whom was only six, when she was licensed in midwifery in 1677.[43] London midwives may, however, have been involved in the child delivery process either as a deputy or unofficial female attendant for many years. By waiting until their children were grown before acquiring a licence, they were able to devote themselves to the needs of their clients without the demands of their own pregnancies.[44]

We know, for example, that Barbara Crowd(son), of St Mary Aldermanbury was married in October 1586, in the parish of St Mary Aldermanbury and that she bore a daughter, Mary, in 1589, who lived only a few months. Crowd was licensed as a midwife some thirty years later.[45] Elizabeth Somner of St Dunstan in the West buried infant sons in 1628 and 1629, and had at least one other child who survived. She was licensed in midwifery in 1639.[46] Mary Benson, also from St Dunstan in the West, was practising as a licensed midwife by 1664. Elizabeth and Henry Benson, both children, were buried in 1638 and 1641 while infant Rowland Benson succumbed in 1655.[47] In the parish of St Anne Blackfriars, Winnifred Allen, wife of John Allen, tailor, bore sons in 1642, 1643, and 1645. Allen's midwifery licence was issued in 1662, some seventeen years after the last recorded birth of her own children.[48]

---

41 Guillimeau, *Childbirth*, 84. Giardina Hess discusses the careers of nine midwives, six of whom waited until their children were at least in their teens before practising, while one of the remaining three began sooner because of unusual life events. Giardina Hess "Midwifery practice," 67.

42 GL MS 10342/63, 69, 73v, 82, 221v, 234; GLRO DL/C 340/211v.

43 GL MS 3556/2 unfol.; PRO prob 11/351/96; GL MS 10,116/10.

44 It was probably for the same reason that training schools for midwives in the Netherlands, established in the nineteenth century, admitted women between the ages of twenty-five and thirty-five, "preferably unmarried women or widows." See M. J. Van Lieburg and Hilary Marland, "Midwife Regulation, Education, and Practice in the Netherlands During the Nineteenth Century," *Medical History*, 33 (1989): 296–317.

45 *Registers of St Mary Aldermanbury*, vol. 61 51, 54, 55. GLRO DL/C/341 (fol.illeg.) The surname was Crowdson in the sixteenth century but was subsequently shortened to Crowd or Croud.

46 GL MS 2968/3/344v, 366. The assessment for 1679 shows widow "Sumner" living on Myter Close with two grandchildren: GL MS 2969/4 unfol; GLRO DL/C 344/61v.

47 GL MSS 9537/17/66v; 2968/3/551, 595; 2968/4/255. At least eleven infants with the surname "Symonds" were buried in the years 1645–59 in the parish of St Dunstan in the West. Two (and possibly more) were the children of Abigail Symonds, licensed in 1667 to practise midwifery. GL MSS 2968/4/8v, 34, 135, 136, 233v, 254v, 258v, 304, 316v, 321v; 10,116/5.

48 Parish Registers of St Andrew by the Wardrobe and St Anne Blackfriars 1560–1837, 1558–1837; GL MS 4502; GL MSS 10,116/2.

Children of London midwives followed a variety of careers: the son of Edith Torshel (1) of St Clement Danes (licensed in midwifery in 1634) was a graduate of Cambridge and clergyman of St Giles Cripplegate. Tutor to King Charles I's two youngest children, Torshel dedicated a treatise to the nine-year-old Princess Elizabeth on her birthday. He was preacher to the House of Commons in 1646. Torshel died in 1650.[49] Charles, the son of Anne Adams of St Anne Blackfriars (who was practising midwifery in 1638), carried on the trade of gunsmith after his father's death in 1638.[50] London citizen and cutler William Garland was the son of Elizabeth Wharton, midwife of St Dunstan in the West, by her first marriage.[51] Anne, the daughter of Isobel Halsey, of Allhallows the Less, was married to citizen and clothworker Thomas Moody. Isobel was predeceased by her son or, more probably, stepson Clement, a brewer at the time of his death in 1663, whose brother John continued to work as a citizen and brewer.[52]

Like parents everywhere, midwives and their spouses strove to provide for the welfare and security of their children. Widow Alice Fox of St Botolph Aldersgate was licensed in 1678 in midwifery. By the time of her death she had appointed a friend and "Aunt Joan Barton" to be executors of her estate and guardians of her three young children. Money for the support of her two sons until they were old enough to be apprenticed (and for providing the apprenticeship premiums) was to come from the interest on bonds and notes totalling £179, with the rest of her estate to be divided among the three children at age twenty-one or at the time of marriage.[53] Elizabeth Gaskar of St Anne Blackfriars was widowed in 1651; as sole executrix of her husband's estate, she was to arrange an apprenticeship for their son and ensure that funds were available for his maintenance until his training was completed.[54] In naming Honor Powell, the widow of a mariner, as the principal beneficiary of her estate, Katherine Carpenter of St Mary Matfellon excluded two other daughters in 1678. Both were married, and possibly well provided for; their mother may have felt they had no claim to the estate.[55] Isobel Glover, midwife of St Katherine Coleman, was widowed in 1642. Her husband Nathaniel, citizen

49 Samuel Torshel, *The Woman's Glorie, A Treatise Asserting the due Honour of that Sexe and Directing wherein that Honour consists* (London, 1645). Sir Henry Ellis, ed., *The Obituary of Richard Smyth, 1627–1674*, Camden Society (1849), 29. A list of Cambridge alumni give his year of death as 1646, but the "Obituary" is quite specific in the date it gives, making it more reliable. I am grateful to Michael Treadwell for establishing the connection between midwife Torshel and son, Samuel.
50 GL MSS 9537/14/35v; 9171/27/42v.
51 GL MSS 9172/70; 10,116/1. I am grateful to Adrian Wilson for pointing out that Percival Willughby mentions a Mrs. Wharton of London. Willoughby *Observations*, 97. Wharton was licensed in 1661.
52 PRO prob. 11/322/163; 312/114.
53 GL MS 9172/70. We believe that the Alice Fox of St Botolph Aldersgate and the Alice Fox of St Bride, whose will survives, are the same person since the parishes lie close to one another (they touch at one point) and the clients who gave sworn testimony for Fox all resided in an area lying between St Sepulchre and St Botolph Aldersgate. LP MS VX 117/11/ 9.
54 PRO prob. 11/217/102.   55 GL MS 9172/67, May, 1678.

and painter-stainer, had made generous provision for his widow and also for his son Richard and his daughters Isobel, Dorothy, and Elen, who were all under the age of twenty.[56]

London midwives were grandmothers, too. At the time of her death in 1646, Elizabeth Whipp left bequests to six grandchildren. Three of the children received £20 each.[57] The remaining three children were orphans. To the two boys she left £30 apiece, and to their sister, £40. Mrs. Whipp also made clear that the orphans were to live with the families of her two married daughters: John Jones was to live with the Shepheards who were the parents of two sons; James and Elizabeth Jones were to live with the Sydeys and their son. Ann Moody, granddaughter of Isobel Halsey of Allhallows the Less, was named the sole beneficiary of her grandmother's estate in 1666.[58]

Helen Ormes, licensed in 1622, made her two grandchildren, James and Elizabeth Ormes, the major beneficiaries of her substantial estate in 1673, bypassing her two sons and two daughters in the process.[59] Temperance Pratt favoured her "loving granddaughter" Temperance Hare, rather than her daughter Hanna, to inherit her estate in 1687, while Susanna Annet was a favourite grandchild of midwife Alice and her husband Nicholas of St John the Baptist.[60] In 1682, Robert Glover, the grandson of midwife Deborah Glover of St Gregory by St Paul, inherited one-third of a legacy, which his grandmother had previously received from her brother, Thomas Strackly.[61] From her modest estate, Anne Parrott of St Sepulchre (formerly of St Clement Danes) left a bequest of £5 to her grandson William Parrott in 1698, with further small bequests of twenty shillings apiece to grandchildren Mary, James, and Elizabeth Parrott.[62] The extremely wealthy midwife Anne Baxter of St Clement Danes left the sum of £400 to her grandson John Seiren, who was also to be her executor, in her will of 1698.[63] Midwife Mary Sherwood of St Martin Outwich was the loving grandmother of three granddaughters and three grandsons at the time she was widowed in 1705.[64]

SPOUSAL OCCUPATIONS/SOCIAL STATUS

Since it appears that all licensed midwives were married or widowed, an examination of their spouses yielded useful information about the women themselves. Early in the century, the recording of spouses' occupations for women who were

---

56 GL MS 9052/11 (original will).   57 GL MS 9052/13.   58 PRO Prob. 11/322.
59 GL MS 9051/9/658.   60 GL MSS 9171/54, 9171/76.
61 GL MS 9172/71. We believe that midwife Deborah Glover of St Gregory by St Paul, licensed in 1672 (GL MS 10,116/7), and Deborah Glover of St Lawrence Jewry, who died in 1682, are one and the same. Glover may have moved to live with her son Joseph Glover, the eventual executor of her estate.
62 GL MS 9172/88. Although we cannot say for certain, we believe that Anne Parrot of St Clement Danes, licensed in 1672 (GL MS 10,116/7), is the same Anne Parrott who was living in St Sepulchre at the time of her death in 1698.
63 GLRO AM/PW 1698/5.   64 PRO prob. 11/485,1705.

licensed was not carried out routinely. In the years 1607–11, we know that three midwives were married to haberdashers and two were married to bricklayers. Others were married to, variously, a mariner, armourer, citizen and joiner, yeoman, painter-stainer, merchant, barber-surgeon, tailor, weaver, and a dyer.[65] In 1617, Grace Allred, the wife of a barber-surgeon from St Andrew Holborn, was licensed, as was Mary Page, the wife of William Page, a leather seller of St Botolph Aldgate. The following year, Elizabeth Bysey, the wife of gentleman Thomas Bysey, was licensed (Bysey's clients also included a gentleman's wife).[66]

In the next decade, we find that Elizabeth Bartlett of St Andrew Holborn was the spouse of a clothworker when she was licensed in 1627.[67] In 1638, Margaret Dodson, St Sepulchre Newgate, was married to a goldsmith. Dina Ireland of St Bridgid and Helenora Evans of St Botolph Bishopsgate, both licensed in 1639, were married respectively to a gentleman and a merchant.[68]

For the period 1661–1700, 106 testimonials out of 521 show the occupation of the husband of the midwife who was applying for a licence. This information is shown in Table 4.1: Occupation/status midwives' spouses.

In assessing the socioeconomic status of Tudor-Stuart midwives, information about the occupational status of spouses provides valuable insights. Occupations associated with clothing production and sales afforded employment to the greatest number of midwives' spouses in the foregoing sample. Of the twenty spouses in the clothing trades, one was a draper and six were haberdashers. Both of these occupations have been linked with significant indications of prosperity in Restoration London.[69] The second-greatest number of spouses (18) were designated as gentlemen. The remainder of the midwives were married to men of moderate status or better, with most engaged in skilled occupations. Of particular significance is the fact that only a few spouses were employed in semi-skilled trades or occupations and *none* were labourers or paupers.

Among midwives with exceptional spouses was Alice Culpeper, widow of Nicholas Culpeper, one of the century's most prolific medical writers and described as having had "a far greater influence on medical practice in England between 1650 and 1750 than either Harvey or Sydenham."[70] She was licensed to practise midwifery in 1665, some eleven years after her husband's untimely death.[71] Alice Field was only fifteen years of age when she married Culpeper and was a widow who had borne seven children (only one of whom survived beyond

65 GLRO DL/C 339, 340.
66 GLRO DL/C 241, fols. 37, 39, 71v. For examples of spousal occupations and women in the paid labour market see Peter Earle, "The female labour market in London in the late seventeenth and early eighteenth centuries," *Economic History Review* XLII, 3 (1989): 348–53
67 GLRO DL/C 343/23v.   68 GLRO DL/C 344/37v, 50v, 55.
69 M. J. Power, "The social topography of Restoration London," Beier and Finlay eds., *London*, 214.
70 F. N. L. Poynter, "Nicholas Culpeper and his Books," *Journal of the History of Medicine* 17 (1962): 153.
71 GL MS 10,116/4. None of the male signatories identify themselves as clergy, which is not surprising given Nicholas's nonconformist bent.

Table 4.1. *Occupation/Status Midwives' Spouses*

		Total
Clothing (19%)	draper, dyer, citizen and haberdasher (3), haberdasher (3), framework knitter, milliner, tailor (7), citizen and weaver, weaver (2)	20
Gentlemen (18%)		19
Distribution/transport (10%)	coachman (2), farrier (2), mariner (5), packer, porter	11
Building (8%)	bricklayer, carpenter (2), glazier, joiner, painter-stainer (2)	9
Metalwork (8%)	citizen and blacksmith, blacksmith, cutler, citizen and goldsmith, gunsmith, silversmith, sword cutler, wiredrawer	8
Victualling (8%)	baker (2), butcher (2), brewer's clerk, cooper, innholder, victualler	8
Misc production (7%)	belt maker, boltmaker, box maker, caliury?, clockmaker, diamond cutter, instrument maker	7
Leather (7%)	cordwainer (5), shoemaker, tanner	7
Professions (6%)	clerk (2), clergyman, barber-surgeon (2)	6
Merchants (5%)	grocer (3), citizen and merchant tailor, merchant	5
Decorating/furnishing (3%)	stationer, upholsterer (2)	3
Land (agricultural)/farm (3%)	farmer, gardener (2)	3
Officials (2%)	majesty's lifeguard, parish clerk	2
Labourer		0

Note: The foregoing percentages were rounded off to the closest decimal point. Occupational categories were adapted from A. L. Beier "Engine of Manufacture," Beier and Finlay eds., *London,* 164.
Sources: GL MSS 10,116/1–14, 25,598; LPL VX 1A/11.

childhood) by the age of twenty-nine. Nicholas Culpeper spent a number of years at Cambridge, but did not complete his studies in preparation for a career in the Church. Instead, he entered an apprenticeship to become an apothecary. His interests led him into the practice of physick and he had a thriving practice in which he treated large numbers of poor patients out of charity or for what they could afford.

Alice Culpeper no doubt assisted her husband in his practice and became familiar with many of the treatments which he carried out. Culpeper's other preoccupation was the translation of medical treatises into English so that the layperson could avail himself of their contents. As a result, he was the author or translator of at least thirty-eight medical treatises, many of which were published after his death. It is no coincidence that in 1651 he published *A Directory for Midwives*.[72] Alice Culpeper was actively involved in the printing and publishing of many of her husband's posthumous works and the "Forward" to one of his 1659 publications was purportedly written by her.[73] Peter Cole of Leadenhall was responsible for printing at least twenty-eight of Culpeper's publications, and it is his name which appears (along with eight other men's names) on Alice Culpeper's testimonial certificate. Widow Culpeper's testimonial also points out her status as a responsible taxpayer of long standing in her community in Stepney.

Extant wills provide glimpses of universal and timeless personal domestic relationships in the families of midwives. In 1633, Solomon Tanfield, husband of midwife Sara Tanfield of St Anne Blackfriars, left his daughter and son-in-law, Elizabeth and Thomas Cooper, the sum of £10 and enjoined them to "avoid my house in Black Fryers London and dwell elsewhere leaving my executrix [the midwife Sara] free from being charged with them."[74] Tanfield also ordered all of the Coopers' possessions removed from his house and delivered to them, and he released Cooper from debts which he owed him both for loans and for "diett." Temperance Pratt, midwife and widow of St Mary Whitechapel, died in 1687. She left to her only surviving daughter, Hanna Hare, "one shilling and no more" because Pratt had already in her lifetime given Hanna goods and money "to the utmost of my ability."[75] We can only guess at the reasons why Margery Hutchins revoked her former will and left her estate to her landlady instead of her "undutiful son."[76] On the other hand, the second marriage of midwife Isobel Sweatman (formerly Ellis), midwife, formerly of St Martin in the Fields and, after her second marriage, of St Andrew Holborn, successfully blended Ellis and Sweatman children who shared equally in William Sweatman's bequests.[77] The spouses of mid-

---

72 See "Introduction," for assessments of Culpeper's publication for midwives.
73 Nicholas Culpeper, *Culpeper's School of Physick* (London, 1659). This treatise also contains an eloquent plea on behalf of the sick poor.
74 GL MS 9168/18/195.
75 GL MSS 9172/76; 10,116/3. Some twenty-four years earlier, Pratt had been described as having had "a great charge of children."
76 GLRO AM/PW 1725/115. Hutchins of St James Westminster was licensed in 1700.
77 GL MSS 10,116/3, 9052/32.

wives who predeceased them and who left wills invariably made their wives their executrices. Susan Amussen has pointed out that when a man named his wife as the executrix of his estate, it indicated his confidence in her administrative ability, while Philip Riden regards the appointment of a wife as executrix as a sign of affection.[78] The spouses of London midwives demonstrated both confidence in, and affection for, their wives.

At least three of the midwives had experienced personal tragedy as a result of the civil war.[79] Rector John Williams of St Peter Paul's Wharf testified in 1662 on behalf of Elizabeth Collins, the daughter of glazier John Baptist Sutton of St Andrew Holborn.[80] He described how her husband, Thomas Collins, had been murdered by Thomas Howard, one of Colonel Pride's soldiers, leaving her with four small children to raise. Elizabeth, who was a lifelong resident of St Andrew Holborn had five years' experience as deputy to Francis Mabbs. Mabbs added a separate statement to the sworn testimony of Collins' five midwifery clients. The following year, the rector of St Martin in the Fields noted that applicant Elizabeth Wharton's husband, cutler Charles Wharton, "suffered very much by imprisonment and otherwise in tyme of the late usurpacon for his loyalty to his Sovereign."[81]

Interestingly, midwife Collins (who had also suffered much because of the actions of the rebels) testified on Elizabeth Wharton's behalf. The important work of midwifery was apparently unaffected by political alliances. Joane Maxey, however, a six-year resident of Hammersmith who became a licensed midwife in 1666, had come upon hard times through her support of the Royalists in Rutland where she had lived some years earlier.[82]

Touched by a later battle, Mary Burnham of Stepney had been a deputy midwife for a year when her husband, mariner Thomas Burnham, was killed in "the May Engagement in 1672."[83] In 1674, she successfully applied for her licence in order to continue to support herself and two children.

IMMIGRANT MIDWIVES

As previously mentioned, not all London midwives were English. The city was a cosmopolitan centre which attracted individuals from overseas, as well as from all parts of the British Isles. French and Dutch Protestants, who fled persecution in their homelands in the sixteenth and seventeenth centuries, established their own

78 Susan Dwyer Amussen, *An Ordered Society* (Oxford: Basil Blackwell, 1988), 81; Philip Riden ed., *Probate Records and the Local Community* (Gloucester: Alan Sutton, 1985), 66–9.
79 A study of the family and the civil wars has concluded that there were two types of damage to the family, one was ideological and the second was personal. The latter was a result of fatalities or through losses sustained by supporting the losing side of the Royalist cause. The three midwives exemplify both types of personal loss. Christopher Durston, *The Family in the English Revolution* (Oxford: Basil Blackwell), 161.
80 GL MS 10,116/2.   81 GL MS 10,116/3.   82 GL MS 10,116/4.
83 GL MS 10.116/8. Known as the "third Dutch War," France and England were allied against the Netherlands in the war of 1672 in which England was defeated.

London congregations. In 1593, at least three Dutch midwives, all members of the Dutch church, were living and practising in the metropolis.[84] Mistress Alores, born in Ghent, was a widow who maintained her own household and employed two English servants.[85] Widow Klerine Molney of Antwerp came to London in 1584. Nine years later, she was living with her eleven-year-old daughter, who had been born in Antwerp, and a Dutch maid servant.[86] A parishioner of Broad Street Ward, midwife Kernell of Louvain had come to England thirty years earlier. Widow Kernell lived alone in her own dwelling place.[87]

By 1593, French midwife Phillis DePort had lived in England for forty years. The widow, who was a member of the French congregation, employed no servants and lived alone.[88] Practising midwife Elenor Gyllam was the wife of diamond cutter Anthony Gyllam, formerly of Antwerp but, in 1593, a London resident for nine years. The prosperous Gyllam household in Bread Street Ward was made up of three children, a Dutch maid servant, and three English men servants in addition to the parents. They were members of the French Church in London. Either Anthony or his wife had been born in Armentiers before going to Antwerp.[89]

At least two French midwives were among the refugees fleeing persecution in France in the next century.[90] Suzanne Piau, widow of Jaques Piau of Rochelle, arrived in London in 1681 with four daughters, aged fifteen to twenty-one, and a niece. The family received a total of more than £8 in relief from the funds administered by the Threadneedle Street Church before they were established in their new home.[91] Midwife Piau may have been the midwife who received five shillings from the relief authorities for delivery of the newly arrived wife of ship's carpenter Samuel Masson.[92] Midwife Madelaine Maillet received only one pound and two shillings in relief assistance after her arrival on May 30, 1682.[93] We have no evidence that these two women were licensed in midwifery by the English ecclesiastical authorities but, as stated above, Piau, at least, seems to have been practising among the Huguenot refugees.

It is unclear whether foreign midwives who served only immigrants in England

84 Anna Cornelys, another Dutch midwife, was practising in London as early as 1561. See R. E. G. Kirk and Earnest F. Kirk eds., *Returns of Aliens Dwelling in the City and Suburbs of London part 1 1523–1571* (Aberdeen: Publications of the Huguenot Society of London, 1900; reprint,1969), 279, 282.

85 Irene Scouloudi, *Returns of Strangers in the Metropolis 1593, 1627, 1635, 1639* (London: Huguenot Society of London, 1985), entry no. 11.

86 Ibid., no. 782.   87 Ibid., no. 639.   88 Ibid., no. 338.

89 There is some confusion regarding midwife Gyllam's origins. One entry states that she was English, but a second entry says that she was formerly Elenor Mulbranck, who was possibly born in Armentiers. A number of years later, midwife Gyllam appears as Gillam in the visitation records of another parish.

90 Under the edict of 1680, which stated that papist midwives must deliver Huguenot women, Huguenot midwives were unable to legally carry out the work of child delivery in France. Hands and Scouloudi, 9.

91 Ibid., no. 155.   92 Ibid., no. 14.   93 Ibid., no. 133.

would have been required to take out a licence. Certainly, the penalty of Anglican excommunication would have been of little consequence to them. We know, however, that at least two other French midwives and a Dutch midwife were licensed by the Church of England to practise midwifery. Jaqueline de la Roche of St Martin in the Fields was licensed in 1678.[94] Her testimonial certificate, which was signed by eight women in addition to a senior midwife and the parish vicar W. Lloyd, noted that she had practised "many years," both in England and France.[95] It also stated that she was "conformable to the Church of England as it is now established."

The minister of the French church, Richard Demonery, and churchwardens Denise and Voisin, signed the testimonial of Mary Des Ormeaux of St Giles in the Fields, licensed in 1680, and whose practice was apparently drawn mainly from among her country women.[96] Although a member of the French church, her testimonial states that she was "in all things" a conforming Anglican, demonstrating the requirement that foreigners who were licensed to practise in England held appropriate religious beliefs. Des Ormeaux may have been able to convince church officials of the sincerity of her beliefs in 1680, but subsequent events, including her arrest and conviction on charges of murdering her abusive second husband, revealed a darker side to her life.[97]

In the last decade of the century, there were no licenses issued to identifiable immigrant midwives but a resident of Stepney, the Dutch woman Catherine Bont, presented a testimonial signed by Samuel Biscope, minister of the Dutch church in London, which confirmed her membership in his church "ever since the year 1685." She was licensed to practise midwifery in 1688.[98]

Recent studies of early modern midwifery in continental Europe have revealed many points of similarity with English practice, but there is no way of assessing how much of a contribution these transplanted midwives, who would bring with them the traditions of home, made toward uniformity in customs and practices. Extant records fail to reveal, moreover, whether the majority of London midwives were London born and bred, although there are frequent references to their lengthy associations with a home parish. Documentation discloses, however, that at least some had come to the city from other parts of the country.[99]

---

94 GL MS 10,116/10.
95 Only one of the eight women had a French name. This demonstrates that she had extended her practice to include English women.
96 GL MS 10,116/11.
97 Helen King has shown that by 1688 she was a Catholic. See King, "The politick midwife," 126.
98 GL MS 10,116/12.
99 For example, Mary Lambert, Surrey, LP MS VX 1A/11/41; Susan Kempton, Hertfordshire, GL MS 10,116/13.

MIDWIVES AND THE QUESTION OF LITERACY

The question of the literacy levels attained by some midwives has been of concern to historians who felt that midwives, as products of a system which blocked women's access to higher education, were at a disadvantage vis à vis male practitioners.[100] In view of our argument that the practice of good midwifery in the seventeenth century was linked far more closely to the practitioner's practical skills than to direct access to the inadequate information provided by midwifery books and pamphlets of the period, in one sense the issue of literacy becomes peripheral.[101] Since, however, we want to know what kinds of women London midwives were, any light which can be cast on the subject of literacy adds another dimension to their lives.

Aside from Thomas Raynald's translation of Rosselin's midwifery book in the sixteenth century, which suggested that literate women of the upper class could take the book to deliveries as a reference manual, most of the seventeenth-century publications on the topic of midwifery were ostensibly directed to midwives themselves, with an implicit acceptance of their literacy or at least the literacy of a substantial number of midwives who could then disseminate the printed information.

One of the midwives' objections to Peter Chamberlen's proposed takeover of midwifery training and licensing in 1634 was based on the premise that they had anatomy texts (in English) "which would direct them better" than his lectures could.[102] This argument attests to the literacy of a substantial segment of London midwives (more than sixty midwives supported the petition) and would lose its validity if midwives were illiterate. Evidence about provincial midwives of the period suggests that many of their number had attained high levels of literacy.[103] This encourages the belief that London, as the centre of the book trade, would have had even greater numbers of literate midwives than the rest of the country. Support for this view comes from Peter Earle's study, based on London court depositions, which has demonstrated a high rate of literacy for midwives. At 86%, their literacy was second only to that of female schoolteachers.[104]

Two outstanding examples of highly literate midwives of the century have received ample recognition. Jane Sharp was the author of a Stuart midwifery text and Elizabeth Cellier was the author of numerous pamphlets on political incidents,

---

100 Smith, 109–13. For a critique of this viewpoint, Harley, "Ignorant Midwives," 6.
101 See "Introduction." I am in agreement with Teresa Ortiz on this point. Ortiz, 98. Ann Giardina Hess has concluded that although Quakeresses generally exhibited a high degree of literacy, they were chosen by clients on the basis of their midwifery skills rather than their literacy. Ann Giardina Hess, "Community Case Studies," 143, 161.
102 Quoted in Donnison, 14.
103 Harley, "Provincial midwives," 34; Giardina Hess relates the high rate of literacy among the midwives of her study to their Quakerism, "Midwifery Practice," 62
104 Peter Earle, *A City Full of People: Men and Women of London 1650–1750* (London: Methuen, 1994), 120.

as well as of a self-aggrandizing scheme for a training school for London midwives. Midwife Sharp made much of the relative importance of practical knowledge over theory acquired from books. Her introduction, however, indicates that there was a need for some basic knowledge of female anatomy, which, presumably, could have been gained through practical experience, or through recourse to a publication such as hers. There may also have been an element of self-interest in her opening remarks, in the hope of greater sales for her book.[105]

Because they have identified themselves only by their initials, the four midwives who wrote a midwifery treatise in 1656, and the single midwife who was almost certainly the author of a 1680 treatise, have been overlooked by historians. But their presence, as well as their publishing activities, lends support for the view of that literate midwives were not a rarity in Restoration London.

While midwives who published were uncommon, hints of literacy can be garnered here and there. The records of the anonymous London midwife are an insight into the world of a midwife with the tools of literacy and numeracy, including basic bookkeeping.[106] An inventory from the home of one midwife disclosed that the family owned twenty books and a bible. The will of Elizabeth Forrest of Chelsea requested that an unspecified number of books be divided between her two sons.[107] Midwives' homes, such as that of Ann Flower of St Martin in the Fields, might predictably contain a family bible and common prayer book but in 1693, Margaret Beighton (Beikon), midwife of St Paul Covent Garden, owned two bibles, her own large bible, and one which had belonged to a deceased woman. Jane Barwick, an aged midwife from the same parish, left her two bibles to a female friend in 1721. Both examples point to at least a small circle of literate women and midwives in that parish.[108]

It is difficult to find evidence of the literacy of the majority of midwives, but based on Cressy's argument that a signature in this period was proof of literacy, indications of literate midwives can be found in records associated with their licensing.[109] Midwives applying for a licence at the Bishop of London's court were not required to sign their names in conjunction with their oath-taking. In some cases, however, senior midwives have signed a statement on behalf of the applicant. As a result, in the period after the Restoration, we have a dozen or so signatures of midwives themselves.[110]

Because a different format was adopted at the court of the Archbishop of Canterbury whereby clients frequently, and midwives occasionally, signed by

---

105 Sharp, 1–3.
106 See also the diary of Kendal midwife Elizabeth Thompson; the records of Frisian midwife Catharina Schrader; Harley, "Historians as Demonologists," 11 and "Ignorant Midwives," 8–9, for other examples of literate seventeenth- and early eighteenth-century midwives.
107 GL MS 9174/43: GLRO AM/PW 1698/24.
108 GL MS 9174/43; GLRO AM/PW 1693/3, 1721/111.
109 Cressy, *Literacy*, 55. See also Earle, "The female labour market," pp. 333–6 on the literacy of London women.
110 In addition to these signatures, there are three or four others which may be those of midwives rather than scribes.

mark or signature, we have the signatures of seven midwives who were applying for licences or supporting applicants.[111] In one case, the signature of the same midwife appears in the records of both courts.[112] Although these figures cannot be taken to represent the level of literacy among midwives as a whole, they are an indication of a literate core among the senior midwives. When all of the evidence is considered, a "best guess" leads to the conclusion that the majority of London midwives had acquired literacy skills, particularly those who were active toward the end of the century.

MIDWIVES' FEES

Enormous fees were paid to royal midwives in the seventeenth century: £100 in 1605 and 1606 to Alice Dennis for the deliveries of Princess Mary and Princess Sophia, and 500 guineas apiece to the two midwives who attended the birth of James II's son in 1688.[113] But what did the commoner pay for midwifery services in seventeenth-century London? The best evidence of the fees charged by London midwives is found in the account book of the London midwife whose records cover the years 1695–1723. Parish records also provide periodic comment throughout the century on what the parish paid to midwives for their services to poor parish women or to transient women who gave birth in the parish (usually despite parish efforts to have them "removed" before the impending delivery!).

The parish of St Dunstan in the West recorded its payment to a midwife in 1633 for bringing a woman to bed: The unnamed midwife received 2s.6d. The same parish paid midwife Carnaby 5s. for two deliveries in 1639, but only 1s.6d. in 1642.[114] The latter fee was paid to a parish midwife in 1649, while, in 1664, midwife Wharton was paid 2s.6d.

In 1674, Mrs. Parrott, a midwife from St Clement Danes, was paid 5s. for delivering a woman in St Dunstan's, which may indicate that in other parishes midwives were paid more generously for their services, or that midwives from other parishes were paid more generously for attending women outside of their home parish.[115] The following year, a midwife was paid only 2s. for delivering Joseph Penny's wife.[116] By 1688, the parish had increased its payment for deliveries to 5s., the amount the midwife received for "delivering a poor woman who fell into labour" in the parish.[117] The fee of 5s. was standard for the rest of the

111 Considering the sizes of the respective collections of testimonials, it would appear at first glance that midwives applying to the archbishop's court were much more literate as a group than their counterparts at the bishop's court. But because signing was not a requirement at the bishop's court, this conclusion is very tentative. Moreover, the practice of having the midwife sign was apparently not a requirement but merely a carryover from the more regularly applied practice of midwives' clients' signing.

112 She is Elizabeth Best of St Botolph Aldgate who signed on behalf of Elizabeth Lewys and Elizabeth Vesey. GL MS 10,116/10; LPL VX 1A/11/52.

113 Aveling, *English Midwives*, 31, 33, 60–62.   114 GL MS 2999/1 unfol.

115 Ibid. Not only did the parish pay this relatively high fee to the midwife, it paid an additional 3s.6d to two women for assisting her. Anne Parrott was licensed in 1671.

116 GL MS 2968/5 /184.   117 GL MS 2968/6/132.

century. That was the amount paid by St Dunstan in the West for at least thirteen women brought to bed in the parish.[118] A fee of only 2s.6d. was paid by St Gregory by St Paul's, considered a wealthy parish, as late as 1677. On the other hand, the prosperous St Mary Aldermanbury was paying 5s. for a delivery early as 1655, and the generous sum of 10s. by 1684.[119]

Although a number of parishes noted specific payments to midwives, in many cases the midwife's fee was included in the total expenditure by the parish for the woman's postpartum nursing and other necessities, making it impossible to establish with certainty how much the midwife was paid. For example, in 1679, the parish of St John the Baptist paid the midwife 10s., her fee, and for "cloths for the child" and, in September 1688, the parish of St Dunstan in the West paid £1.17s.6d. for "a midwife, and nurses and other necessaries for two women who lay in."[120]

By 1653, Hester Shaw, who had been a London midwife for several decades, had amassed a fortune of £3,000, although there is no way of ascertaining how much of her silver and gold was the direct result of her midwifery practice.[121] In the delightfully frank and ribald (at least by twentieth-century standards) so-called "petition to parliament" in 1643, "London midwives" described themselves as "formerly well paid." But now they were feeling the pinch because, with so many husbands called away by the civil war, their clients' chances of becoming pregnant had diminished. Not only were their earnings reduced, their opportunities to "feast high" at christenings had dwindled.[122]

Diaries and letters from the seventeenth century not infrequently mention christening gifts of 10–20s. which could reach a total of £10, paid by the titled and well-to-do, both in the provinces and in London.[123] In 1661, Samuel Pepys

---

118 GL MS 2968/6/172,(January 27, 1690 unfol.) 197, 234v, 257v, 258, 294v, 322, 333.
119 GL MSS 3556/2 unfol.; 3556/3/33v, 47. The last two references are for payments of 10s to Mrs. Whitehorne.
120 GL MSS 7619/147; 2968/6/154. For the provinces, see Harley, "Provincial midwives," 34.
121 Donnison, 10.
122 Anonymous, *The Midwives Just Petition* (London, 1643). Although considered a parody, it reflects the perception of midwifery as a lucrative occupation.
123 See, for example, D. Gardiner, ed., *The Oxinden Letters 1607–1642* (London: Constable and Company, 1933), 251; John Loftus, ed. *The Memoirs of Ann, Lady Halkett and Ann, Lady Fanshaw* (Oxford: Clarendon Press, 1979), 62; F. and M. Verney vol. 2, 21. The Quaker midwife recommended to Edmund Verney charged a fee of five, ten, or twenty pounds, but would not accept christening gifts. Norman Penney, ed., *The Account Book of Sarah Fell of Swarthmoor Hall* (Cambridge: Cambridge University Press, 1920), 241, 335, 439. See also the records of the Earl of Rutland, in E. Upton, *Guide to Sources of English History from 1603–1660: Early Reports of the Royal Commission on Historical Manuscripts*, 2nd edition (New York: Scarecrow Press, 1964), iv, 459, 466, 502. The "new way" of holding christenings without gossips or godparents must have been a threat to at least some midwives' incomes. See F. W. Bennett, "The Diary of Isabella, Wife of Sir Roger Twysden, Baronet, of Royden Hall, East Peckham, 1645–1651."*Archeologica Cantiana* 51 (1939), 117, 121. In 1584, midwife Agnes Bell was left four of Jane Magham's best sheep for her care of the Hull widow in what must have been a difficult delivery; the woman survived, however, long enough to make her will: Borthwick Institute, York, Probate Register 22 part ll, fol. 538v. (I am indebted to Claire Cross for the foregoing reference.)

attended two London christenings. At the first, he gave the midwife a gift of 10s., while at the second, he gave 20s. to be divided between the midwife and two nurses.[124]

The anonymous London midwife of the late seventeenth or early eighteenth century set her fees according to a scale of her own devising. It was extremely flexible and based upon considerations known only to herself. Some of her clients were not charged for their deliveries. Among the latter were a female felon and her own daughter, Mrs. Campion.[125] In total, there are 119 entries in her account book where a fee was not entered. The lowest fees which the midwife charged were 2s. on one occasion, and 2s.6d., a fee which appeared less than a dozen times.[126] On two occasions, the midwife's next-door neighbour, Mrs. Clarke, paid the low fee of 2s.6d.[127] Wealthier clients regularly paid £4, £5, and £6, with one of the Barnardiston women paying £8 for her delivery in 1714.[128] "Madam" Brand paid varying amounts for each of her nine deliveries between 1703 and 1718: The highest, at £4.6s., was for her first delivery in 1703, but she paid almost as much for her last delivery (£4.4s.) and at least £3 for the rest except for the years 1711 and 1716, when she paid £1.1s.6d. (in 1716, the child was stillborn).[129]

The fees paid by less prosperous clients demonstrated a similar lack of consistency: For her nine deliveries, Mrs. Dangerfield paid £1 on two occasions and different amounts ranging from a low of 2s.6d. in 1707 and a high of £1.5s. in 1705.[130] The midwife delivered eight sets of twins according to her records. For two deliveries of twins she received no fee; for the others, she received as little as 10s. (from Mrs. Bromwell the sugar baker's wife) and as much as £3.12s. (from Mrs. Sample of Bread Street). On four occasions, the midwife noted that the children were "dead born" and she was always paid for their deliveries: For two of the stillbirths, she was paid 10s.; for one, she was paid £1; for delivering the wealthy Mrs. Young of a dead child in 1713, she received £8.[131] One suspects, therefore, that the skill of the midwife was never in question in these few instances where the infant was stillborn. The wide variation in fees charged depends upon factors not identified in the account book, but ability to pay was clearly one factor the midwife took into consideration.[132]

---

124 See Chapter 1, n 41. 125 Bodleian Library, Rawl. D 1141/8.
126 Ibid., fol. 66. The midwife charged one Tily Coms, 2s.5d. in 1706, possibly because that was all the woman had, and it was close to the more usual 2s.6d.
127 Ibid., fols. 34, 42v. 128 Ibid., fol. 11.
129 Ibid., fols. 51, 59, 60, 71, 5, 7v, 13, 14, 18. The Quaker midwife, Frances Kent of Reading, reportedly received at least £5 for a delivery, with some clients paying £20. Giardina Hess, "Midwifery practice," 65.
130 Ibid. fols. 35, 42, 50, 58, 65, 71, 2v, 5v, 8.
131 Ibid., fols. 22, 22v, 23, 10. The midwife usually referred to client Young as "madam" and had delivered her on twelve other occasions for sums of £2–£4.
132 Harley has described a similar variation in the fees charged by provincial midwives. Harley, "Provincial midwives," 33. Filippini has also noted that the incomes of Italian midwives were tied to the socioeconomic status of their clients. Filippini, 156. Sixteenth-century Nuremberg

Although the account book of the late seventeenth- or early eighteenth-century midwife provides a good idea of the range of individual fees which were charged, it is less reliable as a way of assessing annual income. It is possible to reorder the entries into a reasonable progression of months and years, but there are obvious gaps in the records.[133] Some pages, as well as individual entries, are impossible to read because of ink blots. The evidence is of variable quality. For example, the first dated entry, in January 1695, recorded the name of the client and the time of day, but no fee. The next entry was not made until May 14, 1695. Of the eight deliveries recorded in this year, the midwife entered a delivery fee in five cases, as well as two christening gifts and a personal gift from "sister Parker" (7s.6d., apparently given as a token of her appreciation). All of the sources netted the midwife £5.5s.[134] In three cases, however, no fee or gift was entered. The account book ends abruptly in 1723 after a single entry for March 27, which shows that Mrs. Maret, a client of long standing, was delivered of a baby daughter with no fee entered. Bearing in mind these limitations, the account book yields some valuable insights into the midwife's income and fee schedule.

Table 4.2: Anonymous Midwife's Earnings, 1695–1722, shows the total annual earnings for this midwife (including gifts presented at christenings) of which we have evidence, and the number of cases recorded. The number of deliveries for which no fee was shown or where the fee is illegible has been specified as unrecorded.

By way of comparison, the casebook of a Kendal midwife, Elizabeth Thompson, who practised in the 1660s and 1670s, revealed an annual income which, at its peak in 1673, yielded £27.5s. for eighty-nine deliveries.[135] The London midwife in her peak year of 1704 earned more than £50 for thirty-seven deliveries, including five infants for whom no fee was recorded. An income of £50 a year for this period has been described in a recent study as one of "reasonable competence," allowing a middle-class London family to eat well, employ a servant, and enjoy a comfortable standard of living.[136] Thirty-seven deliveries meant, on average, one delivery every ten days, so a decent standard of living for an entire family

midwives, who were regulated by the City, charged fees according to their clients' social class and that their incomes compared favourably with those of craftsmen and journeymen. Wiesner, "Early Modern Midwifery," 97. Other areas of southern Germany saw midwives whose earnings combined salary and fees. Wiesner, "Midwives of south Germany," 79.

133 For example, in the year 1698 there were no entries for the first four months and the last month. In 1699 there were almost five months missing. In 1710 and 1711 there were five-month gaps while in 1716 and 1720 there were four and two months, respectively, without entries. In addition, the fee charged has not been entered in a number of cases. It is possible that the midwife did not receive a fee in some of these instances, but there are a number of fees missing in sequence; in the absence of other evidence, it is likely that the midwife recorded the entries at a later date and was unable to remember what she charged. See Lindemann, 181, for the difficulties involved in attempting to assess the incomes of midwives in Braunschweig.

134 Ibid. fols. 4, 5, 6v.   135 CRO MS WD/Cr/1.

136 Peter Earle, *The Making of the English Middle Class* (London: Methuen, 1989), 14. See also Earle, "A Study of the female labour market," 342.

Table 4.2. *Anonymous Midwife's Earnings, 1695–1722*

Year	Total cases	Income (£s)	Fee unrecorded
no date	3	0-19-6	2
1695[a]	8	5-5-0	3
1696	11	6-4-6	1
1697	19	21-12-9	3
1698[a]	12	8-2-6	1
1699[a]	23 (twinsx1)	28-15-0	4
1700	20 (twinsx1)	14-17-10	4
1701	25 (twinsx1)	28-15-6	5
1702	26	18-4-3	1
1703	42	44-9-9	5
1704	37	50-2-8	5
1705	36 (twinsx3)	23-8-11	7
1706	38	44-10-7	4
1707	33	37-9-11	6
1708	34	24-10-6	4
1709	35	33-10-6	12
1710[a]	18 (twinsx1)	16-19-6	3
1711	37	34-12-4	5
1712	27	31-14-9	8
1713	29	37-0-3	4
1714	27 (twinsx1)	29-9-9	5
1715	29	44-8-11	4
1716[a]	22	28-12-6	5
1717	30	43-11-6	6
1718	22	30-12-6	4
1719	23	26-12-9	2
1720	24	38-8-0	3
1721	18	17-3-6	4
1722	13	20-11-6	1

[a]Indicates the years in which the most obvious gaps occurred.
Source: Bodleian Library, Oxford MS. Rawlinson D 1141.

could be secured (and up to five deliveries provided *gratis* for charity) without an exceptionally demanding schedule and without compromising the standard of care provided to clients. Judging from the available but incomplete records, the midwife's annual income was somewhat lower than £50 in most years. We do not know, however, whether this midwife was providing the sole family support, and we do not know whether the years of lower levels of activity (assuming that the account book accurately records the bulk of her practice) were the consequence of personal choice or lack of business. London midwifery clearly could offer a reasonable livelihood for a widow, or a valuable supplement to a family income. At its peak, it could support an entire family at a reasonable, and very respectable level.

The records of midwife Elizabeth Thompson of Kendal extend for only a six-year period, 1669–74, and give her annual income and number of deliveries. The total number of cases which she delivered was 419, or an average of sixty-nine deliveries a year, which was considerably higher than our London midwife's (admittedly imperfect) records show. From a limited comparison of the two account books, it is evident that the London midwife was appreciably better paid for less work than her provincial counterpart several decades earlier.[137]

On at least one occasion, when both a physician and midwife attended a confinement (in 1680), the midwife's fee was substantially higher than that of the physician.[138] Even so, at the end of the century, the parish of St Dunstan in the West paid the sum of £1 for the services of a male midwife described as "doctor" when two midwives were unable to complete a difficult delivery. Unfortunately, there is no indication of whether the child was born alive or whether the male midwife was merely called, according to the custom of the period, to use his instruments to facilitate the delivery of the dead fetus.[139] At any rate, his fee was twice that paid to midwives of the parish when they delivered a child, and an indication of the growing rewards to be reaped from male midwifery.[140]

The economics of Stuart midwifery are important not only in revising the picture of midwives with its connotations of poverty and ignorance, but also in understanding the tangible rewards which attracted male practitioners to midwifery, particularly in the eighteenth century when an increasing number of young surgeons and apothecaries were swelling the workforce and increasing the competition for clients.[141]

Further evidence of economic viability is found in the wills of London midwives. In some instances, generous bequests were left to family members and friends. Mary Baldwin, the daughter of midwife Anne Baldwin of St Clement Danes, was to receive £60 "at the day of her marriage or age 21."[142] Anne

---

137 The London midwife was also less active than the Frisian midwife, Catharina Schrader, whose casebook covers the period 1693 to 1745, and who averaged 120 deliveries per annum in the period 1698–1712. In addition to frequently receiving no fee, the Frisian midwife was paid in kind, a practice to which the rural midwife of Kendal makes no reference. Marland, "*Mother and Child were Saved.*" For other examples of the relatively low fees paid to rural midwives, Forbes "Registration," 238 and Alice Clark, 279.

138 Clark, 280. Wiesner has noted the discrepancies in civic salaries paid to midwives, surgeons, and apothecaries, the latter two groups being much better paid. Wiesner, "The midwives of south Germany," 79.

139 Adrian Wilson has concluded that male midwife Percival Willughby was called in the majority of cases (whether by a midwife, the mother, father, or others) to deliver a *dead* child. Wilson, "Childbirth," 256.

140 GL MS 2968/6/334. The male midwife who delivered Judith Edwards in 1698 is described as "Doctor" Johnson.

141 For eighteenth-century comparisons in Spain, Ortiz, 103; in Holland, Marland, "The '*burgerlijke*' midwife," 203; in Braunschweig, Lindemann, 181.

142 GLRO AM/PW 1692/2.

Somner (Sumner) of St Martin in the Fields divided £95 between three grand-children in her will of June 18, 1678.[143] When she died in 1698, Elizabeth Forrest, the wealthy widow of a Chelsea glazier, left £100 apiece to her oldest son and two oldest daughters, £100 to her second son, and £200 each to her two youngest daughters for a total of £850.[144] While midwife Forrest's will was unusual in the generosity of its bequests, other midwives, such as Sara Nicholson, Rebecca Wiggins, Ann Rampton, and Isobel Gunn of St Martin in the Fields left lists of more modest cash bequests, frequently of £5 or £10, often combined with legacies of personal effects, clothing, and jewellery, as well as household linens and furnishings.[145] Even so, Francis Grant of St Ethelburga left moderate bequests to some forty relatives and friends which totalled the not inconsiderable sum of £450 in cash.[146]

London midwives were not objects of parish relief. Not only did midwives acting as executrices of their spouses' estates distribute charity to the poor of their parishes, they themselves earmarked portions of their estates for the benefit of parish poor. In 1633, the will of Solomon Tanfield instructed his wife Sara, a midwife of St Anne Blackfriars, to give "to evere one of the poore pentioners of Black Friars aforesaid Twelve pence" while the widow of John Grant was to ensure that the poor of St Ethelburga received "a six penny wheaten loaf [each] Whitsunday and All Saints Day."[147] George Seeley, husband of midwife Elizabeth Seeley, left a bequest of 40s. to Christ's Hospital where he had received his education.[148] Margaret Beighton of St Paul Covent Garden also gave 40s. to the poor of Kegworth and the same amount to the poor of Sawley in Derbyshire. Deborah Glover's beneficence was extended in the form of new gloves for everyone attending her funeral in St Lawrence Jewry in October 1682, and Anne Baxter of St Clement Danes wanted poor widow Smith in Drum Alley to have 20s.[149]

The sums of money which midwives allocated for their funerals were, in some instances, indications in themselves of modest affluence. Susanna Skelton's estate was large enough to support the not inconsiderable sum of £30 for funeral expenses, while Isabell Gunn instructed her executor, daughter Jane Hanmer, to spend £20 on her funeral.[150]

Not only were London midwives, in many cases, comfortably well off, they were able to turn an occasional profit by loaning money. The inventory of Elizabeth Heron noted that she was owed £12 in "desperate notes" at the time of her death.(See Appendix E.) In her will of 1691, Sara Nicholson excluded the loans made to her sons, but left other money from other creditors to her daughter. The well-to-do Elizabeth Forrest was owed the huge sum of £400 in notes and

143 GLRO AM/PW 1678/67.   144 GLRO AM/PW 1698/24.
145 GLRO AM/PW 1692/69 (Nicholson), GLRO AM/PW 1678/50 (Rampton), GLRO AM/PW 1670/34 (Gunn), GLRO AM/PW 1687 (Wiggins).
146 GL MS 9052/31.   147 GL MS 9168/18/195; PRO prob. 11, 350/1676/38.
148 GL MS 9172/45.   149 GLRO AM/PW/1693/3; GL MS 9172/71.
150 GLRO AM/PW/1735/34;1670/34.

bonds at the time of her death. The niece of midwife Mary Wood of St Martin in the Fields was to receive the interest on a loan of £30 which her aunt had made to a parish periwig maker "for her better maintenance and education"; at the age of twenty-one or marriage, the young woman was to receive the principal amount.[151] At the turn of the century, the assets of at least two midwives included investments in stocks.[152]

HOMES AND FURNISHINGS

Of the seventy-six midwives who were intensively investigated, at least twenty-eight lived in homes to which criteria such as taxes on rent and the number of hearths can be applied to give us an insight into their accommodations.[153] Judith Newman of All Hallows the Less, and midwives Hensman and Clarke of St Ethelburga, lived in homes with six hearths in 1670, homes classified as medium-sized according to a recent study.[154] Widow Elizabeth Carpin of St Anne Black-friars and Alice Burell of St Dunstan in the West lived in large and spacious dwellings with nine and eight hearths respectively, while Margaret Ward of St Ethelburga lived unpretentiously in a Helmut Court house with three hearths.[155] Earlier in the century, tithe rental records reveal the annual rent which a number of midwives and their spouses from the twelve core parishes paid. Midwife Isobel Halsey and husband Clement of All Hallows the Less paid a rent of £26 annually which placed them in the upper quartile for rents in their parish, while midwife Juliana Cooke's annual rent of £28 indicated an even more substantial, possibly lavish house with only six householders (out of 248) paying a higher rent in her parish of St Andrew Wardrobe.[156] Even the relatively modest rents of £9 paid each year by widow Sension and midwife Ann Clifton's family placed them in the upper half of rent values for their poorer parish of St Olave Silver Street, as did the annual rent of £20 paid by Elizabeth and George Seeley in the wealthy parish of St Dunstan in the West.[157] From later in the century, rental information

---

151 GLRO AM/PW 1713/124.

152 James Alexander "The economic and social structure of London c. 1700" (Ph.D. dissertation, University of London, 1989), listed under occupation "midwife": Widow Albritain was shown as having £50 invested, while Mistress Hassell's investment was £25. Albritain (Albrighton) was the Quaker midwife who carried out at least seven deliveries noted in London Quaker birth notes 1683–89. PRO RG6 1626.

153 Information about the homes of another seven midwives from other parishes has been included in the table below.

154 M. J. Power, 210. See also S. Dowell, *A History of Taxation and Taxes in London* vol. 2 (London: 1884, reprint ed., Frank Cass and Co., 1965), 38

155 CLRO Assess. box 25.9/27/35; Assess. box 25.9/18/4; Assess. box 25.9/34.

156 LP LMS 272/37, 56v. In 1638, records were made of the tithe rents in ninety-seven London parishes. T. C. Dale has compiled the information contained in the Lambeth Palace records under the title *The Inhabitants of London in 1638* (London: Society of Genealogists, 1931).

157 Dale, 169, 234. Seeley's will also mentions his rent as £20. GL MS 9172/45.

for ten midwives (seven of whom lived outside of the twelve selected parishes),[158] has been included in Table 4.3: Midwives' Housing.

Aside from their principal residence, midwives and their spouses acquired other properties which earned rental income for the family. Gentleman William White and his wife, midwife Mary White of St Anne Blackfriars, not only owned their spacious home on Water Street where they accommodated three lodgers and their servant, William was also the owner of the George Inn in West Smithfield, which passed to his wife on his death in 1700.[159] Similarly, gentleman John Grant, spouse of midwife Francis Grant of St Ethelburga, owned the King's Head in Fetter Lane, which he rented out on lease.[160] Midwife Joan Nott of St Katherine Coleman, widowed in 1627, shared her "doctor of medicine" husband's substantial holdings in Farnsborough and Aynsford, Kent, Ratcliffe, and the City of London with her three adult children.[161] Citizen and haberdasher Nicholas Annett, husband of midwife Alice of St John the Baptist parish, held leases on at least three properties, including one at Mile End Green. Gunsmith Thomas Adams of St Anne Blackfriars left property leases of unspecified value to his wife Anne in 1638.[162] Isobel Glover of St Katherine Coleman shared joint ownership with her husband of rental buildings on two acres of land in Stepney, and the income from this property became hers for life in 1643.[163] Elizabeth Wicks (Weekes) was given the task of administering her husband's estate on his death in 1722, a task which involved selling houses in East Street, St Andrew Holborn, and an "Estate" in Hanover Street near Long Acre in St Martin in the Fields. She was to maintain houses in Pallon St near Hanover Square and transfer a house in Crown Street, Hogg Lane to a married daughter.[164]

Other indications of a comfortable way of life enjoyed by a number of midwives are found in references to family servants. Of sixteen midwives who were heads of households at the turn of the century, eight maintained servants: Elizabeth Hassell of St Gregory by St Paul's had three female servants, three other midwives maintained two servants, and the remaining four kept one servant.[165]

In some cases, female "maids" were companions of long-standing, remembered by various bequests at the time of the midwife's or her spouse's death. Midwives Elizabeth Whipp of St Ethelburga and Mary Wood of St Martin in the Fields both left their maids gifts of £2.[166] Whipp took her servant Mary with her when she joined the household of her daughter in her declining years and remembered not only her own maid, but also her "daughter [midwife] Sidays mayd" with a

---

158 The rental information on ten of the midwives was taken from Alexander, occupational group "Midwives."

159 CLRO Marriage Tax 1695 17.17; PRO prob.11/456/108.   160 PRO prob.11/350/38.

161 PRO prob.11/153, 1628, will of John Nott.   162 GL MS 9171/54, 9171/27/42v.

163 GL MS 9052/11.   164 GLRO AM/PW 1722/127.

165 Alexander, occupational group "Midwives." In addition, Midwife Winckles and her family employed the services of servants in their home in St Gregory by St Paul's. CLRO Marriage Assessment, 1695 35.27.

166 GL MS 9052/13; GLRO AM/PW 1713/124.

Table 4.3. *Midwives' Housing*

Name	Parish	Hearths	Rent (£ per annum)
Halsey	AHL		c30
Newman	AHL	6	
Cooke	SAW		c28
Allen	SAW		c5
Carpin	SAB	9	
Whipp	SE		c10
Sydey	SE	6	
Benskin	SE		c12
Hensman	SE	6	
Clarke	SE	6	
Ward	SE	3	
Hughes	SGP		12
Hassell	SGP		40
Glover	SKC		12
Chamberlain	SKC	4	
Whitehorne	SMA		5[a]
Clifton	SOSS		9
Sension	SOSS		9
Griffith	SOSS		10
Wicks	SDW		c42
Seeley	SDW		20
Somner	SDW		c14
King	SDW		12
Croxon	SDW		30 (shared with W. Dickins)
Bradford	SDW	6; 9 (moved)	
Burell	SDW	8	
Mainwaring	SDW		10s.6d.[b]
Senior	SDW	8 (1666)	c52 (1638)
Albrittain[c]	SDB		26
Carter[c]	SLF		8.5
Clapton[c]	SML		10
Kendall[c]	SAA		7
Semcoe[c]	SAA		6
Mordant[c]	SA		10
More[c]	STA		16

Sources: CLRO Hearth Taxes: Box 41.15 (1670), Box 25.9/5, 15, 20, 22, 27, 34, 36 (1672?); LPL MS 272 (1638); T. C. Dale *The Inhabitants of London in 1638.* London: Society of Genealogists, 1931. The additional information on midwives outside of the core parishes (designated[c]) was taken from James Alexander "The economic and social structure of London c. 1700," Ph.D. dissertation, University of London, 1989, occupational group "Midwives."

[a] John Whitehorne, the midwife's husband, was assessed £5 as a tithe assessment on front ground, house, and back ground in 1671, which was very high. CLRO assess. Box 5.7.

[b] In 1689, Thomas Mainwaring, the midwife's husband was assessed as a landlord at 10s.6d., which was also very high. GL MS 3014/1.

[c] Midwives outside of the core parishes. See Appendix H: London Parishes.

modest gift. In addition to a generous bequest of £20 to her maid Hannah Layfield in 1695, Francis Grant left the following instructions:

I give my best Gowne and pettycoate to my cousin Elizabeth Feezy and my next best Gowne and pettycoat to her daughter. And my next best Gowne and pettycoat after the former to my maid Hannah and all the rest of my wearing Apparrell Silke linnen and Woollen I give and bequeath unto my said Cousin Elizabeth Feezy and to her daughter and to my maid Hannah equally to bee divided amongst them share and share alike.[167]

Among her more modest list of bequests, Elizabeth Bincks remembered her maid Elizabeth with the practical gift of a "darke serge petticoate."[168]

Extant wills of midwives and their spouses cast light on the material comforts which London midwives enjoyed and seem to argue that the anonymous midwife whose financial records have survived was not exceptional: silver plate, jewellery, clothing of good quality, well-furnished homes, books, linens, and other niceties, not to mention luxuries, which, at least in part, must have been a result of their professional earnings.[169] Among treasured personal belongings were Susanna Skelton's gold watch, Sara Nicholson's diamond ring, and Ann Rampton's ring with three diamonds. The probate inventory of Elizabeth Heron, senior midwife of St Giles in the Fields, drawn up on April 24, 1667, depicts a spacious house of nine rooms with seven hearths and a cellar, plus a "room in the yard." (Appendix E.)[170] Aside from the kitchen, all rooms were well furnished with beds and bedding, tables, stools, and chairs. Most boasted rugs or carpets, curtains and valances, and fireplace equipment. Other amenities included trunks, cupboards, couches, a desk, striped hangings, tapestry hangings, two settle beds, as well as a trundle bed, nine pairs of sheets, and three dozen napkins plus other linen. A variety of brass pieces brightened the parlour. These included two brass kettles, two brass pots, and two brass skillets. A brass mortar, which the midwife used to prepare her favourite "receipts," was also listed. The kitchen contained two iron pots among its equipment, as well as a cupboard for storage, one rack, and one pair of pot racks. The cellar housed eight barrels of beer. The deceased midwife had clearly possessed a substantial London residence suggestive of the well-to-do middle-class matron.

167 GL MS 9052/31. It should be noted that this bequest also casts light on the close and intimate relationship which could exist between women and their servants. In the wills which I have examined, favourite articles of clothing were generally left to family members.

168 GL MS 9052/15.

169 Detailed evidence of the material wealth of London midwives is provided in Chapter 5. See the wills of Elizabeth Towers, widow of St Michael Queenhithe, 1664, GL MS 9052 Box 14; Elizabeth Bincks, widow of St Botolph Aldersgate, 1665, GL MS 9052 Box 15; William Sweatman, 1683, GL MS 9052 Box 24; Helen Ormes, St James Clerkenwell, 1673, GL MS 9051/9/658. For a provincial midwife who also had a well stocked-linen cupboard, as well as other attractive items in her home, see the will of Joane Norwood of Chertsey, Surrey (probated October 2, 1612), PRO prob.11/120/207.

170 GL MS 9174/19. For a comparison with other seventeenth-century inventories, J. S. Moore, ed., *The Goods and Chattels of Our Forefathers* (London and Chichester: Phillimore, 1976).

Mary Preston of St John Hackney was licensed in midwifery in 1697.[171] She predeceased her husband, Edward, whose probate inventory was taken in 1724.[172] The Prestons had lived in an eight-room house with a cellar, their own brew house, and a stable. Their property fronted the river and they enjoyed fishing as well as the use of two "ferry boats." On warm summer days, the midwife and her family could pass the time pleasantly at the tables and benches placed along the riverside. Inside the house, at least two rooms were furnished with stoves either as an adjunct to, or in place of, open fireplaces. The "best chamber" contained blue Chinese furniture, including six blue chairs, a looking glass, and a tea board. In the great parlour were other touches of affluence: cane chairs, five turkish embroidered chairs, and pictures. Still another room displayed white window curtains, matted chairs, a coffer, a looking glass, an eight-day clock and case, three prints, delftware, glasses, "about twenty books," as well as a bible and a drum. The impressive list of kitchen equipment was valued at more than £7, which was second in value only to the contents of the room which contained the clock and the books (valued at £9.10s.) and bespoke a family which took great pains as well as pleasure with their "diet."

Although more modest in scale, other midwives' homes were obviously furnished with care and well stocked with the "necessaries" such as bed linens and tablecloths, in addition to little luxuries such as looking glasses, comb boxes, pictures, and tapestries.[173] Gentleman Robert Peppet of St Martin in the Fields willed treasured linens and pewter which his deceased spouse, a midwife, had brought to her marriage "marked with her father and mother's name" to his granddaughter (and wife's namesake) Pricilla Peppet.[174] Silver spoons, cups, and "[silver] Plate" were heirlooms not infrequently mentioned in midwives' wills. In some cases, midwives' children had been given silver as christening gifts: The four children of Isobel Glover received a total of fifteen silver spoons at their christenings.[175] Midwife Mary Wood, St Martin in the Fields, left two silver spoons and her silver mug to one niece and two silver spoons (plus £8 and a "second best hood and scarf") to another niece.[176] A silver cup and several silver spoons were carefully distributed among friends and relatives by midwife Margaret Beighton of Covent Gardens in her will of 1693.[177] Elizabeth Forrest placed a high value on a family silver tankard and silver cup and left them in the hands of a friend until her two youngest daughters were twenty-one, at which time they would become part of the young women's inheritance.

Two midwives took such pleasure in the furnishings of their bedrooms, they left the entire contents to relatives. Anne Baldwin mentions in particular her "green bedd with beddstead, featherbedd, curtains, vallences, chairs, stools and all

171 GL MS 10,116/14.   172 GL MS 9174/43.
173 GLRO AM/PI/1696/7, inventory of James Flower, St Martin in the Fields; inventory of John Monger, St Clement Danes GLRO AM/PI(1) 1680/21.
174 GLRO AM/PW/1714/30   175 GL MS 9052/11.   176 GLRO AM/PW 1713/124.
177 GLRO AM/PW/1693/3.

the furniture belonging to the Roome," which is to be her daughter's at marriage or age twenty-one.[178] Ann Rampton wanted her daughter Ursely to have her chest of drawers, bed, and bedding "and the furniture that is in my roome yt I now lye in."[179] Midwife Susanna Skelton was particularly proud of her well-equipped house, leaving all of the kitchen furniture and "utensils in the wash house and the garden" to her sister.[180]

While not all midwives lived as well as the women who have left such rich evidence of their material lives, still it is clear that the midwives who were the subjects of the more intensively focused investigation, whether typical or not, enjoyed many of the amenities and small luxuries associated with a comfortable standard of living.[181] They were women who could feel at ease with the trappings of affluent clients who lived in the grandest of dwellings and yet bring to the humblest settings their abilities to create an orderly and appropriate space for the important events to which their work was central.

Broadly speaking, London midwives were usually of a mature age at licensing and, in most cases, had borne children themselves. They were married to, or were the widows of men who were employed in a wide range of occupations and generally enjoyed some standing in their communities, including that of "gentleman."[182] Midwives charged their clients according to a flexible scale of their own devising and successful midwives could make a substantial contribution to the family income.

To establish with more clarity the full range of the socioeconomic positions of London midwives, the midwives of twelve sample parishes were investigated in as much depth as the records permitted. The next chapter will present a brief description of these 76 midwives in their own parish settings.

---

178 GLRO AM/PW 1692/2. 179 GLRO AM/PW 1678/50.
180 GLRO AM/PW 1735/34.
181 Harley, "Provincial midwives," 31–2 for the social and economic status of a number of Lancashire and Cheshire midwives.
182 Giardina Hess, "Midwifery practice," 68, gives the spousal occupations of a small group of Quaker midwives. It would appear that London midwives as a whole were married to men of higher social status than the Quaker midwives.

5

Midwives of Twelve London Parishes:
A Socioeconomic Case Study

In this chapter are details recovered about the circumstances of seventy-six seventeenth-century London midwives from twelve London parishes.[1] The classification of parishes as "wealthy," "mixed" or "poor" is intended to ensure the most representative sampling of midwives possible. It is not a definitive characterization of the parishes.

ALLHALLOWS THE LESS

The parish of Allhallows the Less contained between sixty and one hundred tithable residences on the eve of the English Revolution.[2] Although it was a poor parish, it was not completely devoid of inhabitants of wealth and influence since its northern end extended into areas where trade and commerce flourished.[3] By 1695, the parish had 455 inhabitants living in seventy-five homes and one-third of the households in the parish were designated "substantial."[4] The following are the midwives which we have identified as resident in the parish in the seventeenth century. In all cases, we can establish the year they were licensed (or appeared on visitation records) and the names of their spouses.

Alice Palmer: Licensed in Stepney in 1612 and All Hallows the Less in 1619. Husband Edward may have been a physician who died c 1631; Palmer parish

---

1 For a list of London parishes, see Appendix F. We have attempted to place these women in the socioeconomic context of their own parishes. See Tai Liu, *Puritan London*; Ronald Herlan, "Social Articulation and the Configuration of Parochial Poverty in London on the Eve of the Restoration," *Guildhall Studies in London History* 11 (1976): 43–53; Emrys Jones, "London in the Early Seventeenth Century: An Ecological Approach," *London Journal* 6 (Winter 1980): 126; M. J. Power, 221.
2 Tai Liu, 31.   3 Tai Liu, 31.
4 P. E. Jones and A. V. Judges, "London Population in the Late Seventeenth Century," *Economic History Review* 6 (1935–6): 58. The term "substantial householders" is defined as heads of households with a personal estate worth not less than £600 or real estate worth not less than £50 per year (as well it includes the titled, certain members of the hierarchy of the Church, doctors of divinity, law and medicine, a gentleman, and a few other special categories). In other words, it encompasses "very much the upper part of society in respect of income and status." See D. V. Glass's introduction to his edition of *London Inhabitants Within the Walls* (London: London Record Society, 1966): xx.

assessment in 1621–23 was one of the highest, by 1631–32, average. John Palmer was possibly a son.[5]

Isobel Halsey: Licensed in 1632; attended the parish visitation of 1637.[6] Husband Clement was previously married to Elizabeth Pyam (1626); assessment for clerks' wages slightly higher than average for 1632–42.[7] High tithe rental in 1638 for Cold Harbour property – within the upper quartile of moderated rents.[8] Clement died c 1642. Stepsons were brewer Clement Halsey and John Halsey, citizen and brewer; granddaughter, the child of Thomas and Anne Moody, inherited Isobel's estate upon her death in 1666.[9] Matthew and the wealthy John Halsey were brothers-in-law of the midwife.[10] Grandson Clement, brewer of St Peter Paul's Wharf, died in 1700.[11]

Mrs. Could: Parish visitation.[12] Husband Humfrey paid an assessment for clerks' wages 1632–42 well above average.[13] Son or grandson William (1681).[14]

Judith Newman: Licensed in 1661; had resided in the parish (6th precinct of Cripplegate ward) more than thirty years at the time of licensing.[15] Husband William's assessment for the subsidy of 1621–23 (on the value of real estate) was above average; assessments for other parish rates 1631–42, average, but showed periodic nonpayment.[16] In 1658, Newman made a generous contribution for "the

5 GLRO DL/C 340/44; DLC/ 341 (fol.no. illeg.); PRO E 179/147/491; GL MS 823/1 unfol. Approximately 100 parish inhabitants paid the same assessment as Palmer; forty-nine paid a higher assessment and one person paid less. Because of the imprecise nature of the sources which follow in this section, and the fact that some assessments were made on the basis of ward, instead of parish divisions, the term "average" will be used occasionally with the understanding that it implies that a particular assessment was shared by at least fifty percent of the persons named on the assessment roll. CLRO tithe rate assessments 1671, Assess. Box 45.17 and 1675, Box 45.11.
6 GLRO DL/C 343/139v; GL MS 9537/15/65.
7 Parish Registers of St Andrew Holborn and St Anne Blackfriars 1560–1837, 1558–1837. Toronto Public Library microfilm no. 96468; GL MS 8231/1.
8 LPL MS 272/37. In 1638, records were made of the tithe rents in ninety-seven London parishes. The figures given were "moderated" rents or three quarters of the actual rent values. Halsey was paying £26 rent annually. T. C. Dale has compiled the information contained in these records at Lambeth Palace Library in MS 272 under the title *The Inhabitants of London in 1638* (London: Society of Genealogists, 1931). I have personally checked these manuscripts, but since I have also made use of Dale, I will cite his work where appropriate. Halsey's name is found on page 15 of Dale. In Halsey's parish, 77 recorded rents were lower, twenty were higher, and one was the same as Halsey's, placing him in the upper quartile of rents.
9 PRO prob.11/312/163; 322/114.
10 M. Fitch, *Index to Testamentary Records in Archdeaconry Courts of London* 2 (London: British Record Society, 1985), 169. Matthew was also a resident of Allhallows; W. J. Harvey, ed. *List of the Principal Inhabitants of the City of London 1640* (Isle of Wight: Pinhorns, 1886), 9. John Halsey is shown under the parish of St Gregory by St Paul.
11 GL MS 9172/90. The prosperous brewer also owned property in St Katherine Coleman.
12 GL MS 9537/15/65. 13 GL MS 823/1. 14 CLRO Box 45.17.
15 GL MS 10,116/1. Newman is also found in the visitation record for 1664: GL MS 9537/17/77v.
16 PRO E 179 147/491 1621–23; GL MS 823/1. Parochial comparisons which would be more precise are not possible in the case of the subsidy of 1623–25 which was done on the basis of wards.

beautifying and amending of the parish church."[17] The Newman family home in Allhallows the Less was probably destroyed by fire in 1666; by 1670, it was replaced by a substantial home with six hearths.[18] William Newman, who wore the livery of the company of coopers, may have been the midwife's husband.[19]

In summary, the four midwives of Allhallows the Less were at least at the parish median or above in their socioeconomic circumstances.

ST ANDREW WARDROBE

By the fourth decade of the century, the parish of St Andrew Wardrobe was a "decaying" parish containing 100–200 homes. Trade and commerce were negligible in a parish where the inhabitants were for the most part "carmen, watermen and other handicraftsmen" and its civic leaders during the revolutionary years were undistinguished. Moreover, two breweries which had previously contributed to the support of large numbers of parish poor had declined.[20] By 1695, slightly more than 500 inhabitants were living in 106 residences in the parish and 6.6% of the parish households were described as "substantial." It would appear that the decline, which was evident at mid-century, may have been halted but not reversed.[21]

Anne Coxe: Wife of Henry, licensed in 1613.[22] She attended the 1636 visitation.[23] Widowed by 1638, her assessment for a moderated rent of £6 was in the upper half of parish rents in 1638.[24] She died in 1644, and her son Charles was granted the administration of her estate.[25] Henry Coxe, a tax collector, was likely a son.[26]

Ellinor Spinner (Widow): Licensed in 1615.[27] She may have remarried.[28]

---

17 GL MS 823/2/74.

18 CLRO Box 25.9/22. According to Power, this would be a medium-sized house.

19 "Members of the City Companies in 1641," Society of Genealogists, typescript, (1935), 121. Three Newman children were buried in the years 1660–3, but it is likely that they were grandchildren rather than children of the midwife. GL MS 823/2/110, 138, 149.

20 Tai Liu, 41.   21 Jones and Judges, 59.

22 CLRO DL/C 340/117v. A Henry Coxe, who was in receipt of a small pension between the years of 1615 and 1621, was probably the midwife's father-in-law since the payment of 1s.4d. was the minimum amount for single pensioners. GL MS 2089/1 unfol.

23 GL MS 9537/14/36.

24 LPL MS 272/58v. Also shown were John Cox (fol. 58) and Mr. Cox (fol. 59), who may have been sons. John Patten has suggested that, in 1664, rent of less than £1 per annum was one of the criteria for being a member of the "exempt poor" who were excused from paying the Hearth tax. See John Patten, "The Hearth Taxes, 1662–1689," *Local Population Studies*, 7 (1971): 18.

25 GL MSS 2089/1 unfol.; 9050/7/172.

26 PRO E179 252/15, records of Bread St., Cripplegate, and Dowgate wards for 1645.

27 GLRO DL/C 340/175v.

28 Barbara Todd has commented on the difficulty of tracing English widows in the early modern period. See Barbara Todd, "The Remarrying Widow," Mary Prior, ed., *Women in English Society*, 57.

Katherine Horner: Wife of Joshua, was licensed in 1619.[29] She was still an active midwife in 1631.[30]

Juliana Cook (John?): Attended visitations in 1636 and 1637. Possibly five children were born between 1599–1612. The oldest son, Matthew, was listed among the leading inhabitants of his ward, Castle Baynard in 1640.[31] In 1638, Mrs. Cook had an extremely high assessment for yearly tithes; her annual rental was seventh highest of 248 rents in the parish.[32]

Winnifred Allen: Married to John, a tailor. She was licensed in 1662 after more than ten years' experience in midwifery.[33] Three children were born between 1642–45. The Allens' assessment for tithes and rents in 1638 was in the middle third of rents for the parish.[34] Widow Allen's parish poor rate assessment was above average in 1681.[35]

Anne Goodwin (Godwin): Licensed in 1663, she attended visitation in 1664. Thirteen women endorsed her testimonial.[36] Her clientele were economically and geographically diversified. Edward Goodwin may have been a son. Goodwin's poor rate assessment for 1681 was above average.[37]

Mary Hodgkinson (als. Osgood of St Giles Cripplegate): Her second husband was Thomas Hodgkinson, a printer. Midwife Hodgkinson was licensed at a visitation of 1669 after being excommunicated in 1667 for failing to show proof of licensing. In 1669, she was living on Purpool Lane, in the parish of St Andrew Holborn; her deputy, midwife Katherine Howell of St Bridgid, applied for a license in 1678.[38]

Margaret Hopkins: Attended the visitation of 1680.[39] Licensed as Margaret Hopkins of Edmonton in 1670, she moved to the City between 1670–80.[40]

Two midwives of St Andrew Wardrobe left indications of family incomes which were in the upper half of parish incomes, while a third midwife paid a tithe on rents which suggested that she was one of the parish's affluent residents. Of the remaining five midwives, one was married to a tradesman whose trade could provide a living of moderate comfort, three were licensed, demonstrating

29 GLRO DL/C 341 (fol. no. illeg.)   30 GL MS 2089/1 unfol.   31 *Principal Inhabitants*, 6.
32 LPL MS 272/ 56v. A Mr. Cook appears on the same assessment roll for St Andrew Wardrobe with an assessment of £1.6.8. and a moderated rent of £14, which was also well above average. He was probably the midwife's son, Matthew.
33 GL 10, 116/2; GLRO DL/C 344/178v.   34 LPL MS 272/56.   35 GL MS 9801 box 1.
36 GL MSS 10,116/3; 9537/62.   37 GL MS 9801 box 1.
38 GL MSS 10, 116/10; 25, 533/1/16v, 91v.   39 GL MS 9537/22 unfol.
40 GL MS 10, 116/7.

at least a measure of economic viability, and one midwife, identified at a visitation, left no other traces.

ST ANNE BLACKFRIARS

St Anne Blackfriars was in a depressed condition by the middle of the century. As one study has revealed, a levelling process occurred throughout the century which resulted in decreased numbers of gentry and titled inhabitants and increased numbers of "lodgers, foundlings, itinerants and foreigners," in addition to a large number of poor.[41] Toward the end of the century, the number of tithable houses in the parish had increased from 200 to 373, but poverty in the parish was still rife with only 1.1% of the households in the parish considered "substantial."[42] The figure of 1.1% was the lowest for eighty intramural parishes in the study by Jones and Judges.[43]

Anne Adams: Attended the visitations of 1636 and 1637.[44] Her husband, Thomas, and son, Charles, were both gunsmiths. She had a married daughter, Elizabeth Conley. Anne was the executrix of her husband's will, probated in 1638. Among the items comprising his estate: household goods (pewter, linen), property leases, gunsmith's tools and equipment (left to his son). Daughter Elizabeth was to receive 50s. for a mourning ring and further provision at her mother's discretion.[45]

Elizabeth Cooper (Richard?): Attended the visitation for her parish in 1636.[46] By 1637 she had moved, died, or remarried. A male infant born to a Cooper family in 1624 may have been a son.[47]

Elizabeth Gasker: Attended visitation in 1636 and 1637 (described as "deputy").[48] The wife of barber William Gasker, she was widowed in 1651. Executrix for her husband's will, she inherited half of his estate. Their only son William's half was earmarked for his education and apprenticeship as a distiller.[49] At his death in 1673, this son, citizen, and distiller, owned property in St Anne Blackfriars containing two tenements which provided support for his widow Mary.[50]

Sara Tanfield (alias Parks): Attended the visitations of 1636 and 1637.[51] Married to Solomon Tanfield, she was widowed in 1633. It may have been a second marriage

---

41 Tai Liu, 41.   42 Tai Liu, 213.   43 Jones and Judges, 59.
44 GL MSS 9537/14/36v; 9537/15/57.
45 GL MSS 9537/14/36v; 9537/15/57. 9171/27/424v.
46 GL MSS 9537/14/36v; 9537/15/57.
47 The registers of St Anne Blackfriars, October 24, 1624, Toronto Public Library, microfilm no. 96468.
48 GL MSS 9537/14/36v; 9537/15/57.   49 PRO prob. 11/217/102, January 31, 1651.
50 PRO prob. 11/344/19, January 22, 1673.   51 GL MSS 9537/14/36v; 9537/15/57.

for both Sara and Solomon. Their daughter was married to Thomas Cooper. Sara was the administrator and chief beneficiary of Solomon's estate.[52]

Anne Alkin: Licensed in 1670.[53] Her husband, Francis, citizen and merchant tailor, owned property in a number of parishes.[54] Anne was deputy to Mrs. Bissick of St Clement Danes and also had an association with midwife Francis Austin. When Francis Alkin died in 1686, his estate was administered by his wife Anne.[55] Two years later, Anne Alkin was living in St Gregory by St Paul and was assessed as a landlord for a poll tax in the middle range.[56] Anne Alkin was still an active midwife in 1692, when she delivered an unmarried woman at parish expense.[57] By 1695, widow Alkin was living in the parish of St Andrew Wardrobe in the same house as her widowed daughter, Elizabeth Brown.[58]

Elizabeth Carpin (widow of Francis): Licensed in 1680. She lived in a commodious house with nine hearths.[59] Mrs. Carpin had borne at least one child, a daughter, Elizabeth.[60] She was an associate of fellow parishioner and licensed midwife Anne Alkin (licensed in 1670), probably in the capacity of deputy midwife.[61]

Anne Fowler (wife of Elias): Licensed in 1689. She was the deputy of midwife Mary Challoner of Stepney.[62] The Fowlers lived in Ireland Yard.[63] On the marriage assessment roll of 1695, Elias and Anne Fowler were assessed at the customary rate for couples of child-bearing age.[64]

Mary White: Licensed in 1689. A gentlewoman and wife of William.[65] Mary White had a working relationship with two senior midwives: Margaret Griffin, licensed in 1677, and Sara Slycer, licensed in 1684.[66] Mistress White drew her clientele, at least in part, from the gentry, some as far away as Surrey. The Whites'

52 GL MS 9168/18/195. Tanfield appointed two overseers to help his wife administer his estate, described merely as "goods, chattels, debts, plate, monies and estate."
53 GL MS 10,116/7. Alkin was licensed in St Anne Blackfriars, but there were also links with St Gregory by St Paul and St Andrew Wardrobe.
54 GL MS 9801/2.
55 GL MS 25,625/4/93, 109v. These documents give the Alkins' parish as St Gregory by St Paul's.
56 CLRO Assess. box 33.17, unfol.
57 GL MS 1337/1. She was paid sixteen shillings, a fair fee for the period. The parish had probably been unwilling to pay for the infant's delivery (which was usually only the first stage of assuming responsibility for the child's long-term support) and the Lord Mayor had intervened.
58 CLRO Marriage Act, 1695 15.7.
59 CLRO Assess. Box 25.9/27/35. According to Power, this would be classified as a large house.
60 The registers of St Anne Blackfriars July 18, 1631, Toronto Public Library, microfilm no. 96468.
61 GL MS 10,116/11.   62 GL MS 10,116/12.   63 GL MS 7770.
64 CLRO Assess. 17.92 (Fryer St.). For a full discussion of these sources, see D. V. Glass, ed., "Introduction," *London Inhabitants*, ix–xxxviii.
65 GL MSS 10,116/12, 9532/1/89.   66 GL MS 10,116/10, 11.

parish rate and tithe assessments for 1674 and 1681 were slightly above average.[67] In 1692, William White, his wife, and child were living in the home of widow Imens on Water St.[68] In 1694, the Whites were landlords in a house on Water Street with a servant and a lodger, Deborah Smith.[69] In 1695, their household consisted of both parents, son Edmund, and their servant Elizabeth Salisbury, as well as three lodgers (a widow and a married couple).[70] William White owned the George Inn in West Smithfield. At William's death in 1700, Mary and son Edmund were the beneficiaries of his estate: half of the house, all of their household goods, furnishings, silver, jewels, and rings were to be hers. Their son was to have half the house in Blackfriars and the inn in Smithfield, as well as debts and money owing to the estate, at age 21.[71]

As the wives of variously a gunsmith, barber, merchant tailor, and gentleman (not to mention the wealthy widow Carpin), more than half of the midwives from this extremely depressed and economically deprived parish were drawn from the small segment of economically privileged inhabitants of the parish. Although some of the midwives were undistinguished, or at least left few traces in the documentation, none were in receipt of parish charity.

ST BARTHOLOMEW BY THE EXCHANGE

The small (60–100 houses) parish of St Bartholomew by the Exchange was situated slightly to the north and east of the City's centre. An observer from the sixteenth century took pains to mention the beautiful homes lining St Bartholomew Lane.[72] In the seventeenth century the parish was a beehive of market activity inhabited, for the most part, by wealthy tradesmen who played leading political and religious roles, particularly in the revolutionary years. But it also contained a significant number of parish poor, which have been estimated at one in every thirty-five inhabitants for the seventeenth century.[73] The parish made substantial contributions to other less affluent parishes in the years 1639–66.[74] By 1695, it was home to some 800 inhabitants living in 114 houses. One-third of its households were considered wealthy.[75]

Elizabeth Lewis: Wife of the parish clerk and sexton, Charles Lewis. Licensed in 1667, midwife Lewis attended the visitation of 1680.[76] In the 1650s, the Lewises paid a low poor rate and their scavenger rate for 1658 was in the lowest quartile

67 GL MSS 9532/1; 9801 Box 1 (tithe assessment).   68 GL MS 7769 unfol.
69 Ibid., (1694).   70 CLRO Marriage Tax 1695, 17.17.   71 PRO prob. 11/456/108.
72 John Stowe, *Survey of London*, C. L. Kingsford, ed., (London: J. M. Dent, 1960 reprint of 1908 edition), 162.
73 Tai Liu, 29. Ronald W. Herlan, "Poor Relief in London During the English Revolution," *Journal of British Studies* 18 (1979): 41 n.27.
74 Herlan, "Poor Relief," 38.   75 Jones and Judges, 59.   76 GL MS 9537/22 unfol.

for the parish.[77] By 1670, Charles Lewis' scavenger rate had soared, indicating an increase in the family fortunes.[78] Aside from Elizabeth's contribution to the family income, by 1662 Lewis was in receipt of wages for his work as clerk and sexton and also of the various additional "perks" which accompanied the position of parish clerk.[79] Lewis was paid at least £20 per annum for his parish work, but, in addition, he shared the donations of cash and bread, cheese, and coal which were given periodically to the parish poor.[80] The principal family residence was in Throgmorton Street; Lewis also paid taxes in 1671 on property containing a shop in Jeley Alley whose assessment was in the upper quartile of assessments.[81] The busy midwife enjoyed the services of a maid servant who helped to take care of several parish infants until they could be put out to nurse.[82] The clients of Elizabeth Lewis were drawn from a group which were above average in literacy. This is not surprising given her husband's, and possibly her, educational attainments.[83] By 1681, midwife Lewis was widowed.[84] In 1689–90, Elizabeth Lewis paid one of the parish's highest assessments for a pew at £3.0.8.[85]

Elizabeth Lewis was the only licensed midwife that left any records relating to this parish in the seventeenth century.

ST ETHELBURGA

The parish of St Ethelburga contained 100 to 200 tithable houses on the eve of the revolution. It was a poor parish in the seventeenth century.[86] Innholders and minor tradesmen made up the parish's leaders in the revolutionary era. In 1659–60, St Ethelburga was one of five parishes (out of 97) that failed to contribute to a special fund for poor relief, presumably because of its own poverty.[87] By 1695,

77 The rate of 4s.4d. paid by Lewis seems to have been the lowest basic rate: of 79 names, 53 were assessed at a higher rate, and 25 at the same rate. One person was assessed a few pence less than 4s.4d., but that may have been an error. Edwin Freshfield, ed., *The Vestry Minute Books of St Bartholomew Exchange in the City of London 1567–1676* (London: Rixon and Arnold, 1980), 49, 65.

78 Ibid., 110. The rate had increased from 1s.4d. to 7s.

79 For an antiquarian and somewhat romanticized study of the parish clerk, based, for the most part, on literary sources, see Peter H. Ditchfield, *The Parish Clerk* (New York: E. P. Dutton & Co., 1907).

80 Freshfield, 96, 102 (a petition for arrears in payment for his work as a sexton, totalling more than three pounds in 1665), 107, 115, 127. Cash from a bequest for parish poor netted Lewis two pounds in 1670. Freshfield, 112.

81 Freshfield, 117. Of 37 assessments, 25 were lower, 8 were higher, and 4 were the same. For Lewis's attempt to get permission to build another shop adjacent to the parish church, see Freshfield, 119.

82 GL MS 4383/1/601. The fact that Mrs. Lewis employed a maid is an indication of her social rank; but she also charged the parish for the maid's work, such as tending the infants or mending clothing for poor parishioners.

83 Four women out of seven signed their own names. According to David Cressy, in the 1670s, only 22% of women in London were able to sign their names. Cressy, *Literacy*, 147. Charles Lewis not only wrote in an extremely fine hand, he seems to have had a knowledge of Latin.

84 GL MS 4383/1/3 (under 1681). Widow Lewis received four cauldrons of coal periodically, while the widow of Mr. Jenkins, the previous parish clerk, continued to receive bread and cheese for an extended period of time. Freshfield, 96, 98.

85 GL MS 4383/1.   86 Stowe, 154; Tai Liu, 38.   87 Herlan, "Social Articulation," 47.

the parish had 133 inhabited houses and a population of 645; one-fifth of the households were headed by prosperous individuals.[88] Parish registers for only the last thirty to thirty-nine years of the century have survived, but eight parish midwives have left traces in wills, tax records, and a variety of ecclesiastical records.

Elizabeth Whipp (Robert): Licensed in 1622.[89] See Chapter 4 for the details of Whipp's career.

Sara Sydey (Waldegrave, citizen and merchant tailor): Licensed in 1663. See Chapter 4.

Elizabeth? Benskin: "Mrs. Benskin" attended the visitation of 1669, but, in all likelihood she had been a midwife since the 1630s.[90] In 1634, she had successfully fought mandatory licensing by the Church.[91] Richard Benskin gave £1 for a voluntary tithe in 1635, an amount which placed him in the upper third of donors.[92] By 1638, the Benskins' moderated rent was above the parish average.[93] Richard Benskin, a resident of Peachen Alley, was assessed in 1666 as a landlord and inhabitant for a sum which was average or slightly below the parish median.[94] Mrs. Benskin, widowed by 1672, was living in a small home.[95] Elizabeth Benskin died in 1673.

Mrs. Hensman (wife of William): Attended the visitation of 1669. Hensman's 1672 assessment on land and movable goods was well above average (see midwives, Clarke, Grant, and Ward, below, for comparison). The Hensman house was of medium size (with six hearths) in Clark's Alley.[96]

Elizabeth Clarke: Licensed in 1673. The wife of haberdasher William Clarke.[97] In 1672, the Clarke family was living in a home of medium size in Clarke's Alley.[98] William Clarke contributed regularly to the poor rate between the years 1679–92.[99] Midwife Elizabeth Clarke died in 1705 and her husband in

88 Jones and Judges, 59.   89 GLRO DL/C 341/267.   90 GL MS 9537/18/65v.
91 See Chapter 1, 47–8.
92 GL MS 4241/1. Of 38 donors, 14 gave a greater amount than Benskin.
93 Of 110 rents, 39 were higher, 4 the same. See chapter 4 for comparison with Whipp and Sydey.
94 CLRO Assess. Box 66.3.
95 The home had four hearths, which would still indicate comfortable accommodations. CLRO MS 25.9/34 1672?. There is some uncertainty about the date of this tax, but the sources at the CLRO state that it was, in all likelihood, levied in 1672.
96 CLRO 25.9/34 1672?   97 GL MS 10,116/8; GLRO DL/C 345/104.
98 It was a home with six hearths: CLRO MS. 25.9/34.
99 His usual contribution was four shillings, four pence per annum. GL MS 4241/2 fols. 42–70, passim. The parish records are fairly consistent in their treatment of William Clarke, but widows Grant and Ward, two parish midwives, paid varying amounts. Widow Ward paid a shilling more than Clarke for two years, and the same amount as Clarke for two years. Widow Grant paid twice as much as Clarke in 1687, the same as Clarke for two years, and no assessment for two years. The civic records, however, appear to confuse William and John Clarke, and one assessment shows a

1710.[100] Unmarried merchant William Clarke, who died in 1672, was probably a nephew, son of John Clarke. He left a bequest of £20 sterling to his sister Sara Sydey, widow of Waldegrave Sydey junior, and to his nephews Waldegrave and John, £10 each (see Chapter 4 for Sara Sydey).[101]

Margaret Ward (wife of Richard Ward): Licensed in 1676, and attended the visitation of 1680.[102] In 1672, the Wards were living in a small house on Helmut Court with three hearths.[103] In 1673, Ward was assessed as a landlord with stocks or investments.[104] Richard Ward died intestate in 1677 and his estate was administered by his wife.[105] By 1678, Margaret Ward and two children had moved from Helmut Court. Church receipts for 1679–80 show contributions which were at the median for the parish.[106] In 1690, Mistress Ward was living alone and contributing regularly to poor relief, indicating her ongoing economic viability.[107] She may have died, remarried, or moved to live with her married daughter, Martha Humphreys, after 1698.[108] Richard Ward, sawyer, was probably the midwife's son.[109]

Francis Grant (widow of John, gentleman): Appeared at the visitation of 1680. Widowed in 1676, she was executrix and sole heir of her husband's estate. Grant was the owner of the King's Head in Fetter Lane, which he had rented by lease.[110] In 1640, his name had appeared on the list of the most prominent or "principal inhabitants" of London.[111] Widow Grant, with no surviving children, was living in her home on Clarke's Alley with a kinswoman, Margaret Head in 1677.[112] Mrs. Grant's contributions to church receipts in 1680 and poor receipts in 1686–88 indicated her substantial personal wealth.[113] In her declining years, contributions to the poor rate were lower (after 1688) and no contributions were made in the three or four years preceding her death in 1694.[114] In 1690, Widow Grant was

William Clarke on Clarke's Alley and one on Helmet Court. The important point is that all of the William Clarkes were self-sufficient individuals who were not on parish welfare, and in some cases were actually wealthy. See CLRO asses. box 20 MS 6 and box 11 MS 4.

100 *The Registers of the Church of St Ethelburga*: burials for 1705 and 1710 (unfol.).
101 PRO prob. 11/340/133: will of William Clarke, merchant, of St Ethelburga, probated June 6, 1672.
102 GL MS 10,116/9; GLRO DL/C 345/161; GL MS 9537/22 unfol.
103 The house had three hearths. CLRO 25.9/34.   104 CLRO Assess. Box 20 MS.6.
105 Marc Fitch, ed., *Index to Testamentary Records in the Archdeaconry Court of London*, Vol. 2 (London: British Record Society, 1985): 146.
106 GL MS 4241/1/569. Of 105 contributors, 39 paid less, 20 the same, and 46 paid higher amounts.
107 GL MS 4241/2/40, 49, 56, 81, 140, poor rates for 1693–94; 4241/2 no pagination for 1696–97.
108 Martha Ward married Robert Humphreys in 1684. *The Registers of the Church of St Ethelburga* (unfol.).
109 CLRO assess. box 7.8 fol.11: Poll tax 1690.
110 PRO prob. 11/350/38: will of John Graunt, gent., St Ethelburga.
111 *Principal Inhabitants*, p. 10, shows Grant in the parish of St Mary Magdalen in 1640.
112 CLRO assess. box 11 MS.4: Poll tax 1677/8.   113 GL MSS 4241/1/571; 4241/2/21,42.
114 GL MS 4241/12/51, 57, 67, 81.

living with her maidservant, Hanna Layfield, a subsequent beneficiary.[115] She left instructions for an elaborate funeral and arranged for a generous bequest to the parish poor.[116] Francis Grant left the bulk of her estate, after numerous individual bequests to relatives and friends, to niece Elizabeth Feezy.[117] Her extensive wardrobe was to be divided among relatives and her personal maid.[118] A small bequest of £5 was left to Barbara Roberts, who was licensed as a midwife in 1684, and had possibly been Grant's former deputy.[119]

Of the six midwives of St Ethelburga, three were at the economic median for their parish or above. Three, possibly four others, were well above the median. Of the latter, three left wills, which indicated substantial wealth and social prominence.

ST GREGORY BY ST PAUL'S

The large and prosperous parish of St Gregory by St Paul's contained more than 200 tithable houses.[120] At mid-century, rich tradesmen formed a sizeable segment of its inhabitants. In particular, well-to-do merchant tailors congregated in the parish; parish inhabitants played an influential role in guild and civic life.[121] In 1658, St Gregory by St Paul's gave the highest amount of 102 parishes to a special collection for the poor.[122] Toward the end of the century, the parish boasted 275 inhabited houses and almost one-third of its households were designated substantial.[123]

Mary Hughes (wife of Richard): Licensed in 1615. In 1638, widow Hughes was living in a modest home on Knightrider Street, but there is no record of her attendance at the visitations of 1636–37.[124]

Deborah Glover (alias Strackly and formerly of St Lawrence Jewry): Widow, was licensed in 1672. She was an associate of two licensed midwives, Elizabeth Sumner

---

115 CLRO assess.box 20, MS. 12: Poll tax 1690.
116 The original will of Francis Grant was probated April 6, 1695: GL MS 9152/31. Grant specified that £30 was to be spent on her funeral; see GL MS 4241/106 for details of how some of that money was spent.
117 Francis Grant left more than sixty individual legacies, which totalled over £400, in addition to bonds, rents from leases, and other assets. Grant calls Feezy her "cousin" at one point, but it appears from her initial remarks that she was her niece, the daughter of the midwife's deceased brother John Sanders.
118 Mrs. Grant left several bonds, which she held to Ferrand, as well as a lump sum of £50.
119 GL MS 10,116/12. Roberts lived in St Mary Whitechapel, which was close to St Ethelburga.
120 Tai Liu, 40.   121 Ibid., 40.
122 The parish gave almost £40; see Herlan, "Social Articulation," 45.
123 Jones and Judges, 59.
124 Although Hughes was paying the substantial sum of £12, in this wealthy parish the house would not be lavish. Dale, *The Inhabitants of London*, p. 67. The rents were shown for 205 inhabitants of the parish: 136 paid a higher rent, 55 paid a lower rent, and 14 paid the same rent of £12 annually.

and Elizabeth Davis, and was probably Davis's deputy.[125] She had two sons, Joseph and John; the latter had predeceased the midwife.[126] Joseph was her executor and her grandson, Robert, the son of John, was the recipient of a legacy of £30, which Glover herself had received from her brother Thomas Strackly. Deborah died in 1682 and her will was signed with her own signature, an indication of her literacy.[127]

Jane Winckles: Licensed May 30, 1679 by the jurisdiction of the dean and chapter of St Paul's.[128] Her husband, Jonathan, was a paver by trade. She claimed at least one client of prominence.[129] The Winckles paid a substantial assessment for church pews in 1686. Jonathan Winckles was well paid for paving the parish church between 1684–98, including £37 received in 1692 alone.[130] In 1694, he was named to the responsible position of churchwarden for his parish.[131] In 1695, the Winckles' household consisted of the parents, two daughters, a son, and a male servant; Winckles also functioned as an "assessor."[132]

In this prosperous parish, two of the three licensed midwives who have come to light were well above the socioeconomic median for their parish.

ST JOHN THE BAPTIST

With 100 to 200 tithable houses, the parish of St John the Baptist, while not a wealthy parish, could claim a number of inhabitants of the "better sort" as well as several civic leaders of note during the revolutionary years.[133] By the closing years of the century, only sixty-nine inhabited houses were tallied, with a population of 419.[134] Groups of craftsmen in wood and textiles, as well as members of semi-skilled building trades, tended to cluster in the parish in 1666.[135] Toward the end of the century, the parish was inhabited by an estimated 221 individuals per acre, and only one-fifth of its households were headed by persons of means.[136]

---

125 GL MS 10,116/2, 7.
126 GL MS 9172/71, original will. An inventory was taken of midwife Glover's possessions but, unfortunately, it has not survived. There is a good chance that Glover moved to live with her son sometime between 1662 and 1672.
127 This placed her in the estimated 36% of women who were literate, Cressy, *Literacy*, 147.
128 GL MS 25,598.
129 Marjorie Carpenter was the wife of brewer John Carpenter, common counsellor for Portsoken (1680) and Without Aldgate (1689). See J. R. Woodhead, *The Rulers of London 1660–1689* (London: London and Middlesex Archaeological Society, 1965), 43.
130 GL MS 1337/1/53v, and see also fols. 30, 43, 45v, 49, 51, 53v, 58v (the year he was churchwarden), 65v, and 68.
131 We note that, in 1664, the parish of St Bartholomew by the Exchange passed a motion that any man nominated to the position of churchwarden must possess personal assets of at least £300 as a security (Freshfield, 98).
132 CLRO Marriage assessment, 1695 35.27.   133 Tai Liu, 36.   134 Jones and Judges, 59.
135 Power, 216.
136 Jones and Judges, 59. Approximately two-thirds of the parishes in their study were less crowded than St John the Baptist in 1695.

Alice Annett: Wife of Nicholas, citizen and haberdasher, licensed in 1676.[137] She had served as the deputy of Anne Penn.[138] The Annetts had three sons, one of whom died as a child in 1673.[139] Tax assessments placed Annett in the comfortable middle income range by 1688, although fifteen years earlier his assessment for parson's maintenance had been low.[140] Midwife Annett periodically delivered poor women and was paid by the parish.[141] Nicholas Annett was the parish's senior churchwarden in 1687–88.[142] Alice Annett predeceased her husband, a man of considerable wealth, whose will was probated in 1707.[143] His property leases, personal goods, linens, and silver were divided between his only surviving son, Nicholas junior, if he returned from "beyond the seas," and his granddaughter, Susanna.[144] Annett senior, who was living at Miles End, old town, Stepney, at the time of his death, requested an elaborate funeral, to cost the equivalent of two years' rents from his various properties, including several tenements at Mile End Green. Alice Annett is the only midwife who has left evidence which places her in the parish of St John the Baptist.

ST KATHERINE COLEMAN

The eastern tip of the poor parish of St Katherine Coleman touched the eastern wall of the City north of Aldgate. Estimated to hold between 100 and 200 tithable houses in 1638, when it was one of the poorest parishes within the walls by its own claim, it was full of lodging houses and alleys, which were home to a population composed mainly of manual labourers and devoid of the prosperity associated with inhabitants engaged in retail trade. By 1695, there were 213 residences within its confines.[145] The parish did, in fact, receive financial assistance to its poor relief fund from the wealthier parish of St Olave Jewry at some point between 1631 and 1666.[146] By 1666, occupational clustering has been demonstrated for craftsmen in wood as well as for carriers.[147] Economic conditions in the

---

137 GL MS 10,116/9.
138 GL MS 25,533/2/6. Since there is no record of licensing for Anne Penn, there is a good possibility that she was a member of the prominent Quaker family by that name.
139 GL MS 5771 extraordinary receipts for 1673–74. See also the will of Nicholas Annett: GL MS 9171/54 probated March 1704.
140 CLRO assess. box 46.12; GL MSS 7619/11; 577/2/26.
141 GL MSS 7619/147; 577/2/46.
142 As a tribute to Annett's honesty or excessive efficiency, it was noted in the churchwarden's accounts for 1689–90, that more than £7 was donated to two charities "being too much collected in Mr. Annet's year." GL MS 577/2/76.
143 Power, 214.
144 Annett had been predeceased by another son, Richard; his son Nicholas was overseas, and his father's will stated that he must return to England if he wished to establish his claim to his father's estate.
145 Tai Liu, 38, Jones and Judges, 59, M. J. Power, 209.   146 Herlan, "Poor Relief," 38.
147 Power, 216.

parish may have improved toward the end of the century, since it was estimated that slightly more than one-fifth of the parish households were wealthy in 1695.[148]

Joan Nott: Married to John Nott, "doctor of medicine."[149] They resided on the south side of Pye Alley. Midwife Nott attended the visitation of 1637.[150] Doctor Nott regularly paid above-average parish assessments 1616–27. After his death in 1627, his wife continued to pay these assessments.[151] The couple had two daughters (Dorothy, unmarried, and Anne Blankett) and one son, Thomas, who were alive in 1627. Joan and Dorothy Nott were the executrices and major beneficiaries of Nott's estate, which included sizeable land holdings in Kent and Middlesex, as well as personal property.[152] Mrs. Nott, a woman of considerable wealth, continued to practise midwifery for at least ten years after her husband's death.[153]

Isobel Glover: Wife of Nathaniel, painter-stainer, lived in Northumberland Alley, moving to Northside in 1632. She was present at the visitation of 1637. The mounting fortunes of the Glover family can be traced in the parish records between 1616 and 1642.[154] Nathaniel was hired by the barber-surgeons, in 1632, to paint the company's coat of arms, as well as the master's and wardens' names on the "great Sunne Dyall."[155] By 1633, Glover paid more than £3 in fines to excuse himself from the office of parish constable.[156] In 1638, the Glovers' rent was in the upper third of rents for the parish.[157] Mr. Glover acted as the church beadle in 1624 and did various repair jobs for the church in 1637.[158] Nathaniel Glover was senior churchwarden of his parish in 1638–39.[159] There were three daughters: Isobel, Dorothy, and Ellen (all under twenty and unmarried at the time of their father's death), and one son, Richard, who became a prosperous goldsmith.[160] Nathaniel died in late 1642. Isobel and son Richard were the chief beneficiaries of his estate, which included occupied buildings on two acres of

---

148 Jones and Judges, 59. More than one-quarter of the eighty parishes in their study had a lower proportion of "substantial" households than St Katherine Coleman in 1695.

149 Although Nott's will describes him as a "doctor of medicine," we have not been able to find him among the graduates of Oxford or Cambridge. Other routes to the M.D. degree were possible, although relatively uncommon.

150 GL MS 9537/15/66v.

151 GL MS 1124/1/22, 31, 40, 56, 58, 64v, 77 (the clerk incorrectly listed the midwife as "Mr." instead of "Mrs." in 1632) but in 1634, she was listed as "midwife" Nott.

152 PRO prob. 11/153: will of John Nott, probated January 7, 1628.

153 Catharina Schrader, the Frisian midwife, also continued to practise midwifery as a well-to-do widow of her second husband. Marland, "*Mother and Child*," 7.

154 GL MS 1124/1/31, 41, 52, 56, 64v, 94v. The rents on Northumberland Alley indicate that the houses there were the most modest in the parish. Dale, 82.

155 Glover was described as a "dyall maker" and was paid £3. 8s. for his work. See Sidney Young, *The Annals of the Barber Surgeons of London* (London: East & Blades, 1890, reprint N.Y. A.M.S., 1978), 400.

156 GL MS 1124/1/101.   157 Dale, 81.   158 GL MS 1124/1/54v, 82.

159 GL MS 1125/1/30v.   160 PRO E179/252/32 no.2, hearth tax for 1666.

property on Broadstreet, Stepney.[161] The girls were to receive small legacies, and all four children were given the silver they had received as christening gifts. Nathaniel Glover, tailor, living in Playhouse Yard in 1692, was probably the midwife's grandson.

Margaret Jay (or Gay): Widow, lived in Brown's Court. She was licensed in 1661, with thirty years' residency in her parish, seven years as a practising midwife.[162] She was present at the visitation of 1664.[163] She made small, regular contributions to the parish poor rates between 1687 and 1690, and to ward taxes in 1688. She died c. 1691, probably after a period of declining health.[164]

Susan Chamberlain: The wife of Robert, clerk (or cleric), lived in Northumberland Alley. She was licensed as a midwife in 1662.[165] Widowed by 1670, she was living in a small home with four hearths.[166] Between 1687–94, Widow Chamberlain's name appeared on poor rate rolls with no assessment: daughter Katherine lived with her.[167] In 1695, they shared their home with four lodgers.[168] Widow Chamberlain and daughter were in receipt of parish relief periodically between 1694–1700, although they were not on the permanent poor relief registers.[169]

Anne Crouch: Attended the visitation of 1680.[170] Husband John Crouch paid a moderately high poor rate in 1678. He died intestate in 1684, and his estate was administered by his widow.[171] The midwife's children, Anne and John, had been the beneficiaries of their paternal grandmother's substantial estate (administered by their father in 1669).[172] While son John lived comfortably with his wife, child, and two servants, widow Crouch was forced in 1692, and also in 1694, to seek

161 GL MS 9052/11, original will of Nathaniel Glover, probated February 13, 1643.
162 GL MS 10,116/11; GLRO DL/C/344/145. It is unfortunate that Jay's documents do not contain any women's names, since the fact that she had practised for seven years suggests that she had been apprenticed to a senior midwife who remains unknown.
163 GL MS 9537/17/79v.
164 GL MS 1145/2 unfol. See also CLRO Assess. Box 6.13, 17 and 18 month assessments.
165 GL MS 10,116/2; GLRO DL/C 344/218v. The bishop's registers have recorded the surname as "Chambers." The Chamberlaine who earlier appeared on the tithe assessment rolls of 1638 may have been the midwife's father-in-law. He was paying a moderated rent of five pounds, which placed him roughly among the lowest third of rents for the parish.
166 CLRO 25.9/5, 36.
167 GL MS 1145/2 unfol. The inclusion of widow Chamberlain's name on the assessment lists, but with the amount unrecorded, suggests that, as the widow of a cleric, she was excused from the tax or, alternatively, she was on the borderline between the well-to-do contributors to the tax and the self-reliant noncontributors.
168 CLRO Marriage tax of 1695 42.11.
169 GL MS 1145/2 unfol. There was a massive increase (almost fourfold) in the number of parish relief recipients in 1694. While the midwife and her daughter were not on the permanent poor relief rolls, they were listed among those "needing frequent assistance."
170 GL MS 9537/22.   171 GL MS 9050/14/86.
172 GL 9052/17: original will of Mistress Crouch, mother of John Crouch, the midwife's husband, probated October 17, 1669.

parish relief along with many other economically disadvantaged of her parish.[173] She died c. 1694.

Mrs. Humton (widow?): Appeared at the visitation of 1680, but no other information has been recovered.[174] She may have remarried or died shortly after 1680.

Mary Bennett, who we believe was the widow of Rubin, a coachman, was licensed in 1690 and lived in Northumberland Alley.[175] Bennett contributed to the parish poor rate regularly between 1687–92, except in 1691.[176] By 1693, she had moved, remarried, or possibly died.

In the poor parish of St Katherine Coleman, the social standings and incomes of two midwives were well above that of their neighbours. Two midwives maintained at least average economic viability, and two were forced to seek parish relief toward the end of their lives. It seems likely that one, and perhaps both of the latter, were no longer practising their profession at that time in their life cycles. Their financial difficulties were also apparently a reflection of temporary, undue hardship in the parish as a whole in 1694. One midwife left no traces, except her name in a visitation record.

ST MARTIN OUTWICH

The small parish of St Martin Outwich had less than 100 tithable houses. In the sixteenth century, its poor had received relief from funds raised on lands owned by the mercers.[177] By the seventeenth century, the small number of tithable houses in the parish posed a problem for parish administration, but these difficulties were offset to a degree by the fact that, by 1638, the majority of its inhabitants were well-to-do tradesmen who lived in fine houses.[178] With sixty-eight inhabited houses and 444 inhabitants in 1695, almost 37% of its households were "substantial," indicating no fundamental change in parish characteristics over the last decades of the century.[179]

---

173 GL 1145/2; CLRO Assess. Box 33.2/61. There is the possibility that the "widow Crouch" who sought relief was not the midwife, but her sister-in-law. There is no way that we can establish her identity with certainty. If our identification is correct, then midwife Crouch clearly suffered financially in her later life by the fact that her husband's parent had chosen to skip a generation and bequeath her estate to the grandchildren. As a London widow, Crouch had the right to enjoy a minimum of one-third of her deceased husband's estate for the duration of her lifetime, but she had no claim upon the economic resources of adult children.
174 GL MS 9537/22 unfol. She was marked present.
175 GL MSS 10,116/13; 9532/1/74v; PRO E179/252/32 no.2.   176 GL MS 1145/2.
177 Stowe, 242.
178 Tai Liu, 36. Because of these two divergent factors, Tai Liu has categorized the parish as "mixed" in economic composition.
179 Jones and Judges, 60.

Mary Sherwood (Ralph, citizen and grocer): Licensed in 1676. For the details of Sherwood's life, see Chapter 4.[180]

Frances Sowden (Southen): Wife of William, was licensed in 1686.[181] She was an associate of midwives Ursula Chesmore and Anne White.[182] Frances married William Sowden, a widower with at least two small children, some time between 1683 and 1685, after his first wife died in childbed.[183] Midwife Sowden herself gave birth to a daughter in 1685. William Sowden's assessment for the scavenger rate, 1678–90 placed him in the upper third of parish scavenger rates.[184] The death of an eminent midwife "Southern" in a house fire at Lord Rochester's house in Richmond, Surrey, where she had gone to preside over the lying in of Lady Essex, Lord Rochester's daughter, was reported in 1721. It was, in all likelihood, Frances Sowden.[185]

In this small parish, both midwives were the wives of prosperous men; one of them, Mistress Sherwood, was also socially prominent.

ST MARY ALDERMANBURY

The small (60–100 tithable houses) but wealthy parish of St Mary Aldermanbury was close by the Guildhall in north-central London. Described as one of the "most important parishes of Puritan London," its beautiful homes and prosperous inhabitants had drawn comment in the sixteenth century.[186] Particularly noteworthy was its lovely parish church with its churchyard and cloisters, as well as the conduit which ran beside the church and carried water from the Tyburne River to supply London inhabitants. Strongly Puritan, it was the parish of the radical clergyman Edmund Calamy who was ejected by the church hierarchy in 1642 for nonconformity.[187] The parish made one of the largest contributions of any Lon-

---

180 GL MS 10,116/9; CLRO DL/C/345/155. According to Calamy, Kidder was ejected as vicar of Stanground, Hunts. in 1662, but was reinstated after proof of conformity. A. G. Matthews, *Calamy Revised* (Oxford: Clarendon Press, 1988), 307.

181 GL MSS 10,116/12, 9532/1/31. We have found three spellings of the surname (Sowden, Southen, and Sowthen) but will use the spelling with which the midwife was identified for the purpose of licensing.

182 GL MSS 10,116/10; 25,598. In 1695, midwife Chesmore and her husband Edmond were living very comfortably in their household in Hand Alley, St Botolph Bishopsgate, employing two servants. CLRO Marriage Act MS. 103.

183 *The Registers of St Martin Outwich, London* vol.32 (London: Harleian Society, 1905), unfol.

184 GL MS 11395 unfol. Sowden paid three shillings annually; the extremely wealthy Ralph Sherwood paid five shillings.

185 *Applebee's Original Weekly Journal*, October 7, 1721. Her unnamed deputy was severely injured when both midwives attempted to escape the flames by leaping from a window. I am grateful to Isobel Grundy for the foregoing reference.

186 Tai Liu, 29, 30; Stowe, 100, 262.

187 Alice E. McCambell, "The London Parish and the London Precinct 1640–1660," *Guildhall Studies in London History* 2 (October 1976): 121. Calamy also compiled a biographical list of all clergy ejected at the time of the Restoration. Matthews, *Calamy Revised, passim.*

don parish to Parliament in 1642. In addition to a hub of wealthy merchants, at least five of its inhabitants were elected as aldermen of the City. By 1695, the number of inhabited houses in the parish had increased to 124 (at least a 25% increase) and the social composition of the parish may have deteriorated since fewer than 29% of the households were considered to be of substance.[188]

Margaret Clark: "Widdow and mydwiffe," appears in the burial register of St Mary Aldermanbury for the year 1610, but details about her life and practice, which belong for the most part to the sixteenth century, have not been uncovered.[189]

Barbara Crowd (or Croud): Wife of Michael, was licensed in 1619.[190] Among her clientele, she numbered women from the upper class. Barbara Croud had been married thirty-three years at the time of her licensing, and she had at some point in her life given birth to two children, one of whom died in infancy. A widow Crowson, probably the midwife, died in 1626.[191]

Mary Manslawe (or Manshawe): Attended the visitation of 1637. She was married or widowed, but nothing further is known about her.

Rebecca Slarke (Clarke): Most likely a widow when she was licensed in 1664.[192] She was an associate of midwife Francis Austin. Her clientele were drawn from a wide area of London.

Elizabeth Whitehorne: Married to John Whitehorne, a carpenter, and licensed in 1677.[193] She attended the visitation of 1680.[194] In 1671, high property taxes and King's subsidy were levied against the Whitehornes.[195] Widowed in 1672, in 1693, widow Whitehorne was still living in her own home with one female servant.[196] Mrs. Whitehorne bore at least two sons, John and Bartholomew, and a daughter, Elizabeth, who, with a cousin, shared the estate of their uncle, Thomas Whitehorne, who died in 1676.[197] Midwife Elizabeth Whitehorne's son John was a

---

188 Jones and Judges, 60.
189 *The Registers of St Mary the Virgin, Aldermanbury, London* vol. 61 (London: Harleian Society, 1931), 86.
190 GLRO DL/C 341 (fol. illeg.).
191 The bishop's registers use the spelling Croud, but the parish registers show the surname as Crowdson or Crowson. See *The Registers of St Mary Aldermanbury* Vol. 1, 51–84, passim, births and burials for 1626.
192 GL MS 10,16/3.   193 GL MS 10,116/10; GLRO DL/C/345/161v.
194 GL MS 9537/22 unfol.   195 CLRO assess. box 5.7, CLRO 57.19 unfol.
196 *Registers of St Mary Aldermanbury* vol.2, 183; CLRO assess. box 14.21 unfol.
197 PRO prob. 11/351/96: will of Thomas Whitehorne, probated July 24, 1676; *Registers of St Mary Aldermanbury* vol. 2, 220.

victualler. He was a widower who died in 1699, only four years after his mother, leaving a young daughter, Elizabeth.[198]

For the small, but wealthy parish of St Mary Aldermanbury, we have recovered evidence about one midwife which places her above the economic median for her parish. Few (if any) details about the lives of the other four women have been uncovered, but we know they were self-sufficient throughout their lives because none were ever in receipt of parish poor relief.

ST OLAVE SILVER STREET

The parish of St Olave Silver Street was included among a group of the five most prosperous London parishes of early seventeenth century London in a study of London charities. Indications from the sixteenth century, however, pointed to a parish with a modest economic base and few illustrious inhabitants.[199] Recent research has concluded that, by 1638, most of the parishioners were poor and that, by the late 1650s, the parish contained "serious pockets of poverty or virtual slums."[200] Unfortunately, St Olave Silver Street was among the seventeen parishes missing from the study by Jones and Judges of the London population of 1695, but Herlan has pointed out that, overall, very little change took place in parochial poverty and social profile between the years of 1658–59 and 1695, leading us to conclude that the parish was a poor London parish throughout most of the century.[201]

Anne Clifton: Wife of Kellam, was licensed in 1619. She was an associate of midwife Joan Sens(t)ion, who may have been her deputy, and claimed a prosperous clientele.[202] In 1638, the Cliftons' rent was in the upper half of rent values for the parish.[203] Kellam Clifton was appointed porter or "under beadle" for the barber-surgeons' company in 1603, suspended, then reinstated in 1617, and, finally, dismissed in 1621.[204]

---

198 GL MS 9172/89: will of John Whitehorne, probated March 1699. John named his brother, Bartholomew, as his executor and the protector of his young daughter, Elizabeth, but Bartholomew must have died shortly after John because his will was probated by Bartholomew's widow, Eleanor.

199 W. K. Jordan, *The Charities of London 1480–1660* (London: George Allen & Unwin Ltd., 1960), 35. Stowe spoke disparagingly of the parish church as "a small thing and without any noteworthy ornaments." Stowe, 274.

200 Herlan, "Social Articulation," 48.

201 Jones and Judges note that the records for these seventeen parishes have disappeared. See Herlan, "Social Articulation," 49.

202 GLRO DL/C/341 (fol. illeg.).

203 Dale, 169. Of 130 rents, 47 were higher, 64 were lower, and 19 were the same.

204 Young, 303. It is not clear precisely what Clifton's duties were, but they seem to have involved ceremonial aspects of the guild. The SOED defines one role of the beadle as an apparitor for a trade guild.

Joan Sension: A widow who was licensed in 1627.[205] She was still active at the visitation of 1637.[206] She was an associate of Anne Clifton, senior midwife. In 1638, as head of her own household, she paid a rent in the upper half of parish rents.[207] Parish records of 1640–41, 1652–53 refer to midwife Sension as she carried out deliveries of parish women.[208]

Elinor Gillam: Married to Anthony Gillam, a Huguenot diamond cutter. She attended the visitation of 1637. She was still practising in 1661. An associate of Joan Cockson, who was probably her deputy.[209] The midwife had two sons. One of them, Thomas Gillam, became a wealthy surgeon.[210]

Mary Taylor: Wife of Thomas, citizen and haberdasher, was licensed in 1661.[211] Widowed in 1663, she was the sole heir and executrix of her husband's oral will.[212]

Elizabeth Bickerstaffe: Wife of James Bickerstaffe. She was licensed in 1679[213] and present at the visitation of 1680.[214] Bickerstaffe's tithe assessment in 1681 placed him in the third quartile for his parish.[215] James was more than likely the son of Anthony Bickerstaffe, a prosperous linendraper, described as a "gentleman," with extensive land holdings in Surrey.[216] In 1679–80, a Bickerstaffe child died, who may have been the midwife's son. The parish records also note the death of a Mrs. Bickerstaffe in 1689–90, who we believe, was a relative of the midwife.[217]

Anne Shorter: Wife of William, attended the visitation of 1680. Widowed in 1683, she was granted an administration for William's estate.[218]

Four parish midwives were probably not wealthy or socially distinguished, but they were self-sufficient householders occupying respectable positions in what

205 GLRO DL/C/343/23v.   206 GL MS 9537/15/63.
207 Dale, 169. Like the Cliftons, she paid a moderated rent of £6, actual rent of £8 a year.
208 GL MS 1257/1/34, 67.   209 Scouloudi, *Returns of Strangers*, 546; GL MS 10,116/1.
210 Thomas Gillam was fined in 1614 for dissecting a cadaver out of this "[barber-surgeons'] Hall," which was located in St Olave Silver Street, the midwife's parish. See Young, 331, 334, 494.
211 GL MS 10,116/1; GLRO DL/C/344/166v.   212 GL MS 9052 box 14.
213 LP VX 1A/11/12; Sancroft Register vol.2, fol. 221.   214 GL MS 9537/22 unfol.
215 GL MS 1262/1 unfol.; CLRO 18.13/5. There is every likelihood that James Bickerstaffe was the son of Anthony Bickerstaffe of Christ Church, London, a prosperous linen draper who was also described as a gentleman: PRO E 320/46, 179/186/437.
216 PRO E320/R46; 179/186/437.
217 GL MS 1257/2, burials for the years 1679–89. There was another Bickerstaffe family in the parish, that of John Bickerstaffe, possibly the midwife's brother-in-law. There may also have been a connection with the gentry since Edward Bickerstaffe, gentleman, of St Clement Danes, was undoubtedly a relative. On Elizabeth's testimonial, her spouse is given as "Edward"; I believe this was an error since the registers and parish records show only a James and John for St Olave Silver Street.
218 GL MS 9050/14/8.

was, admittedly, a poor parish. Gillam was prosperous and married to a skilled tradesman in a luxury craft. Taylor, as the wife of a citizen and haberdasher, in all likelihood enjoyed the material and economic advantages associated with her husband's occupation, one of the most profitable in Restoration London.[219]

ST DUNSTAN IN THE WEST

With more than 400 tithable houses on the eve of the revolution, and 436 inhabited houses in 1695, St Dunstan in the West was a large and prosperous extramural parish.[220] Fleet Street, the most important link between the City and Westminster, ran through the heart of the parish, which was situated in the City's largest ward of Farringdon Without.[221] St Dunstan was an exception to the rule that the wealthy tended to congregate around an early modern urban centre. As Emrys Jones has pointed out, "the entire parish of St Dunstan's in the West was comparable to the city core, and it boasted four titled householders."[222] It was also the home of an unusually high number of professional men, as well as a substantial number of gentlemen. With two Inns of Court situated within its confines, not only legal practitioners, but auxiliary tradesmen such as scriveners and stationers made their home in the parish; surgeons and physicians also congregated in St Dunstan toward the beginning of the seventeenth century.[223] By 1640, many wealthy tradesmen were found among its parishioners, as well as a number of radicals who were active during the revolutionary period.[224] Debtors' prison on Fleet Street and Bridewell for the poor and vagrant were both located within its confines, as was the busy meat market of Smithfield.[225] A recent study of poor relief during the revolutionary years has concluded that St Dunstan in the West was wealthier than several other extramural parishes during that period.[226] With a population of 2,673 in 1695, there were 436 inhabited houses. Slightly less than one-third of the households were considered well-to-do.[227]

The large extramural parish of St Dunstan in the West claimed the services of at least twenty-four licensed midwives over the course of the century. This number appears disproportionately large at first glance, but when compared with the populations of other parishes, the ratio of midwives to inhabitants is roughly the same.

219 Power, 214.
220 Dale, 230–34. In Fleet Street, houses in the wealthy parish of St Dunstan in the West had an average of 7.5 hearths, while in the poor parish of St Bride, the average house had only 5.6 hearths. Power, 174.
221 In 1631, the population of Farringdon Without was 20,846 with the other six extramural parishes having a total population of less than 20,000. William McMurray, "London: its population in 1631," *Notes and Queries* 11:1 (May 1910): 426.
222 Jones, 131.   223 A. L. Beier, "Engine," 155.   224 Tai Liu, 41, 42.
225 Herlan, "Poor Relief," 4–15.   226 Ibid., 30.   227 Jones and Judges, 62.

Isobel Doubleday: A widow of Crown Court, was licensed in 1611 at age sixty with thirty years' experience.[228] She paid a number of parish assessments ranging from above average (1596) to low (1613).[229]

Joyce Megon: The wife of James Megon, who was probably a tailor. She was licensed in 1616.[230] At least two of midwife Megon's children died when they were very young and two others survived childhood. The burial charges for daughter Anne in 1620, as well as the site of burial, suggest above-average income and social status.[231]

Alice Carnell: The wife of cooper Francis Carnell, lived in Three Leg Alley. She was licensed in 1629, and attended the visitation of 1636.[232] Carnells' assessment for scavenger rates was low in 1629.[233] The Carnells had lost at least one child, infant John in 1616.[234] Parish records of the overseers of the poor note two payments to Francis in July and August 1638 "in his sicknes."[235] He died soon afterward and had a respectable, if modest funeral with a knell and pall.[236] Alice Carnell survived her husband and in 1644, was renting part of her home to Jane Fletcher.[237] Despite the financial difficulties experienced at the time of her husband's illness and death, there is no evidence of midwife Carnell becoming a parish charge.

Catherine Wicks: Lived with husband Richard in Bell Lane. She was licensed in 1630.[238] Her attendance at both the visitations of 1636 and 1637 was recorded.[239] In 1638, Richard Wicks paid the extremely high moderated rent of £30 per year, which placed him in the top ten percent of rents for the parish.[240]

Elizabeth Seeley: Licensed in 1622 when living in St Clement Danes. Later, she and husband George moved to live in Sheire Lane "between the sign of the Drume and the sign of the Blackmore" in St Dunstan in the West. She was present at the visitation of 1636.[241] George Seeley died in 1638, the same year that

228 GLRO DL/C/340/11v.   229 GL MSS 2968/1/416, 499; 2968/2/80.

230 GLRO DL/C/340/211v. Three clients were married to tailors living in three different parishes.

231 GL MSS 2968/2/53v, 178v; 10342/63, 69, 73v, 221v, 234. As far as we can ascertain, Anne and James died, and Frances and Thomas survived.

232 GLRO DL//C/343/68v.   233 GL MS 3783/4v.   234 GL MS 2968/2/128.

235 GL MS 2999/1.   236 GL MS 2968/3/549.

237 GL MS 2968/3/549, 661v. Perhaps Fletcher had been a poor woman who had been delivered by midwife Carnell. The parish paid Fletcher's rent of 7s. 6d.

238 GLRO DL/C/343/91.   239 GL MSS 9537/14/37; 9537/15/58v.

240 LPL 272/401v. Only 27 of more than 460 rents recorded for this wealthy parish were higher.

241 GL MS 9537/14/37; GLRO DL/C 431/284 (spelled Ceeley).

their rent of £20 was in the upper half of rents for their parish.[242] Elizabeth was the major beneficiary of her husband's estate.[243] Son Richard Seeley of Clifford's Inn died in 1668.[244]

Alice Carnaby: Probably a widow. Her name was listed among the parish midwives at the visitation of 1637, but she did not attend.[245] She did, however, deliver parish women and was described as "the midwife," in parish records.[246] Midwife Carnaby died in 1649.[247]

Elizabeth Somner: The wife of Fleet Street goldsmith William Somner. Licensed in 1639, she attended the visitation of 1664.[248] As early as 1629, the Somners' parish assessment was above average.[249] Elizabeth Somner had borne and buried two infant sons.[250] By 1638, the family's moderated rent of £9 was below average for this parish.[251] Widowed in 1651,[252] in 1660 Widow Somner and two of her adult sons were living in Ram's Alley. By 1663, son John, a sadler who was married and had a child, Anne (born in 1660), had moved to another residence; he died in 1667.[253] Another son, William, was a goldsmith living in Fleet Street who had at least two children: Mary, born in 1653, and Elizabeth, born in 1658.[254] Widow Somner moved to a larger house in Myter Court some time before 1671 after her home in Ram's Alley was damaged by the fire of 1666.[255] Subsequently,

---

242 Although the rent of twenty pounds was given as a "moderated rent" (Dale, 234), in Seeley's will he mentions his rent as being £20. GL MS 9172/45. Seeley's funeral expenses paid to the parish were 11s.13d. GL MS 2968/3/547.

243 GL MS 9172/45.

244 GL MS 2968/5/46. Richard's burial in the chapel of St Dunstan in the West and the burial fee of £1.5s. are indications of social prestige. It may have been the midwife's daughter, Joan Seeley, who died in 1641, and a grandson, Robert, who died 1654. GL MSS 2968/3/612; 2968/4/216v.

245 GL MS 9537/14/37. The midwife's name is shown as Cranaby in the visitation records, but parish records show her as Carnaby.

246 Carnaby was paid five shillings in 1640 for delivering two poor women of the parish.

247 GL MS 2968/4/109v.

248 GLRO DL/C/344/61v; GL MS 9537/17/66v, 52. This visitation has recorded the parish twice.

249 GL MS 2968/3/455v. There is some question about the date shown in the records. It could well be that the clerk made a mistake and the date was 1634. Somner's assessment at twelve shillings was quite high.

250 GL MS 2968/3/344v, 366.

251 Dale, 231. Although rent of £9 would be above average in many parishes, in St Dunstan in the West, it placed Somner in the lowest quartile of rents.

252 GL MS 2968/4/164. Burial costs suggest a moderate degree of affluence.

253 GL MSS 2961/1/10, 117; 2969/2. I believe that the clerk mistakenly showed two John Somners in Ram Alley instead of widow Somner and son John in 1660: 10,345, October 1663 assessments for subsidies to his majesty: 2968/5 burials, October 1667. John Somner's burial charges of 21s. 8d. were very high; he was buried in the church. The John Somner who was named a parish vestryman in 1689 was probably the midwife's grandson.

254 GL MS 10,345/50, 64v.

255 GL MS 2969/2. A valuation and assessment etc. for 1671 unfol. and list of names of those who were "sufferers in the late fire of Sept. 1666 etc.," unfol.

she paid an assessment on rents set at the extremely high sum of 60s. per annum. Her son Henry was chosen parish scavenger in 1664.[256] Mrs. Somner was paid the substantial sum of £2.10s. by the parish in 1672 for services to Mrs. Adams.[257] By 1679, Widow Somner was joined by her daughter or daughter-in-law (probably newly widowed) and two grandchildren.[258] Somner died in 1687 and was buried in the vault of the parish church, as was her granddaughter and namesake, who died in 1688. She left a generous legacy to the parish poor.[259]

Abigail King: The wife of Thomas. The family lived in Cock and Key Alley. No records of licensing survive, but parish records of 1647–48 refer to her as "the midwife."[260] She was the mother of at least three children: Abigail, born in 1629, Sara in 1631, and Susan in 1632.[261] Their moderated rent, in 1638, placed the young family in the lowest quartile of rents for the parish.[262] Widow King was assessed the modest sum of five shillings for a tax "By the Lord Protector and his Counsell" in 1658, an indication of her continuing self-sufficiency.[263]

Joan Cockson: The wife of Thomas, a tailor, lived in Sheire Lane. She was licensed in 1661 after serving as the deputy of the venerable senior midwife Elenor Gillam.[264] In 1661, a daughter, Arabella, was born.[265] Mistress Cockson made a generous contribution toward repairs of the parish church in April 1665.[266] By August 1665, plague had visited the family.[267] Tragically, no further trace of Cocksons survive in parish or ward records.

Elizabeth Garland: A widow who married widower Richard Wharton, upholsterer, in 1654.[268] Her first husband had been William Garland, citizen and cutler

256 GL MS 2969/2 "A valuation and assessment of and upon the lands, offices and stocks etc.," 1671 unfol. There is confusion over the addresses of the various Somner family members. Although I have no proof to date, Ram Alley was probably an adjunct of Fleet Street, and the two addresses seem to have been used interchangeably. After 1671, Ram Alley does not appear on tax rolls, possibly because of damage sustained in the Great Fire of 1666. Our difficulties were further compounded by the appearance of a second "Mrs. Sumner" in Morecroft Court in 1679 (see GL MS 2969/4), who may have been a widowed daughter-in-law.

257 GL MS 2968/5/131v. We are not told what services midwife Somner (licensed some 33 years earlier) performed for Mrs. Adams.

258 GL MS 2969/4.

259 The parish poor were left £5 per annum. GL MS 2968/6/120v, 129v, 140, 151.

260 GL MS 2999/1 unfol. This is also mentioned in Herlan "Poor Relief," 28.

261 GL MS 1034/2/97v, 101, 103v.   262 Dale, 230.   263 GL MS 2961/1/5.

264 GL MS 10,116/1; GLRO DL/C/344/164.

265 A number of Cockson infants were buried in the years 1659–63 but we have been unable to establish their relationship to the midwife. GL MS 2968/3/331, 350v, 399v.

266 GL MS 2968/4/431v.

267 Thomas Cockson received a small sum of money from the parish for relief from the plague. GL MS 2968/ 455.

268 GL MS 10,345/120v.

of London.[269] She was licensed in midwifery in 1661, with 16 years' experience.[270] Parish visitations in 1664 and 1680 recorded her attendance.[271] Her clientele and references suggest strong ties with the Huguenot community in London.[272] Richard Wharton of Fleet Street was assessed moderate rates in the years 1661–64 for a variety of subsidies.[273] His burial expenses in 1669, however, suggest social prominence.[274] Elizabeth Wharton received the same burial in September 1681.[275] Her will (signed in her own hand), which was probated on October 15, 1681, left her entire estate to her son by her first husband.[276]

Mary Seignior (or Senior): Widow of George, tailor, was licensed in 1663, as a long-time parish resident[277] and attended the visitation of the following year.[278] In 1638, George Senior was paying an extremely high moderated rent, which placed him in the top 5% of rents for the parish.[279] Mary and George Senior had at least four children: Simon, born in 1650, Randolph in 1651, Henry in 1654, and Elizabeth in 1655.[280] At least three infants were buried between the years of 1637 and 1647, who may have been Mary Senior's children.[281] George Senior was collector for the poor in 1656.[282] By 1656, the Seniors were living in Fleet Street and paying a rent of £24 a year. In 1663, "widow Seignior" was maintaining the Fleet Street residence and paying the same high rent for the parish-owned property.[283] The Senior house on Fleet Street was damaged by the Fire, and discussions

269 GL MS 9152/70.

270 GL MS 10,116/1; GLRO DL/C/344/167. Wharton's testimonial was signed by Matthew Haviland, who was to be deprived of his charge the following year for nonconformity. See Matthews, 252. Haviland was shown as the rector of Holy Trinity the Less in 1662, but there is no question that he signed Wharton's certification in 1661.

271 GL MSS 9537/17/52, 66v; 9537/22 unfol.

272 One of the men who signed the testimonial was Charles Walsh "de Savoy," which could be a reference to the French Church; clients Aleyn Reade and Elizabeth Delovs bore French names as possibly did Elizabeth Mount, Elizabeth Crayle, and Grace Lawrence. One woman was married to a milliner, a traditionally French craft.

273 GL MS 2969/2 unfol.

274 GL MS 2968/5/61, 274. For purposes of comparison it should be noted that the burial charges for Sir John Bowring the following month were the same as Wharton's.

275 GL MS 2968/6/9.   276 GL MS 9172/70.

277 GL MS 10,116/3; GLRO DL/C/345/15. Her husband, too, was a long time resident. John Senior, the midwife's father-in-law, was parish churchwarden in 1637. GL MS 2968/3 /421.

278 GL MS 9537/17/52,66v.

279 He was paying £35. Dale, 230. Only fifteen individual and noncommercial rents were higher, and seven others out of 440 paid the same rent.

280 GL MS 10,345/44, 47, 53, 58v.

281 GL MSS 2968/3/423, 666; 2968/4/57v. Because the name appears to be "Semor," we cannot say for certain that they were the midwife's babies, but the fact that one of the children was named George is a strong indication that they were.

282 GLMS 2968/4/243.

283 GL MSS 2968/4/268, 279, 287, 261v, 412; 2969 unfol. Rates, Taxes, etc. for 1661, 3016/2/40v; 2968/5/7. The house on Fleet Street was a gift to the parish from Dr. White. Another example of Dr. White's largesse was the distribution of twenty shillings to twenty poor people on December 26, 1657, out of his former residence at which George Senior presided. GL MS 2968/4/279, 284v.

about its fate were prolonged.[284] In the meantime, the midwife was living in a spacious house with eight hearths in Two Crane Court.[285] Mary Senior was buried in the church in 1669.[286]

Mary Benson: The wife of John, citizen and stationer, as well as parish clerk. She attended the visitation of 1664.[287] Parish records contain many references to the popular parish clerk, who was paid £10 a year for his work as a scribe. In addition, he received sums such as £2.10s. paid to him in 1646 "for his paines taken in the busines of Sion Colledge"; or collected the premium for taking an apprentice.[288] Benson, a shop owner, borrowed £20 from the parish in 1654 and repaid it (interest-free) within a year.[289] The family employed two servants.[290] Two Benson children were buried in 1638 and 1641, but son John, born in 1629, survived.[291] The wife of the Bensons' son, John, bore them two grandchildren, Roland and John.[292] There is the possibility that Daniel Benson, who rented land which was owned by the parish, was also a son.[293] John Benson died in 1666.[294] The widow Benson, who broke her leg in 1696, and was afterward lame, might have been the midwife's daughter-in-law, but there is the possibility that it was the midwife, now very aged. The parish paid the invalid two shillings a week for seventeen weeks, paid her rent of £3 per annum, and gave her several small sums of money by way of relief.[295]

Mrs. Hobby: Attended the visitation of 1664. The recording scribe has noted that she was licensed in December 1661, but no testimonial certificates have survived, and her name has not been entered in the bishop's registers. There is the strong likelihood that widowhood and remarriage had intervened in the years between licensing and visitation, and that she was licensed under her first husband's surname.

Abigail Symonds: licensed in 1667.[296] We believe she was the widow of Abraham Symonds who died in 1665, and who was predeceased by infant Abraham in

---

284 GL MS 3016/2/40v, 42, 50v. Well into 1667, parish records refer to Mrs. Senior's "problem" with no mention of how it was resolved. Evidently, the midwife had some claim to the ground on which the house stood. The parish decided to rebuild at least one of its houses in Ram Alley.
285 PRO E179/252/32 (unfol.).
286 GL MS 2968/5/61. The fee was 18s.4d., which was substantial. The family used its own pall. A barber-surgeon of Fleet Street was related to George Senior.
287 GL MS 9537/17/66v. Mary Benson's name appears on the second part of the visitation, which commenced October 2, 1664 and duplicated some of the work of the first part. Midwives Wharton, Senior, and Somner were listed under both parts.
288 In 1646, Benson received £6 to apprentice a poor parish child. GL MSS 29868/4/65v; 3016/1/213, 318v, 349.
289 GL MS 2968/4/238. 290 GL MS 2961/1/121v.
291 GL MSS 2968/3/551, 595; 10,345/120.
292 GL MSS 2968/4/255; 10,345/60. Roland died in 1655. 293 GL MS 3016/2/42v.
294 GL MS 3016/2/37. 295 GL MS 2968/6/295, 306, 307, 307v, 323, 324.
296 GL MS 10,116/5.

1662. Mary Symonds, born in 1654, was possibly a daughter.[297] Abigail, whose testimonial certificate failed to mention a spouse, may, however, have been the widow of Robert, Frances, or William Symonds.[298]

Mary Duckett: Licensed in 1667, the deputy of Mrs. Hatton, licensed midwife.[299] Her husband, John Duckett, B.A., was the parish curate.[300] Shortly after Duckett's appointment, the family sustained losses in the Great Fire and got almost £3 from the various funds allotted to the parish for relief of fire victims.[301] In 1667, a son, William, was born; John junior had probably been born before Duckett's appointment as parish curate. John Duckett augmented his modest wage in 1666 and 1670 by giving commemorative sermons at ten shillings a sermon.[302] The occasional christening or burial paid 1s.[303] John Duckett was buried November 25, 1670, in the chancel of the church, as befitted his position as a member of the parish clergy; there was no charge for his burial.[304] Mary Duckett's difficulties in maintaining herself and her children were alleviated from time to time by the parish. Several payments of five shillings may have been paid for services as midwife to poor parish women in 1675, but at least two payments were made at the request of curate Franklin, John Duckett's successor.[305] Other small sums of money were given to her, in 1675 when she was ill and, in 1677, by "order of the vestry."[306] By 1683, an ailing Mary Duckett had joined the ranks of poor clergymen's widows when a petition netted her twenty shillings. In 1685, another petition resulted in her receiving bread on Wednesdays and Fridays and being presented as a candidate for Sion College, a home for the invalided poor.[307] The burial of Mary Duckett, "pensioner," was recorded on April 13, 1687.[308] The name of John Duckett, her son, appeared on a parish tax roll as a contributor to the Orphans' Tax in 1695.[309]

297 GL MSS 10,345/53v,236; 2968/4/381v.
298 If she was the widow of William Symonds, she was an extremely wealthy woman living in an enormous house with twenty-six hearths. See PROE 179/252/32 and E 179/147/627.
299 GL MS 10,116/6.
300 John Duckett had signed Abigail Symonds' testimonial certificate (see above), while Joseph Thompson, parish vicar, had signed Mary Duckett's. Vicar Thompson (who had signed John Duckett's testimonial three years earlier) mentioned Mary's apprenticeship, but not the fact that her husband was the parish curate. Again, this can be taken as an indication of the Church's emphasis on the practical qualifications of a midwifery candidate.
301 GL MS 2969/2 unfol.   302 GL MS 2968/5/4v, 40, 88.
303 GL MS 2999/1 unfol. Duckett was paid a shilling for burying a poor widow pensioner in September 1667, and for christening a poor woman's child in August 1668.
304 GL MS 2968/5/85. Although the churchwardens' accounts show a payment to Duckett for a sermon after the date of his burial, I believe that, as frequently happened, it had been paid earlier and not recorded at the time.
305 GL MS 2968/5/196, 197, 197v.   306 GL MS 2968/5/197v, 225.
307 GL 3016/2/164, 173. Parish records are full of evidence regarding the plight of the widows of clergy. Mary Duckett was probably prevented from practising her profession of midwifery full time by chronic ill health.
308 GL MS 2968/6/96v.   309 He was living on Bolt and Ton Court: GL MS 2996/1.

Anne Bradford: Licensed in 1672.[310] In 1669, Anne and her husband William were living in Fewter Lane, and their son William was born that year.[311] By 1679, the Bradfords and their five children, William's mother, two apprentices, and a servant lived in a large house in Nevill's Alley with six hearths.[312] In this year, Bradford paid one of the highest parish assessments levied for the French war.[313] Bradford employed two apprentices. At least one Bradford child died in infancy and was buried in the church at a cost of seven shillings which was high for an infant's burial.[314] William Bradford paid the substantial fine of £12 in 1686 to be excused from serving as parish constable and questman.[315] By 1695, the Bradfords were living in St Sepulchre parish with two servants; only one daughter, Rebecca, was still at home.[316]

Mary Benet: Wife of John, limner, was licensed in 1674 in the jurisdiction of Canterbury.[317] Hugh Chamberlain, "Med. Regius," had signed her testimonial. Wives of a gentleman and schoolmaster were listed among her clients.[318]

(Elizabeth? or Mary?) Farewell: Attended the visitation of 1680. The midwife may have been Elizabeth Farewell, the wife of Henry Farewell, Red Lyon Court, mother of two children, who died and was buried in the chancel of the parish church in 1689.[319] Or the midwife was Mary, wife of John Farewell, gentleman and attorney of Fleet Street, who was living with her husband and son John in 1695.[320] Lady Katherine Farewell (possibly the mother of both Henry and John) was buried in the parish church vault in 1692. For both women, there are indications of a socially prominent family.

Mrs. Carter: Appeared at the visitation of 1680. With no indication of a Christian name for the midwife or her husband, it is impossible to cull specific details of her life from the myriad of references to "Carters" of the parish. At least three

---

310 GL MS 10,116/7.   311 GL MS 10,345/91v.
312 PRO E 179/147/627/29v. An earlier hearth assessment (probably for Fewter Lane) showed the Bradfords living in a house with nine hearths. CLRO Assess. Box 25.9/9 fol.3.
313 GL MS 2969/4.
314 GL MS 2968/5/44v. A number of Bradford children and infants were buried in the years 1663–73, but some were from a family which was living in "Sheere" Lane.
315 GL MS 2968/6/95v.
316 Marriage Tax CLRO 109.80. The child who was buried in 1668 was also named Rebecca.
317 LPL VX 1A/11/6; Sheldon Register vol. 2 fol. 255. Limning was the skilled craft of illuminating manuscripts in gold (SOED).
318 It is impossible to chart Mrs. Benet's family status more precisely since there were at least four other families with the same surname. We are not certain whether she was widowed or not at the time of licensing, as the records are not clear on this point; a John Benet had died fifteen years earlier, who may or may not have been the midwife's husband. GL MS 2968/4/336v.
319 GL MSS 2969/4 (1679), 2968/6 burials (1689). Farewell was still living in Red Lyon Court in 1699, GL MS 3015.
320 CLRO Marriage Tax 106.2 When all relevant factors are considered such as age, children's ages, and longevity, I believe that Mary Farewell was the midwife.

Carters, John, Ralph, and William, were prominent in parish affairs and, with a fourth, George, a grocer, have left indications of personal wealth. The midwife may also have been the wealthy widow who lived in Red Lyon Court with her maid in the 1660s and 1670s.[321]

Jane Cooke: The wife of gentleman John Cooke, lived in Bell Yard. She was licensed in 1684.[322] Her testimonial statement, from Hugh Chamberlen, implied both a long acquaintanceship of Chamberlen with Cooke, as well as an acknowledgement of her experience and competence as a midwife.[323] She numbered at least one gentlewoman among her clients.

Alice Burrell: The wife of William, citizen and haberdasher, was licensed in 1686.[324] In 1666, they were living in Nevill's Alley in a house with eight hearths.[325] By 1679, they had moved to Hercules Pillars. Their assessment, in 1689, was higher than average.[326] Burrell had a number of literate clients. Widowed by 1699, and living in Water Street, her assessment reflected modest economic resources.[327]

Sarah Mainwaring: The wife of Thomas, lived in Falcon Court, and was licensed in 1690.[328] A Dr. Mainwaring, possibly the midwife's father-in-law, lived in a substantial house in the parish in 1670. The midwife had at least one child (Edmund) who died in 1689.[329] Thomas Mainwaring's 1689 assessment as a landlord was extremely high.[330] Widowed by 1695, Sarah was living in her own home, which she shared with Edward Hatton and his wife Sara, possibly the midwife's daughter, and a servant.[331]

Ellinor Wallis: The wife of Solomon, believed to be a clergyman. She was licensed in 1693.[332] "Mr. Wallis" was assessed for the rectory of St Dunstan's in 1699.

---

321   GL MSS 3016/2/210, 211, 234v, 213v; 2968/5/8, 105v; 2968/5/289v. William Carter, who was a"clarke," died in 1679; 2968/6/120v. John Carter was buried in St Anne's Chapel, June 8, 1687; GL MSS 2969/2 (1671), 2969/3 (1973), 2969/4 (1679).

322   GL MS 10,116/11. There is also the possibility that notary Edward Cooke of Nevill's Alley was the midwife's husband since the baptism register records the birth of a child, Anne, in 1654, who was the daughter of Jane and Edward Cooke, gentleman. In that case, the testimonial certificate which gave her husband's name as John, was incorrect (GL MS 10,345/54). The names of both John and Edward Cooke appear in parish assessments with both paying above average assessments (GL MS 2969/3).

323   GL MS 10,116/11. Chamberlen does not say, as he did for other midwives, that he had "examined" her; it is likely that their association was social, rather than professional

324   LPL VX 117/11/38; Sancroft Register vol. 2/262.

325   CLRO 25.9/18/4. According to Power's classification, a house with eight hearths was a large house.

326   William Burwell was given the title "esq." on the tax roll of 1689, which was unusual, deferential. GL MSS 2969/4, 2969/2 unfol.

327   GL MS 3015 unfol.   328   GL MSS 10,116/13; 9532/1/75.

329   GL MS 2968/6/48v, 164, 285v.   330   GL MS 3014/1.   331   Marriage tax CLRO 106.4.

332   GL MSS 10,116/13; 9532/1/94v.

Wallis was probably a member of the clergy, which would explain the absence of clerical testimony among the midwife's testimonial documents, an omission which was unusual in this particular parish.

Joan Beadnell: A widow, licensed in 1694. One of her clients was a gentlewoman from Hertfordshire.[333]

In summary, one woman listed in visitation records remained untraceable; four others, about whom we have few details, were probably in modest circumstances or better. Three midwives were at the median, or slightly above, in their socio-economic circumstances within their prosperous parish. Two midwives experienced financial difficulties; one apparently as a result of a spouse's illness, and the other as the widow of an educated, but poorly paid professional. The remaining fourteen women were all married to men who were prosperous members of their parish community. They were gentlemen, skilled tradesmen or craftsmen, and professionals with evidence of substantial income and in some cases, real wealth.

OVERVIEW

Of the seventy-six midwives we have uncovered in the twelve parishes, the occupations of thirty-three (43%) spouses are known. See Table 5.1: Identified Spousal Occupations for Midwives of Twelve Parishes.[334] At least eight (11%) of the women were married to gentlemen or individuals in the professions; five (7%) were married to officials; ten (13%) were married to dealers (citizens and haberdashers, grocers, or tailors); eight (11%) to skilled craftsmen or tradesmen, including a goldsmith, diamond cutter, and a limner; and two (3%) to workers in semi-skilled trades (carpenter and paver).[335]

The occupations of twenty (26%) of the spouses who were alive at the time the midwives were licensed are unknown; these must be accepted as minimum figures. In addition, the occupation of only one spouse of the group of nine women who were designated as widows is known. Similarly of the fifteen women not specifically designated as widows, but whose husbands' names are not given, we know the occupation of only one spouse.[336] If we were to assume for the moment that the sources which provided evidence on spousal occupations are not biased in favour of particular occupations, then a calculation based solely upon the known occupations of midwives' spouses produces the following (based,

---

333 GL MS 10,116/13.
334 This figure assumes that midwife Farewell was married to John Farewell.
335 The term "professional" is used in the twentieth-century sense as an aid to categorization. Paver Jonathan Winckles is classified as a semiskilled tradesman, a label which belies his high standing in the parish as churchwarden.
336 The two men who were married to women in the last two groups were included in the total of 32.

Table 5.1. *Identified Spousal Occupations for Midwives of Twelve Parishes*

Professional/Gentry	Attorney (gentleman), barber (surgeon?), medical doctor (2,) clerics (2), gentleman (2)
Officials	Beadle, clerk (2), clerk and stationer, tax collector
Dealer	Citizen and grocer, citizen and haberdasher (4), haberdasher, merchant tailor (2), tailor (2)
Skilled trades	Cooper, diamond cutter, goldsmith, gunsmith, limner, citizen and painter stainer, printer, upholsterer
Semiskilled trades	Carpenter, paver

Sources: Midwives' testimonials and parish records. See notes for individual midwives.

admittedly, on a relatively small number of cases): 24% professional and/or gentlemen; 15% officials; 30% dealers; 24% skilled trades; 6% semiskilled. We do not need to assert the accuracy of these specific figures in order to demonstrate that all available evidence indicates London midwives were drawn from the well-to-do and middling levels of London society. Poverty hit them, if at all, only at the end of the life cycle, and then only infrequently. They were discovered to be mainly individuals of influence and respect within the parishes.

On the evidence of the sample derived from the research for this study, it appears that Donnison's suggestion that "most 'professed' midwives came from the skilled artisan class" with a modest representation from the middle ranks of society including "gentlewomen," could be revised to show that the majority of licensed London midwives were likely women who were married to men of the more affluent professional (including gentry), or official or entrepreneurial (including merchants) segments of society.[337] David Harley similarly has cited examples of midwives who were married to affluent and educated men in the provinces, and indicated that a preliminary survey in Lancashire and Cheshire has revealed that "many [midwives] were the wives of prosperous merchants and yeomen."[338] His findings are clearly supported by this study of twelve London parishes. Four of the seventy-six women in this study were married to churchwardens. The latter held the most influential and prestigious position in the parish, while two others were married to men who held the respected and demanding post of parish clerk.

In seven of the twelve parishes under investigation, we have found evidence in tithe, tax lists, and/or wills which give a firm indication of the economic viability or, in some cases, affluence of *all* of the midwives and their families of those parishes (for a total of sixty-one midwives). In the remaining five parishes, there

337 Donnison, 9.   338 Harley, "Ignorant Midwives," 8, 9.

were eleven midwives for whom we have evidence in testimonials and other ecclesiastical and parish records, which places them among the financially secure inhabitants of their parishes.[339] Indeed, among these eleven midwives, there are strong indications of at least upper middle class links by way of their husbands' occupations and the status of individuals giving testimonial evidence. Of the four remaining midwives, three names appeared on visitation records and we have uncovered no further information about them. There is the possibility that these three women were deputy midwives or unlicensed midwives, which, as David Harley has argued, does not reflect upon the quality of their practice.[340] It does, however, preclude the type of information provided by testimonial certificates and bishop's registers. The fourth woman was identified as a midwife in parish burial records from early in the century, but the details of her life belong to sixteenth-century records outside of the confines of this study. Since, however, it was highly unusual for midwives to be identified in parish registers by their occupation, midwife Clark of the wealthy parish of St Mary Aldermanbury was in all likelihood a respected member of her profession and valued member of her parish community. Seventy-two of the midwives, or approximately 95%, have left evidence, then, about their socioeconomic positions in their parishes. They were women of good standing in their communities, and most were wives and widows who enjoyed at least a comfortable standard of living and, in some cases, one of affluence and prestige as the wives or widows of prosperous London citizens. In many cases, their children and grandchildren have left their mark as substantial London inhabitants.

Although one or two women received occasional financial assistance from the parish toward the end of their lives, and usually in connection with deteriorating health, only one woman, the widow of a clergyman, became a permanent charge of the parish. The midwives of seventeenth-century London bore little resemblance to the stereotypical ignorant and poverty-stricken midwife of earlier representations.

---

339 We have included midwife Carter here since all of the Carter males who were potential spouses were economically secure or well-to-do.
340 Harley, "Ignorant midwives," 8.

Conclusion

This exploration of the lives of seventeenth-century London midwives has led to a new and different perception of this important group of women who lived and worked in the rapidly changing milieu of one of Europe's major centres. Based on a variety of contemporary sources, the revised picture reflects more clearly the realities of midwives' lives and practices in seventeenth-century London than the more narrowly based traditional view.

Although the ecclesiastical licensing process was not concerned with supervision of licensed midwives, it did ensure that certain standards of competence and good conduct were met before a midwifery licence was issued. It also encouraged the supervision of inexperienced midwives or deputies by experienced midwives, and the interchange of knowledge and assistance among licensed midwives when difficult deliveries were encountered. The substantial outlay of cash which was required to obtain a midwifery licence was, in itself, a form of insurance against the temptation to dabble in midwifery on a whim or merely to avoid the pangs of poverty. Many of these women were career professionals who dedicated years to training and who went on to practise for decades.

Not only did midwives extend their practices beyond the boundaries of their home parishes, within their own parishes they were generally well known, long-time inhabitants, who were customarily respected both as practitioners and as members of their own community. Writing in the Early Restoration years, the minister of St Giles Cripplegate expressed this sense of a midwife's commitment to the greater good of society as he described the long years that Ann White of St Giles Cripplegate had "studied to assist and comford the King's majestyes subjects." Two years later, Elizabeth Ayr of the same parish was perceived as "very fitt for that [the practice of midwifery] as a publick employment."[1]

The midwife was a "specialist" whose expertise was concentrated in the area of child delivery.[2] In some cases, however, her skills and knowledge uniquely

---

1 MS 25,598, 1662 and 1664.
2 In some cases, the midwife might ensure that poor women received parish assistance during their postpartum or lying-in period. GL MS 2089/1, unfol. overseers of poor accounts for St Andrew

qualified her for other tasks – determining whether a woman was actually pregnant,[3] swearing bastardy depositions[4] or testifying about various forms of sexual impropriety.[5] Midwives were credited with having basic knowledge of common diseases, particularly since their clients were at risk when outbreaks occurred. The chemical physician George Starkey noted that every midwife knew that a laxative would be fatal to a smallpox victim.[6] There are a few prescriptions for gynaecological problems in English medical compendia by seventeenth-century female authors, but the indications are that these were the preserve of the midwife, who drew on a fund of orally transmitted knowledge in treating her clients, particularly during pregnancy and in the postpartum period.[7] Reluctant to discuss matters connected with menstruation with male physicians and apothecaries, women sought the advice of midwives.[8] Occasionally midwives were credited with the knowledge of medicines: to "breake and heal sore breasts of women"[9] or of abortifacient agents.[10] The midwifery treatise, published in 1656 by four London midwives, identified only by their initials, includes a section on women's disorders and children's diseases, while Jane Sharp also provides a brief section on children's diseases in her midwifery book.[11] There is the occasional reference to midwives

Wardrobe 1631. David Harley has given examples of midwives who went beyond child delivery in their provincial practices. Harley, "English Archives," 152.

3 GL MS 4409/2. Churchwardens' Accounts for St Olave Jewry for 1650 (unfol.). Mrs. Latin the midwife was called by parish officials to verify pregnancy in a woman "pretending to be in labour." Overseers of the poor in St Andrew Wardrobe paid Mrs. Cox, "the midwife," 1s. in 1635 for confirming the pregnancy of a woman who was then expelled from the parish. GL MS 20819/1, May 19, 1635. See James C. Oldham, "On Pleading the Belly: A History of the Jury of Matrons," *Criminal Justice History* 6 (1985) 1–64 for a discussion of this female jury, which frequently included one or more midwives.

4 Of the 24 cases before the London Consistory Courts in which midwives giving evidence were specifically identified by their occupation in the years 1672–98, 16 cases involved disputes over paternity, 3 related to spousal abuse, 4, to defamation and 1 to bigamy. I am grateful to Jennifer Melville for identifying these midwives. For provincial examples, see Harley, "Provincial midwives," 36–8 and "The scope of legal medicine in Lancashire and Cheshire, 1660–1760," Michael Clark & Catherine Crawford, eds. *Legal Medicine in History* (Cambridge: Cambridge University Press, 1994) 50–2.

5 Giardina Hess, "Midwifery practice among the Quakers," 49–50. See also GL MS 6552/3 August 7, 1711.

6 George Starkey, *Nature's Explication and Helmont's Vindication or a short and sure way to a long and sound life* (London, 1656), 257.

7 Evenden Nagy, *Popular Medicine*, 68–9; T. C. et al, 58, 59, 89, 102.

8 Male physicians had been trying for decades to encourage women to abandon their "ignorance and modesty" and consult them about gynaecological problems. John Sadler, *The Sicke Woman's Private Looking Glass* (London, 1636), "Dedication"; Patricia Crawford, "Attitudes to Menstruation in Seventeenth-century England," *Past and Present* no. 91 (May 1981): 69.

9 A seventeenth-century medical compendium contains the prescription for breast abscesses "used by midwives and other skilful women in London." B.M., *The Ladies Cabinet Enlarged* (London: 1654), 90.

10 T. C. [Catherine Turner] et al. *The Compleat Midwife's Practice*, 120. See also the case of midwife Elizabeth Francis, below.

11 In the Verney papers, a midwife was mentioned who prescribed medication for sick Verney children. Other midwives are also credited by Ralph Verney with treating infants and children. *Verney Memoirs* vol.1, 362; vol.2, 270. See also GL MS 4409/2, unfol., 1650.

who prescribed for children or were called by parish officials to view the bodies of dead children.[12] But in London, at least, midwives apparently concentrated their main efforts on child delivery. Parish records make a clear separation between nurses (who were frequently poor elderly widows) and midwives. During the plague years, when the parishes were hard pressed to care for the dead and dying, there is no suggestion that midwives carried out work other than that of child delivery.[13] In addition, the account book of the anonymous London midwife contains no hint of a fee for services other than infant delivery. Only occasional references credit midwives with other areas of expertise, real or perceived.

London midwives, the spouses of artisans, skilled tradesmen, and gentlemen, were not the rag tag group of poor, elderly females which, until recently, were subject to disapproval and dismissal: they were a proud sisterhood, aware of the responsibilities and obligations of their midwife's oath and committed to honouring its terms. In many communities, the midwife was regarded with respect as a type of "social authority." No more so was this the case than in early modern London.[14] Describing the actions of an abusive husband who was assaulting his wife in the midst of her labour, a witness noted that midwife Anna Emerson warned the man that he would lose his wife and child if his interference continued. When that failed to stop the buffeting, the midwife "cryed out again, Mr. Bauer I must swear in conscience and my oath will goe as far as twelve men." Acknowledging the powerful position of the midwife, and the respect accorded her by the community, as well as the courts, the man finally "gave over and went into the next room."[15]

Since midwives were held in high esteem for the most part, it is not surprising that there were only two cases in the London consistory court records 1672–99 where midwives defended themselves against defamatory attacks. Aware of the importance of protecting her reputation, midwife Maddison charged Mrs. Smart of The Unicorn in consistory court in 1680 after it was reported to her that Smart had called her a drunkard who "has lost a fingar and had spoylt a woman." Four years later, midwife Griffith brought a charge of defamation against a Mr. Wilcox

---

12 Midwives were called occasionally to view the bodies of dead children. GL MS 4409/2 (unfol.) churchwardens' accounts for St Olave Jewry 1650. Mrs. Latin the midwife was paid two shillings for this task.

13 GL MS 2968/4/443. Parish accounts of St Dunstan in the West for September 1665 list seven nurses, none of whom can be identified as midwives. The situation was different in Nuremberg where midwives were expected to act as auxiliary medical attendants during outbreaks of the plague: Wiesner, "Early modern midwifery," 105. In the Netherlands, "plague midwives" were employed. Marland, " 'Stately and dignified'," 276. In rural areas, the midwife may have been more active in prescribing medication. Kendal midwife Elizabeth Thompson's diary contains a prescription, but there is no indication of how it was used and the ingredients, typical of nonspecific receits (variously receipts or recipes) of the day, give no clue. Presumably it was used to treat conditions associated with pregnancy. For prescriptions offered by French midwife Louise Bourgeois, see Perkins, *Midwifery and Medicine*, 54–6.

14 Shorter, 44.

15 The unfortunate woman had already experienced one miscarriage after her husband had kicked her. GLRO Consistory Court of London Deposition Book DL/C/244, 1695. I am grateful to Jennifer Melville for this reference.

after he slandered her, calling her a "whore." Testifying on the midwife's behalf, her son-in-law protested "she lives very well, and is of good repute among her neighbour . . . such scandalous reports may be of great prejudice to the sayd producent in her practise."[16] London midwives appearing in the courts of London were, in almost all cases, respected or "expert" witnesses.

SEVENTEENTH-CENTURY MIDWIFERY: A WOMEN'S WORLD.

One hundred women were invited to the funeral of Elizabeth Dyer in the early 1680s. Each woman was given a pair of new gloves, according to funerary custom of the period. The colourful occasion was to include six midwives supporting the decorative pall which covered the coffin. Dyer, who was in all likelihood a midwife herself, wished her coat of arms to be displayed on the pulpit. The prominent role of the midwives was both a mark of the respect and high esteem in which they were held, and also a remarkable tribute to the deceased woman.[17]

At the close of the seventeenth century, the midwife still wore her red mantle of office with pride as she made her rounds to every corner of the City and its suburbs, at all hours of the day or night.[18] Susanna Kent of St Dunstan in the East wrote her last will and testament in 1712; her most detailed instructions concerned her midwife's mantle:

Item I give and bequeath unto my said granddaughter Elizabeth Skinner my midwifesmantle upon this condition and it is my will and desire that my said Daughter Susanna Read have the use of it dureing her life on condition shee comes up to London to practise midwifery either before or after the Death of her husband my will and meaning is that it shall not goe unto the Country but be for use of my said Daughter for life as aforesaid and then to my Granddaughter Elizabeth.[19]

16 GLRO DL/C/239, 241. I am grateful to Jennifer Melville for the foregoing references. See notes 4 and 5 above. In addition to the two midwives who defended themselves, two midwives testified on behalf of individuals who claimed to have been slandered.

17 CLRO MS AM/PW/1683/23. Will of Elizabeth Dyer.

18 The archival evidence which we have found is at odds with the conclusions reached by Kirstin Evenden re the status and position of midwives in seventeenth-century London. Because none of the depictions of Cellier show her with the traditional midwife's mantle, it appears that she was perceived as undeserving of this privilege, thus setting her apart from the majority of licensed and respected midwives who served London women. Images of Cellier cannot be taken as representative of London midwives in general; she was clearly an exception whose religion was the main point of denigration. Her occupation, coincidentally, lent itself to various parodies of the birthing process. Kirstin Evenden, " 'The Popish Midwife': Printed Representations of Elizabeth Cellier and Midwifery Practice in Late Seventeenth-Century London," *Racar*, XX (1–2, 1993): 44–59.

19 LP VH95/1136. The famous caricature of the midwife by Rowlandson shows her wearing a red cape and the inventory of a midwife's son's estate mentions "an old red cloak." GLRO AM/P1(2) 1745/1. In June 1699, a special committee of St Bride's approved a payment of 10 shillings to redeem midwife Henley's "mantle" with no indication of why she had lost it. GL MS 6552/2. The term "mantle" was apparently reserved for apparel worn by the medical profession, as was the colour red. Beryl Rowland refers to the "splendid scarlet academic gown of the fully trained M.D." Rowland, xv. Nurses wore white linen capes (introduced in 1686). See Phillis Cunnington and Catherine Lucas, *Occupational Costume in England from the Eleventh Century to 1914* (London: Adam and Charles Black, 1967), 309, 310, 320.

In London, women were still self-consciously and proudly in control of the whole birth process at the end of the century. Beginning with attendance at a neighbour's, relative's, or friend's delivery, deciding to become a deputy to a well-experienced, older midwife, and finally acquiring the license which entailed responsibility and commitment both to sister midwives as well as clients, the strands of midwives' lives became uniquely and inseparably woven into the fabric of London life and the lives of the women they served in the most intimate of circumstances. The birth process was a female ritual over which the midwife presided; the "mysterious office of women" remained relatively intact and apart from that of men.[20] To read the records of the anonymous London midwife is to step into a world of women where the male is alien. In contravention of the customs of the period, except in a few instances, women's identities in this account book are not conferred through their husbands or their husbands' occupations, but instead through the date and time of day which they were delivered and, in many cases, where they lived. Women bear the children (whose sexes are given) and women's names are credited with the payment of the delivery fee. With the women of London so firmly in control of childbearing throughout the seventeenth century, how was the citadel stormed and the traditionally female role of midwife appropriated by the male practitioner?[21]

THE DECLINE IN THE LICENSING ROLE OF THE CHURCH

In London, by 1720, the licensing system began to break down. With its demise, the midwives lost a significant legitimisation of their professional qualifications and childbearing women lost an important avenue, not only for expressing their views, but for asserting some measure of control in the choice of the women who would be their midwives through the granting or withholding of their testimonial assent. In the last decade of the century, there are some hints of the impending cessation of midwifery licensing reflected in the quality of testimonial evidence. Previously, it was the confidence that women who had experienced childbirth expressed on behalf of their midwives, which was the most telling proof of the high esteem in which many of the midwives were held. Both the direct statements contained in the testimonial certificates and the evidence of the anonymous midwife's account book with its record of repeated visits to the childbed of former clients bespeak the confidence and trust which many London wives and mothers placed in their midwives.

By the closing decade of the century, however, the Church appears to have relaxed significantly its rules requiring the testimony of six women as well as a state-

---

20 The phrase "The mysterious office of women" is the title of the first chapter of Jane Donegan's study, which deals with the history of midwifery in early America but begins with a brief account of English midwifery up to the 1730s.

21 For an account of the way in which the highly competent and respected midwives of medieval Flanders were gradually deprived of their authority by physicians and surgeons, see Myriam Greilsammer, *L'envers du Tableau: Mariage & Maternité en Flandre Médiévale* (Paris: Armand Colin, 1990).

ment from clergy. Not a single midwife of those licensed by the Bishop of London between 1695 and 1700 had the testimonial support of six women and a statement from the clergy. In two cases, twelve and sixteen women, respectively, gave a statement on the midwife's behalf, but were not sworn before the ecclesiastical official. In addition, no statement from the clergy accompanied these testimonials. In another seven cases, women were granted licences without the benefit of a clerical statement. Even more revealing are the records of the Archbishop of Canterbury, where the eighteen midwives licensed between 1687 and 1700 were given licences without a clerical statement even though, between 1669 (the date from which the first testimonials survive) and 1687, every midwife who was licensed produced a testimonial certificate from her parish clergy. This suggests that although female clients were still strong in their support of their midwives, the Church hierarchy, beginning with Canterbury, was no longer as concerned with the function of midwives beyond establishing a basic competence in their profession. With the testimony of the parish clergy no longer central, the voices of the female clients, no matter how urgent or sincere, lacked the public authority and respect commanded by a minister, vicar, or curate. While the change was not as abruptly reflected by the testimonial certificates accepted by the Bishop of London's representatives, the relaxing of Church control under this jurisdiction can also be seen in the paucity of licenses issued to midwives living in London: Of eighty-two licences issued in the years 1690–1700, only four were granted to midwives living within the city proper; thirteen were issued to midwives from extramural parishes; and the rest to midwives living in suburban parishes.

The breakdown in the ecclesiastical licensing of midwives has been linked to the declining power of the Church.[22] The evidence, however, indicates less a decline in power than a changing attitude toward the role of the Church in the licensing of midwives. This change began in the closing years of the century in the centre of the metropolis, and spread to the outlying areas until, by 1720, midwifery licensing was apparently virtually defunct. Ecclesiastical licensing was not central to the expertise and competence of what was fundamentally a self-regulatory system of training and apprenticeship, but it does appear to have been important for the societal respect and credit of the traditional profession. Why else would so many hundreds of midwives go to the considerable trouble and expense of being licensed when the only penalty was excommunication? Both the Church and London's female population had no quarrel with the traditional system of midwifery training and practice, but once the role of the Church was diminished, and with it the status attached to licensing, the seeds of decay were sown. By the 1750s midwives' traditional, practical skill proved no match for the claims of the male midwife, waiting in the wings with his shiny instruments and promises of "scientific expertise."[23]

22 Donnison, 22.
23 For an account of the way in which women's traditional skills were replaced by scientific knowledge, see Anne Oakley, *The Captured Womb* (Oxford: Basil Blackwell, 1984). Another brief summary of the exclusion of women is found in Barbara Brandon Schnorrenberg, "Is Childbirth

176 *Conclusion*

THE RISE OF THE MALE MIDWIFE

Pressure from medical practitioners may have, indeed, been a factor in the Church's loss of interest in the licensing of midwives. There is evidence of increasing competition among the male medical practitioners, particularly in the second half of the century, with apothecaries, barber-surgeons, and physicians, as representatives of "professional" medicine, all jostling for space in the health care system.[24] In addition to the medical "regulars," Phyllis Allen has noted that unlicensed medical practitioners were "worming their way into lucrative London practices" at the end of the century.[25] Young surgeons and apothecaries, struggling to become established, were enticed into midwifery as an untapped, pseudo-medical area of expansion and by the prospect of acquiring the family of the new mother as prospective patients for their general practice.[26] In describing the efforts of Dr. John Maubray to gain support for the male midwife in the opening decades of the eighteenth century, Beryl Rowland has remarked: "Except among the poor, the business of the accoucheur was too lucrative to be passed over by the male physician."[27] The aggressiveness of surgeon-apothecaries as they sought ways of increasing their incomes and expanding their practices also contributed to the growing number of male midwives after 1730.[28]

When Elizabeth Francis, whose parish is unknown, applied for a London licence in 1690 to practise surgery as well as midwifery, she may have seen the

Any Place for a Woman? The Decline of Midwifery in Eighteenth-Century England," *Studies in Eighteenth-Century Culture* 10 (1981): 393–408. See also Elizabeth Harvey, *Ventriloquized Voices*, and Jonathan Sawday, *Body Emblazoned*, on the masculinisation of scientific knowledge. For striking parallels with the unequal struggle between American midwives and the medical profession for control of child delivery in the nineteenth and early twentieth centuries see Charlotte G. Borst, *Catching Babies: The professionalization of Childbirth, 1870–1920* (Cambridge, Mass.: Harvard University Press, 1995).

24 See R. S. Roberts, "Medicine in Tudor and Stuart England: part 2, London," *Medical History* 8 (1964): 217–34. Roberts documents, in particular, the aggressive stance of the apothecaries in moving into general practice. For the opening up of the professions, see Christopher Hill, *Change and Continuity in Seventeenth-Century England* (London: Weidenfeld and Nicolson, 1974), chapter 7.

25 Phyllis Allen, "Medical Education in 17th Century England," *Journal of the History of Medicine* 1 (1946): 141.

26 Donnison, 23. On the continent as well, surgeons were envious of the incomes and status of midwives. Schama, 520. The competition between young medical officers and midwives for the "lucrative business of midwifery" extended into the nineteenth century. Noel Parry and Jose Parry, *The Rise of the Medical Profession* (London: Croom Helm, 1976), 144–5.

27 Beryl Rowland, 18. Ironically, another study has noted that in 1724 John Maubray had little empirical experience, but was called in on occasion for advice of a "theoretical" nature. See H. R. Spencer, *The History of British Midwifery from 1650–1800* (London: John Bale, Sons & Danielsson, Ltd., 1927), 7–8. Despite this limitation, and the fact that he was censored by the College of Physicians in 1726 for practising without a licence, Maubray is described a few pages later as "the first teacher of practical midwifery," thereby discounting at one stroke the traditional system of midwifery training in which countless women had been instructed since time immemorial. Schnorrenberg, 398; Spencer, 14.

28 Loudon, 90. Loudon sees this aspect as more important than the proliferation of obstetrical forceps. See below, "Epilogue" for a more detailed discussion of the men midwives.

handwriting on the wall. Her testimonial certificate was signed by two M.D.s, a surgeon, and Robert Johnson, "surgeon and man-midwife of London." There is no testimony from women or parish clergy. Henry Newton administered the oath and noted that she was licensed in surgery and midwifery, March 31, 1690.[29] Although Mistress Francis acquired her knowledge of midwifery through the practical experience from which the male practitioners who signed her testimonial certificate were largely excluded, the four men attested to the following statement:

These are to certify whom it may concern having examined Mrs. Elizabeth Francis I find her to be very well instructed and practiced in the art of midwifery and also in the knowledge of medicines which may be of use to women in their several maladies . . . [30]

Midwife-surgeon Francis was, evidently, unique. The dual licence, however, would offer an ideal combination of traditional female skills and the capacity to employ the instruments of the surgeon if the necessity arose.[31] Perhaps if more women had been afforded the opportunity to train in both fields, the history of obstetrics would have been written in a completely different way.[32] As it is, Mrs. Francis' testimonial stands as an ominous portent of the way in which the male practitioners were assuming, with the consent of prospective midwives themselves, an authoritarian role in midwifery practice. In another instance of the way in which authority in midwifery was being linked to the male professionals, the records of the Royal College of Physicians note that in December 1689, "Mrs. Wolverston came to have our hands to her being a Licentiate in Midwifery. She was examined and modestly and prudently answered to our satisfaction."[33] The changes were slow and affected only a handful of individuals during the seventeenth century itself, but with the benefit of hindsight, we can see that they foreshadowed the more dramatic changes to come.

Aside from the difficulties inherent in his intrusion into a traditionally female event, the surgeon attempting to establish himself as a male midwife was faced with the problem of his inexperience in normal deliveries as well as the taint of

29 This surgeon and man-midwife was no doubt the same "Doctor Johnson" who was paid by St Dunstan in the West after two midwives experienced difficulty with the delivery of Judith Edwards in 1698. See above, 130, n. 140.
30 GL MS 10,116/13. No connection between Mrs. Francis and the Barber-Surgeons Company has been found, which suggests that her training as a surgeon was not by way of serving a full apprenticeship. A handful of women received ecclesiastical licences in surgery under particular circumstances, but to date no evidence has been found of female surgeons (as opposed to barbers) who were bound and made free as surgeons of the London Barber-Surgeons Company. D. Evenden "Gender Differences," 195–7.
31 The highly-successful Dutch midwife, Catharina Schrader, had been married to a surgeon which undoubtedly influenced her own practice. Marland, " 'Stately and dignified'," 272.
32 Most women would have found the difficulties insurmountable, even if they were permitted to apprentice as surgeons to members of the Barber-Surgeons Company: the double training would involve virtually two apprenticeships.
33 Clark, 363. Mrs. Wolverston may well have taught her examiners something about midwifery. There is no trace of an ecclesiastical licence for midwife Wolverston, who may have merely used the backing of the College to enhance her reputation as a midwife.

an association with instrumental deliveries of dead fetuses and, in some cases, the death of the mother.[34] As early as 1611, barber-surgeon James Blackborne "was found fitt" and allowed to practice "in that Chirurgicall p'te of Surgery touching the generatyve pte of women and bringing them to bedd in their dangerous and difficult labours."[sic] Blackborne had been given specific permission by the Barber-Surgeons Company to intervene surgically in difficult labours by using their hooks and crochets to remove the child, thus sacrificing the infant to save the mother.[35] In 1671, William Sermon's advice manual to midwives offered a number of "medicines" for use in difficult labours. If these failed he notes:

... there are several other ways, but more severe and violent; as the Crochet, Hooks, Tongs and other instruments made for the same purpose. But seeing such remedies are most commonly made use of by men, called to women in such a deplorable state, I shall here omit to make any further mention of them ... [36]

Members of the Chamberlen family, who touted their services as male midwives, ran into trouble with the College of Physicians on several occasions. The Chamberlens had their instruments, but their knowledge of normal childbirth, like that of other male professionals of the day, was inadequate.[37] During the reign of James I, Peter Chamberlen senior faced "a complaint of *mala praxis* in child-bed women" and was forbidden to practice for an unspecified period of time.[38] In 1634, the College decreed that Peter Chamberlen's use of "iron instruments" was allied more to surgery than medicine and was not a part of normal midwifery.[39] More than 50 years later, Hugh Chamberlen was faced with a charge of malpractice after a woman whom he had treated miscarried and died.[40] A contemporary of Hugh senior aptly described him as "Doctor, Projectir, man-midwife and cheat."[41] Although the College prosecuted a number of female empirics for malpractice in the pre-revolutionary period, none of them were midwives, either unlicensed or licensed.

A new alternative to forceps arrived on the scene with the Leiden publication

---

34 For one mother's reaction, see Houlbrooke, 10.

35 Sidney Young, *The Annals of the Barber-Surgeons of London* (London, East & Blades, 1890, reprint N.Y.: A.M.S. Press, 1978), 330.

36 Sermon, 141.

37 The Chamberlens' entrepreneurial bent extended into the eighteenth century, when Paul Chamberlen advertised, stressing the family name, a "wonderful necklace," the wearing of which would relieve the distress of teething children, ailments of the head, and women in labour. BL E112/169.

38 At the same time, an unidentified midwife successfully proved charges against a surgeon, Mr. Douglas, whose "inhumane and unskilful" handling of a woman in labour resulted in the death of mother and child. Charles Goodall, *The Royal College of Physicians of London. An Account of their proceedings against empirics* (London, 1684), 367, 368. The surgeon was required to post a bond of £200 against practising midwifery in the future, as well repaying £5, presumably his fee.

39 Sir George Clark, *A History of the Royal College of Physicians of London* vol.1 (Oxford: Clarendon Press, 1964), 162.

40 Ibid., 362. In 1670, Chamberlen's reputation had led Mauriceau to call on him to assist in a difficult delivery while visiting in France. He was unsuccessful in his attempt to use forceps, and the woman died. Fred J. Taussig, "Chamberlen and Mauriceau: an unsuccessful Forceps application in 1670," *Interstate Medical Journal* (vol.xxii, 1915), 5–62.

41 Quoted in a letter by Bryan Hibbar, *Acta Belgica Historiae Medicinae* (vol.5, no.2, 1992), 84.

of the work of Hendrik Van Deventer in 1701 and its translation into English in 1716 and 1724. Relying mainly on hand manoeuvres of the child, uterus, and coccyx, the techniques appealed to London practitioners who opposed the use of forceps.[42] Married to a midwife with whom he worked, Deventer's theories and practice bore the stamp of the less invasive deliveries carried out by traditional midwives.[43]

THE ROLE OF MIDWIFERY FORCEPS

William Giffard has been credited with the first recorded use of forceps or "extractor" as it was called in April 1726 and, by 1733, when the design of obstetrical forceps was published, surgeons were offered an adjunct to their destructive instruments when called upon by midwives in complicated deliveries.[44] In theory, at least, when judiciously applied by a knowledgeable operator, the baby could be safely delivered as a happy alternative to the previous destructive interventions. Several recent studies have attributed women's choice of the male midwife over the traditional female to their perception that a living child could be delivered by the use of forceps should complications arise. Forceps have been seen as key to the decline of the midwife, but it is a tenuous claim at best when the evidence is examined.

In his study of the problems facing twentieth-century midwives in North America who are currently fighting for legal accreditation, Raymond DeVries has linked the midwife's noninterventionist convictions and the key role of technology "from the invention of the forceps to the development of the fetal heart monitor" to "the midwife's loss of independence."[45] But was the use of forceps a critical factor in ensuring safer deliveries for mother and child?

The eminent eighteenth-century practitioner and male midwife William Hunter noted, "I am clearly of the opinion . . . that the forceps (midwifery instruments in general I fear) upon the whole, has done more harm than good." Blunter yet was his rejection of forceps on the grounds that "Where they save one, they murder twenty."[46]

---

42 For a full explanation of Deventer's methods, as well as a discussion of political divisions, which fostered pro forceps or pro Deventarian camps, see Wilson, *Making of Man Midwifery*, 79–87.
43 Ibid., 80.
44 William Giffard, *Cases in Midwifry* (London: B. Motte and T. Wotton, 1734). There is no indication of where Giffard received his instruction in midwifery.
45 Raymond G. DeVries, *Making Midwives Legal; Childbirth, Medicine and the Law* (2nd ed. Columbus: Ohio State University Press, 1996), 28.
46 His opposition possibly sprang from his loss of a patient whose uterus was fatally ruptured at the Brownlow Street Lying in Hospital. Herbert Spencer, *The History of British Midwifery*, 73; R. Hingston Fox, *William Hunter* (London, 1901), 44. Adrian Wilson, "William Hunter and the varieties of man-midwifery," W. F. Bynum and Roy Porter, *William Hunter*, 343, 362. Wilson's final position is that forceps were a key factor in the obstetrical revolution. For a discussion of Giffard's work, see Wilson, *Making of Man-midwifery*, 91–103. As to the question of why midwives did not use forceps, the Chamberlen forceps were kept secretly for family use only, throughout the seventeenth century. Midwives were also bound by the terms of their oath, which implicitly

Jean Donnison has pointed out the way in which "unnecessary and careless use of instruments by male practitioners attracted continual condemnation from leading men in the field," not only in the early modern period, but into the present century.[47] Laurel Thatcher Ulrich has compared the record of an eighteenth-century New England midwife with those of contemporary New England physicians (with access to forceps) who delivered infants as part of their practise. Martha Ballard's rate of 1.8 stillbirths per 100 live births was lower than that of either of the physicians with whom her practice was compared while all rates were lower than "impressionistic" data of the period normally cited by historians.[48]

By analysing the anonymous midwife's account book, we find that of 683 births, only four were "born dead." There is no way of telling whether these accounts are a complete record of all of this woman's deliveries. If they can be taken as at all representative, they yield a stillbirth rate of 0.6 per 100 births.[49] There is no mention of a maternal death in her records.[50]

On the other hand, *Cases in Midwifery*, the records of eighteenth-century male midwife, William Giffard, published in 1734, three years after his death, chronicle an astonishingly high failure rate. Even given the fact that he was called into obstetric emergencies, the catastrophic losses he experienced, in terms of infant and maternal deaths, while attempting to become adept in the use of forceps, would have been enough to discourage any perceptive, prospective clients. In the last 12 months of his recorded practice, when his skills should have been at their peak, he recorded 66 cases (including the delivery of twins). When we take into

forbade the use of destructive instruments (early forceps could well be perceived to fall into this category), as well as the long-standing taboo against the use of surgical instruments in female hands.

47 Jean Donnison, "The Development of the Occupation of Midwife: a Comparative View," *Midwifery is a Labour of Love* (Vancouver, B.C.: Maternal Health Society, 1981), 5. The debate among the doctors themselves regarding the safety of forceps deliveries has continued throughout the nineteenth and twentieth centuries. See, for example, "Mortality in Childbirth," *The Lancet* (1866), 269; "Epilogue."

48 Laurel Thatcher Ulrich " 'The Living Mother of a Living Child': Midwifery and Mortality in Post-Revolutionary New England," *William and Mary Quarterly* 46 (January 1989): 31–3. The doctors would have access to forceps to assist them in delivering a living child (by their own claim) in complicated cases. The twentieth-century Alabama midwife, Onnie Lee Logan, could recall only three stillbirths in her practice, which spanned four or five decades. Logan, 124.

49 BL Rawlinson MS D 1141. This is an extremely low rate of infant mortality at the time of delivery and we do not know if the pregnancies were full term. Since the midwife was keeping these records as an account of earnings, there is no reason to believe that she would hide any obstetrical disasters. If they are an accurate reflection of her practice, and we have no way of telling this, then they are an indication of her great skill in managing abnormal, as well as normal deliveries. We are unable to compare this rate with, for example, Schofield's and Wrigley's work on infant mortality, which includes death from all causes and is not restricted to perinatal or neonatal deaths. Schofield and Wrigley, "Infant and Child Mortality" in Webster. The Frisian midwife, Vrouw Schrader, had a perinatal mortality rate (single births) of 4.5%, which Marland states compares favourably with European and American figures before 1945. Marland, "Mother and Child," 37.

50 Donnison reports that after hundreds of years of perceived abuse of forceps intervention, in the 1930s the Ministry of Health for England and Wales confirmed the fact that forceps deliveries resulted in higher maternal and infant death rates. Donnison, "The Development of the Occupation Midwife," 5.

account the deliveries which were actually carried out by midwives, of the resulting 56 deliveries for which Giffard was personally responsible, 21 children were "born dead" and 37 live births were recorded, including 5 infants who, by his admission, suffered various injuries from the forceps.[51] Giffard's shocking rate of 37 dead infants per 100 deliveries could hardly have been a persuasive argument for calling for a male midwife and his forceps.[52] In addition, there were four maternal deaths recorded with an inevitable fifth unrecorded (Giffard thought it "more prudent" to leave some afterbirth in the uterus).[53]

In commenting on eighteenth-century midwife Elizabeth Nihell's criticism of Smellie's use of forceps, Wallace B. Shute has noted that the "undependable and primitive forceps of the day gave her plenty of ammunition for her comments."[54] A few years after Nihell's assaults, Philip Thicknesse attacked the institution of male midwifery in *Man Midwifery Analysed*. His attack was mounted on several fronts. Siding with Nihell's assessment of forceps in the hands of male practitioners, he accused male midwives of indiscriminate, frequent, and "injurious" use of forceps whose use they concealed from everyone in attendance so that they could not be charged with any resultant injuries.[55]

A recent study of the rise of the man-midwife eulogises the forceps noting "that we implicitly regard its existence as inscribed in the natural order."[56] However, obstetricians and gynaecologists are still divided as to their appropriate and safe use. In 1992, Wallace B. Shute, a leading obstetrician and designer of the forceps which bear his name, set forth nine criteria for forceps which render them safe in all situations for mother and child. He further notes that no forceps were clinically proven to meet all of these criteria until the 1960s, despite the "three hundred year litany of . . . frequent tragic failures."[57]

---

51 These figures are derived from Giffard's records covering November 1730 to October 1731. William Giffard, *Cases in Midwifery*, revised and published by Edward Hody (London 1734). In 7 of the 66 cases, midwives had already delivered the mother, but Giffard was called to remove the placenta (2 cases), because postpartum haemorrhage had occurred (2 cases), for reasons unspecified (2 cases), and one case where he instructed the midwife in the removal of a hydatid mole because the mother, a gentlewoman, refused to have him touch her (437–8). In an eighth instance, Giffard removed a retained placenta with no mention of a midwife. My findings are at odds with those of Adrian Wilson, who concluded that Giffard's rate of stillbirths in the latter phase of his practice was "one-in-ten." Wilson, *Making of Man-midwifery*, 98.

52 These rates are disastrous even if taking into consideration that Giffard, predictably, blamed the midwife in at least one case, for the infant's death. Giffard, 511, October 1731, the last month of his recorded practice.

53 Giffard, 502–3. Not all male midwives embraced the forceps with such rash and misplaced confidence: William Waylett of Kent, who practised in the late eighteenth century, used the forceps only five times in his twenty-year practice, which involved almost 2,900 births. F. William Cock, *The Life Work of an Eighteenth-century Man-Midwife* (London, 1907), 387.

54 Wallace B. Shute, "History of Obstetrical Forceps from 1750 to the present era," *Acta Belgica Historiae Medicinae* vol. 5, (no. 2, 1992): 66.

55 Philip Thicknesse, *Man Midwifery Analysed* (London 1764), 3, 9.

56 Wilson, *Making of Man-midwifery*, 71. This type of assumption has informed Wilson's study and resulted in the implicit, if unintended, approval of the displacement of traditional midwives by men.

57 Shute, 68.

If forceps did assist male midwives in the displacement of the traditional mid-wife, the assistance could only have arisen with the connivance and dishonesty of the men who not only falsely claimed their efficacy, but justified their use when they were unnecessary.

THE APPROPRIATION OF FEMALE EXPERIENCE

In any discussion of the fate of female midwives, the question must be addressed of how the surgeons, called to only the occasional difficult delivery, acquired the necessary experience to supplant the highly skilled and competent midwife with her previously unassailable authority in female matters.[58] Only tenuous links between midwives and members of the Barber-Surgeons Company have been found. In 1611, Laurence Higginson of St Martin Ludgate, husband of Anne, a licensed midwife, was licensed as a barber-surgeon.[59] There is no evidence that Higginson was a male midwife, but he may have learned midwifery techniques from his wife or they may have operated as a husband and wife team. Despite his family's monopoly of forceps, in 1634, Peter Chamberlen endeavoured to become the only surgeon upon whom the midwives could call because he real-ized that the key to not only gaining the monetary rewards of the situation but, more important, to gaining practical knowledge of the parturient female anatomy and physiology lay in frequent access to women in labour. A close association, or better, an exclusive association with the experienced London midwives would give him the entrée to what he sought. Percival Willughby described a delivery which his daughter was supervising, and for which she wished a second opinion. Willughby was obliged to crawl into the room and carry out the examination shrouded by sheets to avoid detection by the woman, so strong was the taboo against male invasion of the childbed chamber. Willughby became the highly visible author and midwifery "authority" and, although it has been commonly assumed that his daughter obtained her expertise from her father's instruction, there is every likelihood that the reverse is true and his most valuable experience and training were gained through an association with his midwife daughter.[60] Willughby also had the expertise of a Mrs. Willughby to call on. She was a kinswoman, a midwife living in London, whom Willughby described as "long experimented . . . of much practice, and of good repute with women."[61]

58 This question remains unanswered in the recent book by Adrian Wilson, *The Making of Man-midwifery*.
59 Bloom and James, 20. Not all members of the barber-surgeon's company were licensed in surgery; many were accredited as barbers only. See Doreen Evenden "Gender differences in the training and licensing of female and male surgeons in Early Modern England," *Medical History* (April 1998).
60 Aveling, 54–8.
61 Ibid., 59–60. Willughby ostensibly moved to London for reasons involving his "children's" edu-cation. Since his children were adults at the time of Willughby's move (he himself was 60 years old), and he remained only three or four years in London, there is a good chance he came to London to work with this woman and learn from her. In the sixteenth century, a German

When Alice Flewelling of St Peter the Poor was licensed in midwifery in 1687, she gave her husband's occupation as surgeon, establishing another link between female midwifery knowledge and the male practitioner. Aside from the occasional instance of a liaison between a surgeon and midwife, however, male practitioners were hard pressed to gain practical experience in midwifery.[62]

There are scattered references in the literature of the period to private maternity hospitals which were located in homes in the City which, in some cases, had their own midwives.[63] In the seventeenth century, at the parish level, midwives were still called to deliver poor women at parish expense.[64] With the advent of the lying-in hospitals in the 1730s, however, poor women no longer remained in the parish where they had frequently been accommodated in private homes.[65] Instead, they were admitted to the hospitals, which were presided over by male practitioners, who now had access to the labours of poor women. As a study by Versluysen has similarly concluded, this would prove to be the critical factor among the complex issues which contributed to the displacement of the midwife from her position of authority in matters of child delivery (see Epilogue, below).[66] In her study of childbearing in America in the eighteenth, nineteenth, and twentieth centuries, Judith Walzer Leavitt has argued that the childbirth experience remained essentially female as long as the delivery took place at home; this changed when birthing moved to the hospital.[67] Although midwives in London still carried out most of the deliveries in the lying-in hospitals, the birth process had passed into the control of males.[68] Moreover, the traditional knowledge of the ancient

physician was burned at the stake for attending deliveries dressed as a woman in a desperate effort to learn about delivery processes. See E. Burton, *The Jacobeans at Home* (London: Secker and Warburg, 1962), 228.

62 Hilary Marland has noted that the noted author and authority on midwifery, Hendrik van Deventer, married a midwife, thereby gaining an advantage in terms of midwifery practice. Marland, " 'Stately and dignified'," 282.

63 MacLeod Yeardsley, *Doctors in Elizabethan Drama* (London: John Bale Sons and Danielsson Ltd. 1933), 88–9.

64 In all of the parish records which have been examined, the single exception was the entry about Dr. Johnson being called upon for assistance in a difficult delivery, in 1698, in St Dunstan in the West. See above, n. 29.

65 See, for example, GL MS 2999/1 Account Book of Overseers for St Dunstan in the West, 1634 (unfol.) when the parish paid Goodwife Holden for a month's lodging and postpartum care of Margaret Crowder. In 1658, the parish paid for a room for Jane Waters' lying-in and for a woman to look after her for a month, as well as the midwife's fee. See also Wilson, "Childbirth," 4–5.

66 Donnison, 26–7. This argument will be developed more fully in the Epilogue. I wish to acknowledge the work of Margaret Connor Versluysen, whose insightful study "Midwives, medical men and 'poor women labouring of child': lying-in hospitals in eighteenth-century London," Helen Roberts, ed., *Women, Health and Reproduction* (London: Routledge and Keegan Paul, 1981), 18–49, supports many of my own conclusions arrived at independently through archival research.

67 Judith Walzer Leavitt, *Brought to Bed* (New York, Oxford: Oxford University Press, 1986), 115, 202–3.

68 Judith Walzer Leavitt has argued the case for America and sees that female loss of control of the birthing situation coincides with the hospitalization of virtually all deliveries in the twentieth century. When doctors carried out home deliveries in the eighteenth and nineteenth centuries, they were "invited" into the women's homes, and women remained in charge since the prospective mother was usually attended by "birthing companions" with considerable experience. Leavitt, 4–5. Today there is a growing awareness of the need for the attendance of an advocate to help

midwives was no longer the exclusive preserve of women. Once men became seriously engaged in entering the field of midwifery, women could not possibly mount an adequate defence of their territory; the whole weight of tradition and history ensured what the outcome would be.[69]

The replacement of the traditional midwife by a male practitioner during the eighteenth century can be seen as the result of the convergence of a number of factors.[70] The Church's declining role in the process of licensing, the availability of forceps to male practitioners, and their promotion by men who were motivated by the desire to enjoy some of the monetary rewards of child delivery, the intellectual climate of the "Enlightenment" generally receptive to the claims of "scientific" knowledge, and, most important, the advent of the lying-in hospital, all contributed to the demise of the complex and effective system in which London midwives proudly functioned in the seventeenth century.[71] Ahead lay the sordid chapter on puerperal sepsis (childbed fever) as well as other forms of iatrogenic disorders.[72] Despite male protestations to the contrary, women and their infants were to be the losers for generations to come.

In conclusion, our study of seventeenth-century London midwives has not only identified hundreds of previously nameless women who carried out the important task of child delivery within one of Europe's most rapidly expanding cities, it has brought to light information about a great many of them which was

women delivering in hospital to make informed decisions and retain some sense of dignity and autonomy in the experience of childbirth.

69 See Lorraine Code, *What Can She Know?: Feminist Theory and the Construction of Knowledge* (Ithaca: Cornell Press, 1991), 68–9, 206, 225. For a discussion of the enduring legacy of the ancients' "scientific" writings regarding women's perceived mental and physical inferiority, see Vern L. Bullough, "Medieval Medical and Scientific Views of Women," *Viator*, vol. 4 (1973) 485–501.

70 For a "whig" interpretation, see William F. Mengert, *Annals of Medical History*, NS 4 (1932): 453–63.

71 Anne Giardina Hess has noted with regret the loss of Quaker midwives' "unique partnership with the pre-industrial community" that came with their declining role. Giardina Hess, "Community case studies," 346–7.

72 Loudon describes the early lying-in hospitals as "a disaster" because of the epidemics of puerperal fever, which they engendered. Irvine Loudon, ed. *Childbed Fever: a documentary study* (New York and London: Garland, 1995), xxxvi. See Donnison for the long-term developments of the struggle between the midwives and the medical profession. Donnison's observation that the "United States' maternal mortality rate is higher than that of comparable European countries where midwives attend a majority of births" is supported by Leavitt's work; see Leavitt, 24, 183–4, in particular. More recent support for our contention is found in C. G. Pantin, "A Study of Maternal Mortality and Midwifery on the Isle of Man, 1882 to 1961," *Medical History*, 40 (1996): 141–72, which concludes that fewer maternal deaths would have occurred if deliveries had been left in the hands of midwives. In Great Britain, New Zealand, and Scandinavia in the 1920s, deliveries attended by nurses and midwives (or completely unattended) generated lower death rates than those attended by physicians. In the years 1921–27, the maternal death rate in Manitoba (Canada) hospitals was 8.6%. For the same period outside of hospitals (where women attendants frequently assisted), it was 2.65%. Both of the foregoing examples are from "Doctoring the Family," CBC radio, April 4, 1985. (We do not know if the physicians were called to deliver women at higher risk for complications, nor if the hospital figures include women who were hospitalized in anticipation of difficult labours.) Iatrogenic illness is produced by medical treatment. Its agents are treatments, physicians, and hospitals. Ivan Illich, *Limits to Medicine* (Toronto: McClelland & Stewart, 1976).

previously unknown. We now have a better appreciation of how the ecclesiastical licensing system functioned. We know the way the unofficial apprenticeship system produced a supportive network of more experienced midwives who worked alongside trainee midwives. We have a better idea of the fees they charged and the distribution of their practices. The picture which has emerged is one of mature married or widowed women who have themselves borne children, and have acquired years of practical experience. These women were respected and acclaimed for their expertise not only by their clients, but by members of their parish communities, both rich and poor. Almost without exception, their spouses, as well as their children, were responsible parishioners who were economically self-sufficient. In the case of widows, the majority continued to support themselves throughout their lives. Indeed, a substantial number of midwives (including widows) enjoyed a socioeconomic position which befitted the well-to-do. It is our hope that, at least for London, the ghost of the indigent, slovenly, and maladroit midwife has finally been laid to rest.

Epilogue[1]

Because in former times, men were only calld upon extraordinary occasions; some of which (however skilful and ingenious) had not the opportunity of Laying a woman perhaps in many months.. . . .they must have been at a loss in not understanding thoroughly the Practical Part. John Maubray M.D. *The Female Physician* (London, 1724), 180.

Childbearing London women were not completely deprived of the services of accredited female midwives in the eighteenth century, even though after the 1720s the midwives themselves no longer operated within the self-regulating, cooperative and ecclesiastically based network of the seventeenth century. But midwives had lost their self-confidence as they came increasingly under the supervision of male physicians and surgeons. Midwives were no longer undisputed "experts" in infanticide trials; male medical practitioners increasingly dominated court hearings in the eighteenth century.[2] Physicians and surgeons assumed control of the training and accreditation process, and, in so doing, began flooding the market with male practitioners claiming competence in the art of midwifery. By 1745, surgeons were virtually "compelled to practice midwifery" (as well as pharmacy) in order to survive.[3] Writing in 1748, a critic of William Smellie, the

---

1 The foregoing conclusion relates to a study of seventeenth-century midwives in London and stands as a summation of my research on that remarkable group of women. The following discussion is an attempt to answer questions which arose during that study, but required further examination of different archival records relating to the *eighteenth* century. The result is a broadening, strengthening and enriching of the conclusions which were reached earlier. I wish to acknowledge the assistance of the Social Sciences and Humanities Research Council of Canada and Trent University for partially funding the research undertaken for this "Epilogue."

2 Mark Jackson, "Developing Medical Expertise: Medical Practitioners and the Suspected Murders of New-Born Children," Roy Porter, ed., *Medicine in the Enlightenment* (Amsterdam: Rodopi, 1995), 147.

3 Bernice Hamilton, "The Medical Professions in the Eighteenth Century," *The Economic History Review* Second Series (4, 1951): 151. Competition was not as stiff in the provinces and, as late as 1780, the majority of women in Warwickshire were delivered with the help of midwives and neighbours, although the parish surgeon would be called in to terminate complicated labours much as he had done a century earlier in London. Joan Lane, "The Provincial Practitioner and his Services to the Poor, 1750–1800," *Society for the History of Medicine* Bulletin 31 (1982): 12. For the high cost of a medical education, James Axtell, "Education and Status in Stuart England: the London Physician," *History of Education Quarterly* 10 (1970): 141–59.

prominent eighteenth-century male midwife, claimed that there were then five times more surgeons than jobs resulting, in "more men-midwives than streets."[4]

THE FOUNDING OF THE LYING-IN HOSPITALS AND THE ROYAL MATERNITY CHARITY

Although the takeover was the result of a number of converging circumstances, the establishment of the lying-in hospital was, arguably, the single most important factor in the demise of the authority and superiority of the female midwife. Records of the first lying-in hospitals reveal the role of physicians and surgeons in appropriating the knowledge and experience of female childbirth practitioners (the matron and her assistant), and in conferring their approval on males and females alike seeking to practice midwifery. This approval was usually gained through courses offered at the hospital under the doctors' supervision or a series of private lectures, and then practical experience in the lying-in facility. Charles White, a physician writing in the eighteenth century, candidly described a lying-in hospital in the London area in this way: "It was instituted for the purpose of instructing young gentlemen. . . ."[5]

JERMYN STREET

In 1739, Dr. Richard Manningham opened a small private lying-in hospital in a house on Jermyn Street claiming that his concern was:

poor women . . . who very often perish in labouring of Child, together with their infants, for want of timely and skilful Assistance in their Labour, and proper Care and Necessaries during their Lying-in . . . [6]

But a closer examination of his proposal reveals another agenda. Very few, if any, poor women would actually benefit from the services of the tiny hospital: His real motive was to provide midwifery students with live bodies on which to polish the skills learned in Manningham's lectures and on his glass machine designed to simulate a female pelvis, complete with fetus.[7] Manningham would provide some

---

4 W. M. Douglas, *A Letter to Dr. Smellie* . . . (London: 1748), 6. Douglas was a physician and male midwife.
5 C. White, *A Treatise on the Management of Pregnant and Lying-in Women* (London, 1773), 337.
6 Sir Richard Manningham, *The Institution and Oeconomy of the Charitable Infirmary for the Relief of Poor Women Labouring of Child and during their Lying-in* (1739). Reprinted in *An abstract of midwifery for the use of the Lying-in Infirmary* (London: 1744), 27.
7 Only women sponsored by a benefactor (subscriber) could be admitted to the hospital. All others must pay two guineas *before admission*. Poor women without a sponsor could only be admitted free of charge if, after the expenses of rent, etc., had been covered, there was a surplus in the coffers. Moreover, if London or Westminster parishes wanted to send a poor woman, they must pay her maintenance during the lying-in period with Manningham and his staff providing only free delivery and any necessary medical care (including prescriptions). Manningham *Abstract*, 34–5. Poor women had long been seen as suitable candidates for aspiring male midwives to deliver. Percival Willughby noted his early London practice (1656) "among the meaner sort of women." Willughby, 238.

sort of certification to pupils taking his midwifery courses, which were geared and priced according to gender. Male students, particularly medical students, were to be given a compendium of midwifery published in Latin, reflecting perceptions of their greater intellectual capacity and more sophisticated education, and would pay a total fee of twenty guineas for their course, which included instruction in a "genuine delivery." Female students, using an English publication, would pay ten guineas with no mention of hands-on instruction in the hospital, the implication being that female midwifery students already had adequate experience in child delivery. Discounting generations of competent midwifery practice by women within their remarkable peer networks, Manningham condescendingly wrote that the practice of midwifery had improved in his time:

since the Women . . . have admitted the Assistance of both sexes; and the Men being more skilful in Anatomy, and better disposed to find out Help in unforeseen Cases, are therefore more capable of bringing it to a greater Perfection.[8]

At odds with Manningham's assertions were the claims of Jane Sharp, who had specifically charged that male midwives, unlike female midwives who worked within a network of midwives, bound by oath to seek the help of other, more experienced midwives if necessary, did not call in help when in difficulty in order to hide their deficiencies. Despite their inadequacies, traditional midwives would deliver all clients at Manningham's hospital except "difficult and dangerous cases" in which case the physician purportedly would deliver them "gratis," ostensibly using various instruments at his disposal.[9] Little else is known about this institution but, in all probability, it failed to survive after 1744.[10]

THE MIDDLESEX LYING-IN HOSPITAL

A few years later, at a meeting of the governors of the Middlesex Hospital in April 1747, a Dr. Cox introduced a proposal drafted by a Dr. D. Layard: it was agreed that a few beds would be set aside for married women in their last month of pregnancy for their delivery and for care "during their indisposition after their delivery." Layard was subsequently appointed male midwife in ordinary to the hospital with Dr. Sandys to be summoned in "all doubtful cases" in his capacity as male midwife extraordinary. It was further stated that no woman midwife could be named or designated the official "midwife to the hospital," that is, as the top midwifery expert or consultant. This did not mean that female midwives would not be in attendance, but that they would be relegated to the less prestigious rank of "matron." This position entailed hard work, including most of the deliveries, as well as responsibility for the domestic details of the institution, with little or no recognition or authority.

The exclusion of women from the key midwifery positions speaks volumes about the increasing ambition of the medical men in their attempts to secure for

8 Manningham, 31.   9 Ibid., 34.   10 Versluysen, 37.

themselves control of the childbirth process and the denigration of traditional midwives, both inside and outside the hospitals.[11] At this first meeting, it was also decided that for the present, no "pupils whatsoever be permitted to attend the lying in ward." Underlying this regulation (but left unspoken), was the doctors' actual lack of competence and confidence in their midwifery skills. The learning process would take place unobserved by outsiders. Only the matron/midwife and her male counterparts who were staff physicians and surgeons would be privy to a situation where a matron imparted traditional knowledge and skills garnered by generations of midwives. In this way, the doctors would not lose face. As contemporary John Maubray, M.D. noted in 1724, men could easily learn midwifery from well experienced women if they were "more docile and not such obstinate creatures."[12]

Moreover, there were no advocates for the poor, female recipients of the doctors' initial attempts at delivery who would bring to light the bungled births. A glance at the Lying-in Register of the Middlesex Hospital for the years 1747–54 reveals the humble status of its maternity admissions: wives of tradesmen, soldiers, mariners, servants, and even the wife of an unfortunate in prison for debt. Women married to soldiers, mariners, or prisoners would have no male at hand to protest or protect them, while other clients of lowly stature would be unlikely or unable to voice any complaint about the invasive procedures of the male staff or against the controlling male hierarchy.[13]

Preparations began immediately to ready beds for lying-in women and the first midwifery patient was admitted June 30, 1747, with the first baptism of a child born at the hospital taking place July 21. The first year saw twenty-six admissions with twenty-five live births.[14] The first matron and midwife was Mrs. Page, who held the position for two years. Page resigned and was succeeded by Mary Dinning in October 1749.[15] On August 1, 1749, ten beds were designated for lying-in purposes but, by September 1749, Drs. Sandys and Cox were expressing dissatisfaction at the small number of beds set aside for expectant mothers. By October 1749, Dr. Sandys had left and been replaced by Dr. Douglas, while in December, Dr. Cox resigned from his position.[16] In December also, Mary Stephens was appointed matron (and midwife) to replace Mary Dinning, who died in December, barely two months after her appointment.[17] Stephens' work apparently gained the approval of her superiors who granted her a gratuity of ten

---

11 Vesluysen sees this establishment of an occupational hierarchy as a key point in establishing male superiority in the practice of midwifery. Versluysen, 32, 38–9.

12 Erasmus Wilson, *The History of the Middlesex Hospital during the First Century of its Existence* (London: 1845), 6. John Maubray, *The Female Physician*, 178.

13 See also the valuable insights of Versluysen on this point. Versluysen, 32–3.

14 Ibid., 8; Middlesex Hospital Fair Minute Book (after MFMB), 1748–50, 95. Surviving archival sources for the Middlesex Lying-in Hospital are housed in the present Middlesex Hospital archives.

15 MFMB 1748–50, 193. We know that Mrs. Page was a midwife because she left the Middlesex Hospital (along with other staff) to become the first matron of the British Lying-in Hospital in 1749. The specifications for her position at the British Lying-in required that she be a midwife. See below, 190.

16 MFMB 1749–50, 140, 181, 202   17 MFMB 1748–50, 245.

guineas in July 1752, a substantial sum, and double that given the apothecary, Mr. Douglas.[18] Aside from this evidence relating to the matron, there is no reference to the women who carried out the important work of midwife in a lying-in ward in the early years. Generally referred to as "the Matron," she was excluded from the weekly board meetings of the hospital which were, on the other hand, attended by the male midwifery staff.

BROWNLOW STREET

Dissatisfied with the small number of beds, disgruntled medical staff of the Middlesex Lying-in decided to found another hospital with expanded quarters for lying-in women and, by November 1749, had purchased a house on Brownlow Street, Longacre, which would afford 20 beds for their purposes. At the first meeting on November 3, former Middlesex staffers Drs. Sandys and Cox, as well as Mr. Hunter, surgeon, were in attendance.[19] A lengthy appeal for the support of gentlewomen was drafted, asking them to recall their "own fears and sufferings" and support the new institution by becoming subscribers or governors. By the third meeting, November 17, four "gentlemen who practice midwifery" were appointed to staff the hospital. Three of the four were formerly at the Middlesex Lying-in: Dr. Daniel Layard, Dr. Francis Sandys, and Mr. William Hunter.

The defectors were joined by Stephen Degulhon, chaplain, Thomas Yeard, secretary, Nicholas Page, steward, and Mrs. Page, matron, all formerly employed in the same capacities at the Middlesex. The Duke of Portland, patron of the Middlesex Lying-in, was swayed by arguments that the "lying in wards were not getting their fair share of money," resigned and moved to become "president" of the new hospital on Brownlow Street.

The hospital would have two physicians "who practice midwifery, who in difficult cases are to deliver the women" in the weeks they were in attendance. The physicians were also "to prescribe necessary medicines *and give direction to the matron concerning the management of women and children*" [emphasis mine]. Two surgeons who "practice midwifery" alternated their attendance to provide surgical help where needed. The key figure in actual practice was, however, the matron whose duties were described as follows:

A matron, well skilled in midwifery, who is to deliver the Women in easy Naturall Labours, is to take care of the Linnen, to superintend the nurses, and to see that everything necessary for the women & children be provided according to the direction of the physicians & surgeons. But on the approach of any labour, she is to send to the Physician or Surgeon whose week of attendance it is, that he may judge whether the case requires his assistance or may be left to the Matron.[20]

18 MFMB 1752–54, 44.
19 Minutes of the Lying in Hospital for Married Women in Brownlow St near Longacre, Inst. 17th day of November 1749. GLRO H14/BLI/A1/1/1 (unfol.).
20 GLRO H14/BLI/A1/1/2. The staffing and structure of the hospital were outlined in the minutes of November 17, 1749.

It was soon decided that the busy matron needed an assistant, and midwife Barbara Godfrey was appointed to the position at about the same time as the death of Mrs. Page.[21] The vacancy created by Page's death was advertised in the *Daily Advertiser* and eventually, six candidates were considered for the matron's position. With the demise of the ecclesiastical licensing system, the six women had been forced to seek a variety of referees to confirm their midwifery skills.

Elizabeth Blunt was supported by Dr. Sandys, who attested to her skill and character. Esther Butler's letter of recommendation from the apothecary at St Thomas hospital was sent to staff surgeons/male midwives Torr and Hunter. Jane Duncan, who had been the assistant to Bell Alley midwife, Mrs. Usher, for a year, presented a certificate from her mentor stating that she "behaved exceeding well." Mrs. Waite, a midwife of Salisbury Court who had practiced for thirty years, personally spoke (along with an unidentified "lady") on behalf of a former pupil, Ruth More, who had eleven years' experience. Elizabeth Jackson brought along one of her clients who had used her services to deliver eight children over a twenty-five year period and had known her forty years. Ann Rea of Peckham, the final candidate under consideration, brought along her record of deliveries.[22]

Four of the candidates on the ballot, including the eventual appointee, Mrs. Esther Butler (hired at a salary of £26 per annum), were widows. Butler resigned less than two years later and was replaced by Mrs. Frances Oaks in May 1752.[23]

Stung by criticisms of the hospital which had been published in 1751 charging that one in fifteen babies died during delivery by the staff male midwives (described as "wicked men"), the hospital governors instructed that the following statement be published in 1752 along with figures showing deliveries and numbers of stillbirths:

Two experienced midwives constantly reside in the hospital. They deliver the women in all natural labours and the male midwives are called in where these cannot deliver them, which does not happen on the whole above once in 30 to 40 cases: so that the midwifery business of this hospital is certainly as much in the hands of women midwives as it can or ought to be.[24]

It goes on to say that instruments had been used only twice in the 545 deliveries, which took place between November 1749 and January 23, 1752. Obviously, if the published figures were correct, female midwives were carrying out the majority of deliveries and surgical intervention was seldom employed. Unfortunately,

21 Ibid., September 20, 1750.
22 Ibid., September 20, October 4, 1750. The unfortunate Catherine Pott failed to present any testimonial and was excluded from consideration. It is interesting to note that remnants of the system, whereby experienced women taught other women their midwifery skills, were still in existence but, except in a few isolated cases, there is no information about these women.
23 GLRO H14/BLI/A3/1 (Rough Minute Books) October 15 1751, May 1, 1752.
24 GLRO H14/BLI/A3/1/16. The hospital was responding to *The petition of the unborn babes to the censors of the Royal College of physicians of London* published in 1751 by F. Nicholls, a medical practitioner.

there is no way of telling whether the male midwives were, indeed, responsible for the bungled deliveries.[25] As in other lying-in hospitals, women were dying from puerperal fever. For the years 1749–58, the maternal death rate was 1 in 42 at the Brownlow Street Hospital with more than 20 women succumbing to puerperal infection in one particularly disastrous three-month period.[26]

Possibly as a further response to criticism, in June 1752, the board entertained a proposal for the training of female midwifery students. By the end of August, the program was outlined whereby four females, either widows or married women at least twenty-five years of age, would train for six months. They would be instructed by the gentlemen of the faculty in "everything that is necessary for women to know relating to the theory of midwifery regarding both natural and difficult births." After this, they would carry out deliveries under the supervision of faculty or the matron or deputy matron. Upon successful completion of the course, the gentlemen of the faculty would issue a certificate. In this way, the male staff of the hospital could preserve their control of the midwives while satisfying the demands for more female midwives.

In addition to the public perception that male midwives were less competent than their female counterparts, there is a good possibility that the active role played by the female governors at this hospital played a part in the decision to increase the number of female midwifery staff.[27] It was, moreover, spelled out that only females midwifery students would gain admission to the hospital.[28] Ostensibly motivated by the best of motives – to save lives by supplying well-instructed and experienced midwives for the benefit of "this great metropolis" as well as "the remotest parts of the kingdom" – the male midwives would be paid twenty guineas by each pupil whom they instructed. In addition, the students would pay 10s. weekly for board and lodging. The total cost of their training would be the substantial sum of more than £13.[29]

Over the next few years, a steady trickle of candidates came for training, entering at irregular intervals, and usually one at a time. Proud of its program, the board decided that advertisements listing the children baptised at the hospital should also contain the following note:

At this hospital Ladies have an opportunity of supplying themselves with good wet nurses and Female Pupils are here properly instructed in Midwifery.[30]

---

25 I suspect, because of their silence on this point, that the male midwives were, indeed, in attendance when bungled deliveries occurred. The doctors never hesitated to place the blame on female attendants whenever possible.

26 Martin Buer, *Health, Wealth and Population* (London: Routledge, 1926), 145; Spencer, 73; Anon, *An Account of the British Lying in Hospital for Married Women, Situated in Brownlow St, Long Acre from its institution in Nov. 1749 to Lady Day, 1756* (London, 1756).

27 Female subscribers or governors could vote by proxy, or by letter. As an indication of their active participation, in July 1751 at a Quarterly General Court, 88 men attended and voted, 58 women voted (57 by letter, 1 by proxy). For women of the period, this suggests an unusually high involvement in administrative matters. CLRO H14/BLI/A3/1/16.

28 Anon, *An Account of the Rise, Progress and State of the British Lying-in Hospital for Women. . . . ,* 13.

29 Ibid., 148. See also Minutes for August 27, 1752.   30 Ibid., November 17, 1755.

By April 1756, the hospital was renamed the British Lying In Hospital for Married Women.

THE CITY OF LONDON MATERNITY HOSPITAL

The lying-in hospital that contributed in no small part to the public's acceptance of the new institutions was the City of London Maternity Hospital (later City of London Lying-in) which opened in Aldersgate Street in 1750. This acceptance was based, not on lower mortality rates for mother and infant, but on better public relations. Whether accidentally or intentionally, the board and governors, in their efforts to maintain the economic viability of the hospital, did all the right things to present to an admiring public the image of grateful mothers and healthy, cherubic infants. Richard Brocklesby was appointed as the first physician and male midwife with Richard Ball, surgeon and male midwife. Thomas Meadows offered himself as resident male midwife, but his proposal was rejected by the governors who declared that it was "not their intention to have a man midwife within the hospital as the matron will be a midwife ready at any sudden call."[31] Three matrons held office between May 1750 and April 24, 1752 before Ruth Moore took on the task.[32]

At the hospital's board meeting in November 1751, it was resolved that "for the satisfaction of the public," women who had been delivered at the hospital should "repeat their thanks before the congregation at the baptism of the children." What better way to demonstrate the safety and efficiency of the new institutions than mass churchings of grateful mothers (the occasional unfortunate mother who failed to survive would hardly be missed) and rows of newborns in baptism finery?

The emotional appeal of these public ceremonies, regularly advertised in the newspapers, was not lost on the crowds that flocked to get a glimpse of the tiny darlings. Few, outside of the hospital board, would grasp the implications of the agreement with Peter Batt, undertaker, who took care of burials for the hospital at the competitive rates of £0.16.0 for women, £0.8.0 for baptised infants, and £0.3.6 for unbaptised infants.[33]

Christening tickets were printed in the thousands, and burgeoning attendances required structural changes to the chapel.[34] Fixed windows were replaced by casements to afford more air to the sweltering congregation; tables were removed from the chapel to make more room; new lighting was installed in the passageway

---

31 GLRO MS H10/CLM A1/1 (unfol.) Minute Book, May 20, 1750.
32 The three were Mary Coverly, Hanna Manning (who died after serving six months), and Katherine Evans. All were paid £15 per annum. The same salary was paid to Moore initially, but she was granted an increase to £20 less than a year later. Moore or More, had been an unsuccessful candidate for matron at Brownlow Street. See 191 above.
33 Minutes for July 15, 1752. Batt won the competition over William Carter, whose fees were slightly higher.
34 One thousand christening tickets were printed in July 1752, and another thousand were ordered eight months later in April 1753.

between the hospital proper and the chapel; and one side of the chapel was raised
to allow "more commodious seating" at the public christenings.[35] In addition to
music provided by a newly purchased organ, anthems were sung by a choir of
young gentlemen reading their notes from a stand especially constructed for them.
The appreciative audience rendered their thanks for the entertainment by contributing substantial sums to voluntary collections.[36]

THE CHARITY FOR ATTENDING AND DELIVERING POOR MARRIED WOMEN

Aside from the lying-in hospitals, the entrepreneurial bent of the male midwives
and the degraded status of traditional midwives are perhaps best illustrated by the
organization described as "the Charity for Attending and Delivering poor Married
Women in their Respective Habitations; Set on Foot March 25 1757," and later
known as the Royal Maternity Charity.[37]

A Mr. Tooley, whose qualifications are not known, had been serving the
Charity as male midwife (apparently at no cost to the Charity) when it was
proposed, in 1761, that he should be paid an annual salary of £40 and be given
an assistant to cover home deliveries in the Southwark area. Tooley, who was
plagued with creditors, was not satisfied with what the Charity offered and his
rudeness, coupled with an admission that he was asking some of his charity clients
to pay him a fee, resulted in his dismissal in August 1761.

The newly appointed assistant, J. Ford, moved into Tooley's position. Ford had
offered his services without pay until the Charity could pay him, but his motivation was not entirely altruistic. Ford's practical experience had come from an
association with a surgeon and male midwife in Ipswich. His surgical orientation
included "dressing" experience and anatomy lectures. Ford had attended midwifery lectures given by a Dr. Mackenzie, but like most aspiring male midwives
of the period, his practical experience of normal childbirth would be limited. The
Charity provided the ideal setting for gaining "hands-on" experience at the
expense of poor women, safely hidden from the gaze of onlookers who might
note his lack of expertise.

A year later, Ford's confidence waxed even as his charity waned, and he asked
for five shillings a delivery, a request which the Charity board of governors
refused. Instead, he was offered and accepted a salary of £50 a year. Barely sixteen
months later, in January 1764, Ford presented a proposal to the board whereby he

35 See minutes for September 20, October 13, December 11, 1752, May 23, 1753.
36 The public christenings continued to draw crowds to the hospital chapel while back in the wards,
the staff were trying unsuccessfully to eliminate the bugs which infested them, much to the distress
of the lying-in mothers. The attempt of one John Williams, in the summer of 1754, failed to
eradicate the infestation, and the board refused to pay him. The following June 24, bug traps were
purchased whose efficacy is unknown.
37 RCOG Minute Book of the Charity, no. 1. This source is unfoliated. The ensuing information in
the text will be cited by reference to the date. For another perspective on the Charity male
midwives, see Stanley A. Seligman, "The Royal Maternity Charity: The First Hundred Years,"
Medical History (24, 1980): 404.

would train women to serve as midwives in the Charity "intirely under my Direction, I would educate them myself and warrant them capable before they are employed by the Charity."

Their training was to be at no cost to the Charity and would last for two years. At the end of that time, they would be qualified to "do the bussiness in Common Cases" with Ford's assurance that he would "always assist them in extraordinary ones." The board consented to Ford's plan, and more than a century after the feisty London midwives of the 1640s successfully fought a similar scheme for their control by the ambitious Chamberlen enclave, Ford launched his self-serving enterprise under the guise of assisting the Charity.

It soon became apparent that Ford intended to charge the women who wished to be instructed by him. When the board learned that several women had applied for instruction but could not raise the required fee of ten guineas, they voted at an extraordinary meeting to give Ford thirty guineas for instructing three women. Candidates like Ann Green (or her husband Thomas) were required to sign an indemnification promising to pay the Charity ten guineas if they failed to serve the organization "gratis" for two years. I suspect that Ann Green was already competent at deliveries since her indemnification was dated May 4, 1764, and Ford pronounced her properly qualified to attend Charity patients barely seven weeks later. By September, Ford was demanding more "help" and thereafter a steady trickle of women presented themselves for instruction at the Charity's expense, and to Ford's profit.

Faced with complaints by several of his midwife assistants that they were in dire economic straits, in January 1765 Ford persuaded the Charity to pay the women 1s.6d. per delivery. Not one to miss a good thing, Ford changed the terms of his salary the next year: He would forgo his annual wage of £50 per annum and accept 1s.6d. for every woman delivered by the Charity (including those delivered by his female assistants who would continue to receive their 1s.6d. as well) plus ten guineas for instructing each midwife. The canniness of Ford's decision was immediately seen when his monthly salary for the delivery of 120 women by the Charity staff in the month of June soared to £9.

By the summer of 1766, the midwives of the Charity were firmly under the control of Ford. After two years of service, he would issue a "proper certificate" to the women, but in the meantime the women must live in designated areas at the convenience of the Charity and would be under his direction. They must go to assigned deliveries and account to Ford in writing for deliveries which they missed because of sickness or because they were already attending a labour. If the women needed to consult the doctor, they were to send him details of the case in writing. The Charity was always to be informed of the midwife's whereabouts in town, and the midwife could only leave town with permission of the Charity. Failure to go to a labour when called could result in a fine.[38] For all this, the

---

38 Mrs. Cecil was dismissed in November 1766, but she had two previous complaints regarding unavailability. She apparently had some private clients whose needs preempted those of the Charity patients.

Charity midwives were paid a pittance compared with other midwives who were in some cases charging 5s.5d.[39] By April 1767, however, the Charity agreed to pay midwives who had completed two years service and obtained their certificate the sum of 2s.6d. for each delivery.

Although Dr. Ford was still collecting 1s.6d. for each woman delivered, and his payment for the month of October 1767 alone was £16.4s., he sought and received permission to hire another woman to bring the complement of Charity midwives to four adding the caveat: "no woman be chosen to act as midwife who has rec'd instructions in the art under any other practitioner than Dr. Ford male midwife of this charity."[40]

It is not clear how many women chose to remain as Charity midwives after completing their two-year association. In addition, some who stayed on ran into conflicts of interest with their own private patients. Other midwives, like Sarah Wood, "being now in a capacity to support myself comfortably," chose to leave and practise privately.[41]

When the yearly accounts for expenditures showed that Ford had been paid £215 in 1769 for the deliveries of 2,868 women, several of the Charity's governors wanted Ford to disclose how many deliveries he had actually assisted in. As it turned out, of the almost 3,000 labours, he had attended only 152. Ford attempted to justify his salary by stating that he had been consulted in clients' illnesses and lyings-in on 565 occasions.[42] He also pointed out that by training the fledgling midwives, he had saved the Charity £69.[43]

By the 1760s women who aspired to midwifery training, which afforded some sort of accreditation were limited to the training offered to a few "students" by a handful of lying-in hospitals or the Lying-in Charity where they were at the mercy of entrepreneurs like Ford. Training at the lying-in hospitals was costly and out of the reach of many women, while the Charity offered free "training" but required two years of unpaid service on terms which would be untenable to most.

The growing population of London required more midwives than hospitals and charities could provide, and women were forced to turn more frequently to male midwives who were acquiring the training and confidence which made child delivery more attractive and lucrative. The dwindling numbers of accredited midwives lacked the autonomy and self-regulation they enjoyed in the seventeenth century, but at the end of the eighteenth century, they continued to offer, at least to Charity clients, the skills and services traditionally associated with

---

39 The minutes for October 31, 1766, note that the Charity had to pay an outside midwife this sum when one of its midwives was busy and unable to deliver a Charity patient.

40 Of the 216 women delivered, 106 were delivered by midwives who had certificates. I suspect most of the remaining 100 women were delivered by the trainee midwives so that Ford was receiving a tidy sum for acting solely in a "supervisory" capacity.

41 Minutes, June 24, 1768.

42 Evidently Ford counted the advice he gave to poor women during morning consultations in this figure.

43 The rookie midwives had delivered 1,380 women and saved a shilling on each delivery.

practically trained women who carried out their deliveries in a home setting. Serving far more women than the lying-in hospitals, Charity midwives enjoyed a lower maternal and infant mortality rate than the hospitals where the doctors were still polishing their child delivery skills, and where the mothers were exposed to deadly germs.[44]

"DOCTOR LEAKE'S HOSPITAL"

The foundation stone of the New Westminster (later General) Lying-in Hospital was laid August 15, 1765. By April 1769, there was one "female House pupil" who was paying £5 a quarter for board and lodging at the hospital founded by John Leake.[45] No mention is made in the hospital minutes of male midwifery students. Leake's own publications, however, set out a fee schedule for lectures and supervised instruction at the hospital. Any "gentleman" who paid the fee of ten guineas could attend all lectures for one year and then be permitted to practise under Leake's supervision on lying-in hospital patients for six months.[46] Leake explicitly argues the advantages the male midwifery trainee enjoys by training in "his" lying-in hospital. He compares the training his pupils receive with that available to male midwifery candidates not having an association with a hospital in a manner reminiscent of Richard Manningham almost thirty years earlier. It is doubtful that Leake's founding impulse was sincerely motivated by a desire to help poor married women in their childbed experience while there is no question, he sees male midwifery students as beneficiaries of the lying-in facility, noting that previously:

. . . it was extremely disagreeable to seek after labours at a great distance among the *very lowest class of people* in alleys and Remote parts of the town where a number of pupils were obliged to attend the same patient the Gentleman often exposed to insults and could acquire little practical knowledge. . . . [47]

There is scant surviving evidence about female midwifery training at Leake's hospital, aside from the reference to the lone female pupil of 1769.[48] Women paid

44 In addition to lower mortality rates, by 1772, almost one-third of the annual baptisms recorded in the Bills of Mortality were of Charity infants, Seligman, 418, 408.

45 GLRO H1/ST/K10/23, April 25, 1769. This sum was increased to twenty guineas per annum by September 4, 1770.

46 John Leake, *A Syllabus of Lectures or the Theory and Practice of Midwifery* (London: 1776).

47 Leake, *Syllabus*. The humiliation of poor women in labour exposed to the curious gaze of a roomful of young "gentlemen" escapes Leake completely.

48 GLRO H1/ST/K10/23 (unfol.) April 25, 1769, September 4, 1770. It is not clear from the hospital records who taught these female pupils, but evidently the male staff issued the certificates to midwives who had completed some course of training in the hospital. In July 1800, Dr. Thynne (physician and man-midwife at the hospital since 1792) was reprimanded for granting a certificate to a midwife who had not attended any labours in the hospital. In Leake's *Syllabus of Lectures* (London, 1776), which deals primarily with the training and instruction of "gentlemen," who were his own private pupils, Leake writes "Female Pupils–women will be privately instructed, and duly qualified for their own Practice, by being allowed to reside in the Hospital." I suspect the in-hospital instruction was done by the matron/midwife.

their twenty guineas for living at the hospital, but there is no mention of a fee for courses as there was for male candidates. Presumably, women were given practical instruction only.[49] The mandate of Leake and his fellow male midwives/founders of lying-in hospitals for training male midwives is plainly stated in Leake's own words:

The privilege of attending a PUBLIC LYING-IN HOSPITAL has long been wanting in this great Metropolis, to perfect students in the true practical knowledge of midwifery; and it affords me much pleasure, that I have been able to obtain this singular advantage for my Pupils at the Westminster NEW LYING-IN HOSPITAL . . . [50]

The minute books from the early years of the hospital chronicle chronic shortages of operating funds as well as a great number of maternal deaths from childbed fever. Four women died in the month of December 1769 alone.[51] By May 15, 1770, there had been fourteen deaths among the sixty-three admissions in the previous six months.[52] The bewildered staff physicians and surgeons (male midwives) tried to find an explanation for the deaths. By the end of January 1770, the order was issued for chimney pots to be placed on the chimneys in a desperate attempt to prevent further deaths, possibly caused by unhealthy downdraughts.[53] The skilled and well-paid matron, Elizabeth Greenham, did not escape censure as the doctors sought a scapegoat on which to place the blame for at least some of the puzzling deaths. She was found negligent because she had not made "proper enquiry and examination" whether women were suffering from infectious diseases on admission. The doctors must have known it was a charge with tenuous links to the many deaths, and the matron retained her position.[54] Four years later, the ongoing struggle to cope with the baffling deaths resulted in Leake's report to the Board:

. . . . . .that as a contageous order prevails in some wards of this Hospital, that the old mattresses should be destroyed in Hopes of preventing the contagion remaining.[55]

Although we know that the matron and her assistant carried out deliveries without recourse to male staff, Leake goes on to state that more than 5,000 women have

49 Margaret Stephen, author of *The Domestic Midwife* (London: 1795,) received her instruction from a "gentleman" who had been a pupil of William Smellie. With more than 30 years of successful midwifery practice behind her, she chides male midwives for their denigration of female midwives based on male jealousy and economic concerns. She accuses male midwives of charging female students more than male students, but withholding important knowledge from the women. Stephen, 18–20.
50 Leake in Philip Rhodes, *Dr.John Leake's Hospital* (London: Davis Poynter, 1977), 61
51 GLRO H1/GLI/A3/1/224, 225, 230.   52 Spencer, 105.   53 GLRO H1/GLI/A3/1/230.
54 Mrs. Greenham resigned as matron at Christmas 1774 because of ill health, and was succeeded by Mrs. Claverly early in 1775. GLRO H1/GLI/A3/1/299, 324. She was paid £25 per annum as compared with a nurse who was paid £8 per annum (fol. 374). In addition to her other duties, the matron was responsible for hiring nurses, conditional on the final approval of the board who read the rules regarding their position to them.
55 GLRO H1/GLI/A3/1 Board Minutes October 18, 25, 1774 (unfoliated for this year). In addition, wards in the wings of the hospital were to be fumigated.

been delivered "under my direction." Leake used his hospital to train pupils whose substantial fees swelled the doctor's income. Although he has been eulogized in some quarters, Leake reveals in his writings his self-seeking motives, thinly veiled by platitudes professing concern for poor women.[56]

The latter were now being given the opportunity of dying in male-managed lying-in hospitals in the eighteenth century whereas 100 years earlier, they were delivered at home by competent midwives at parish expense and far less risk. As a measure of the doctors' desperation, when a small private lying-in hospital was plagued by puerperal sepsis in the summer of 1761 and lost 20 patients in June alone, the "shocked" male midwives had two corpses placed in one coffin "to conceal their bad success."[57]

Ironically, by 1786 Leake's course of study included participation in postmortem examinations as an added inducement for the recruitment of prospective male midwives. Postmortem examinations, conducted by male practitioners whose unwashed hands transferred infective organisms to women during delivery, have been blamed by historians for the high incidence of puerperal sepsis, or childbed fever, in the eighteenth and nineteenth centuries.[58]

THE END OF AN ERA

It has been suggested that poor pregnant women had been ill served by the care provided under the poor laws and that the opening of lying-in hospitals had been a boon to that segment of the population. Even so, evidence from parish records demonstrates a continuing high level of commitment to the needs of settled parish poor women. The costs of delivery and traditional support during the lying-in period were, however, high, and parish officials would welcome alternatives such as the charity-financed lying-in hospitals.

In 1649, the cost of delivery and care for Elizabeth Cage, a poor woman of St Olave Jewry, totalled £2.12s.11d.[59] Mrs. Cage was in the home of widow Bull, who evidently made her home available for the deliveries and lyings-in of poor parish women. In 1698, although the parish of St Botolph Aldgate approved

56 Philip Rhodes, *Dr. John Leake's Hospital* (London: Davis Poynter, 1977).
57 Charles White, *A Treatise on the Management of Pregnant and Lying-in Women* (London, 1773), 161. Practices such as this help to explain why women failed to realize the potential dangers afforded by male midwives and lying-in hospitals.
58 It is unlikely that the midwives washed their hands after attending women infected with organisms which had been introduced by the instruments and hands of the doctors, thus continuing to spread the malady. Other factors which may have contributed to the high incidence of childbed fever were the probable low standards of hygiene in a communal setting, which resulted in a foreign environment that made the women more vulnerable to certain organisms. As early as 1560 regulations for midwives of Paris mentioned handwashing and the removal of rings in preparation for delivery. Carole Rawcliffe, *Medicine and Society in Later Medieval England* (Stroud, Gloucestershire: Alan Sutton (1995), 202
59 GL MS 4409/2 unfol. (1649). The cost included bed linens and clothing for lying-in, cost of board in Mrs. Bull's house, and midwife Lattyn's (Latin) fee of £0.2.6.

payment for the lying-in of Goody List, who had been abandoned by her husband, they were not forthcoming with Ursula Davis's support for her lying-in at a cost of £1.11s.16d. until ordered to do so by the justice.[60]

The same parish supported the lyings-in of no fewer than six women in 1699. As late as 1721, parish poor women like Ann Crossbrook could expect a month's lying-in at parish expense, as well as payment of the midwife's fee.[61] At the time of Elizabeth Marshall's delivery and lying-in, her husband was in prison, but the cost of her delivery and lying-in was assumed by St Bride's in 1701.[62] Earlier in the year, St Bride's subsidized the lyings-in of three women in a six-week period.[63] Moreover, St Bride's occasionally adopted a humane policy toward non-resident women which also proved costly: In 1722, the records note that midwife Wheeler was paid 5s. for "laying a casual found in the street."[64] In 1709, parish officials of Vedast's approved the cost of five weeks' lying-in for Mrs. Whitehead and two weeks for another woman at 12s. per week per woman, while St Dunstan in the East spent more than £4 on Elizabeth Nash for delivery, nursing, lying-in (five weeks), and clothing in 1705.[65] Poor parishes, in particular, would find these expenses heavy and be open to options such as lying-in hospitals, which would transfer responsibility from the parish to the charity-supported institutions.[66]

In attempting to answer the question as to why male midwives gained wider acceptance and eventually usurped the dominant role of the traditional midwife in the eighteenth century, there are several factors, aside from the lying-in hospitals, which played a part. Male entrée into the birthing chamber was through the midwife, who was confronted with an obstructed or abnormal delivery. With the breakdown of the ecclesiastical licensing system and midwives' dwindling self-confidence, an increasing reluctance on the midwives' part to deal with these problems helped to open the door to the men in the eighteenth century. That was the argument of Sarah Stone, the acclaimed eighteenth-century midwife from

60 GL MS 2626 Churchwarden's accounts (unfol.)
61 GL MSS 9235/3; 1/21/6. The cost of Crossbrook's lying-in was £1.1.0. Payment for what must have been a difficult delivery was £0.7.6 at a time when the going rate seems to have been £0.5.0.
62 GL MS 6552/2 unfol. June 26, 1701.   63 GL MS 6552/2 January and February 1701.
64 All parish records report the insensitive treatment of unfortunate women who were removed from parishes where they were not settled residents, virtually in the throes of labour. This was done to save the parish the expense of delivery and lying-in, and also the long-term cost of caring for the infant until old enough to be apprenticed.
65 GL MS 778/1. (unfol.) February, March, 1709. In addition, the parish paid for the unnamed woman's midwife (£0.2.6) and travel expenses (£0.3.0). GL MS 7882/3/287. The midwife was Susanna Kent.
66 Although these examples relate to the end of the seventeenth century and the first three decades of the eighteenth century, and slightly predate the rise of the lying-in hospitals, there is no reason to believe that parish arrangements and costs that had existed for the previous century were abruptly terminated, thereby making new facilities mandatory. For poor migrant women who flocked to the City and could claim no parish support, the lying-in hospitals, appalling though they may appear to twentieth-century sensibilities, offered an alternative to giving birth in a hovel or out of doors. Versluysen, 40.

Bristol, and later London.[67] Stone argued strongly, in 1737, that women, with the right training and instruction, could manage even the most difficult labours without the assistance of a male. She prefaces her more than forty case studies, demonstrating her management of a variety of obstetrical emergencies and written in the hope that it "may prove instructive to some Women Professors in the Art of Midwifery," with the following observations:

For I cannot comprehend, why Women are not capable of completing this business when begun, without calling in of men to their assistance, who are often sent for, when the work is near finish'd; and then the midwife, who has taken all the pains, is accounted of little value, and the young men command all the praise.[68]

Stone goes on to say that after a midwife calls in a male practitioner several times, for subsequent deliveries her pregnant client will engage the male midwife initially.[69]

According to a treatise published in 1751, the unethical behaviour of hospital nurses was furthering the male midwives' ambitions. Dr. Frank Nicholls was highly critical of lying-in hospitals and the doctors who staffed them. He accused nurses in the hospitals of aiding and abetting the male midwives by terrifying the mothers "by Lyes and false Representations" to discourage their employment of midwives while enhancing the reputations of the male practitioners. In return for their collusion, the nurses received the fee which the "gossips" formerly gave to the midwives. While Nicholls may have been exaggerating, there was probably a germ of truth in the tract which stressed the doctors' emphasis on personal appearance and charm in order to attract female clientele: "comeliness," "polite and tender behaviour," and "wit and lively imagination" were the ploys the men used, according to Nicholls.[70]

Further evidence of the male midwives' entrepreneurial bent is provided by the career of William Smellie who, like the staff doctors of the lying-in hospitals, found the instruction of primarily male students in midwifery highly lucrative and, to that end, paid poor women to permit him to use their deliveries for the purposes of instruction.[71] Thicknesse believed that national characteristics such as "vivacity and the love of novelty," as well as increasing sexual liberty, permitted male midwives to gain a foothold, particularly among upper-class women.[72] Philip

---

67 Sarah Stone's signature appears on a London Quaker birth note from 1704 when she delivered Elizabeth Harrison of St Bartholomew by the Exchange of a son. PRO RG 6 1626/200.
68 Sarah Stone, *A Complete Practice of Midwifery* (London: 1737), Preface, x.
69 For interesting insights into Stone's work and writing, see Isobel Grundy, "Sarah Stone."
70 F. Nicholls, *The Petition of the Unborn Babes to the Censors of the Royal College of Physicians of London* (London: 1751), 8.
71 Smellie's active career in obstetrics encompassed the 1740s and 1750s. Smellie's fees of 20 guineas for a course were similar to those charged by staff doctors in the lying-in hospitals. Smellie's students, however, paid additional sums for deliveries attended and performed. These were rated on a scale based on the number of courses the student took. Glaister, 58–9; Versluysen, 26–7.
72 Philip Thicknesse, *Man Midwifery Analysed* (London: 1764), 13–15.

Thicknesse also agreed with Nicholls that the male midwives had made a conscious effort to create an image which would appeal to those impressed and wishing to impress by ostentation:

. . . . a tawdry chariot, a still more tawdry doctor with a black velvet coat lined with pink silk stopping at their door . . . but that people of fashion should be amazed and cajoled by such external trapping, is very amazing. . . . [73]

The aristocratic tradition of having a resident physician, or at least one close at hand, who supervised deliveries of women of rank by their midwives, may have also been an important factor in the male move toward acquiring expertise in normal labours.[74] While middle-class women might be tempted to emulate their betters for appearances' sake, lower-class women could be induced to use the services of a male midwife on practical grounds. Not only were poor women paid by male midwives seeking experience in child delivery, as an added inducement, free medicines would be supplied. If a traditional midwife attended, an extra charge for prescriptions would necessarily be incurred.[75]

There is also the whole issue of "scientific expertise." Excluded from universities and deemed to lack the capacity for understanding the mysteries of science, women were faced with an insurmountable obstacle when confronted by male midwives' appropriation of child delivery ostensibly based on scientific knowledge or the knowledge of anatomy. In 1744, Sir Richard Manningham, arch foe of traditional midwives, advocated that "women with child, their parents or other discreat Persons" should learn the bones of the pelvis as a way of testing a midwife's competence. If she cannot tell them where "the mouth of the womb" is, then they should send for "better help" (a male midwife?).[76]

The best response to criticism like Manningham's was to come more than a decade later from a midwife herself. Elizabeth Nihell refuted the claim that women cannot be good midwives unless they can recite textbook anatomical terms, the science which is "the province of man, of a physician, not a woman."[77] She points out that if a woman simply understands the "structure and mechanical disposition of the female anatomy," she can perform her task competently. Nihell tellingly adds that the ladies "who want assistance at their lyings-in want someone who can deliver them not dissect them."

By the eighteenth century, midwives' testimonials from London show that the women were attempting to lay claim to possessing "scientific" abilities. In the last

---

73 Thicknesse, 25.   74 Versluysen, 27.
75 Elizabeth Nihell, *A Treatise on the Art of Midwifery* (London: 1760), 58.
76 Richard Manningham, *Abstract of Midwifery for the Use of Lying-in Infirmary* (London: 1744), 21–2.
   A recent study has concluded that better maternal nutrition in the second half of the eighteenth century was the main reason for a decrease in stillbirths and neonatal deaths. Male midwives, however, could seize upon this decrease to argue their own expertise. E. A. Wrigley, "Explaining the rise in maternal fertility in England in the 'long' eighteenth century," *Economic History Review* LI, 3 (1998): 435–64.
77 Nihell, 32–3.

dozen years or so for which ecclesiastical licensing survived in the eighteenth century, more than half the applicants, correctly gauging the prevailing climate, mentioned the term *scientia* in their documentation.[78] But the feeble claims of the midwives were lost in the welter of activity surrounding men intent on gaining control of child delivery. With the "discourse of science and reason" firmly in the control of men, the choices about childbirth that women could make were really not their own.[79]

---

78 GL MS 10,116/18. While 14 women claimed the traditional *arte and experientia*, 16 claimed expertise relating to *scientia*. One woman, Elizabeth Adams, widow of a Kensington surgeon, gave evidence "*de scientia et experientia*," neatly covering both ends of the spectrum.

79 Sawday, 230. Other support for the this view of the male appropriation of childbirth is afforded by analysis of eighteenth-century literature. See Lois A. Chaber, " 'This Affecting Subject': An 'Interested' Reading of Childbearing in Two Novels by Samuel Richardson," *Eighteenth-Century Fiction*, vol. 8 (January 2, 1996): 193–250. My conclusions on this point are in complete disagreement with those reached by Adrian Wilson in *Making of Man-midwifery*, 192. As a former registered nurse, mother, and historian, I make no apologies for presenting and evaluating the evidence as I have found it.

Appendix A: A Sixteenth-Century Midwife's Oath (Canterbury)

I, Eleonor Pead, admitted to the office and occupation of a midwife, will faithfully and diligently exercise the said office according to such cunning and knowledge as God hath given me and that I will be ready to help and aid as well poor as rich women being in labour and travail of child, and will always be ready both to poor and rich, in exercising and executing of my said office. Also, I will not permit or suffer that women being in labour or travail shall name any other to be the father of her child, than only he who is the right and true father thereof; and that I will not suffer any other body's child to be set, brought, or laid before any woman delivered of child in the place of her natural child, so far forth as I can know and understand. Also, I wil not use any kind of sorcery or incantation in the time of the travail of any woman; and that I will not destroy the child born of any woman, nor cut, nor pull off the head therof, or otherwise dismember or hurt the same, or suffer it to be so hurt or dismembered, by any manner of ways or means. Also, that in the ministration of the sacrament of baptism in the time of necessity I will use apt and the accustomed words of the same sacrament, that is to say, these words following, or the like in effect; 'I christen thee in the name of the Father, the Son, and the Holy Ghost,' and none other profane words. And that in such time of necessity, in baptizing any infant born, and pouring water upon the head of the same infant, I will use pure and clean water, and not any rose or damask water, or water made of any confection or mixture: and that I will certify the curate of the parish church of every such baptizing.

Source: This oath is reprinted by kind permission of Yale University Press, from Thomas Forbes, The *Midwife and the Witch*, New Haven, Conn.: Yale University Press, 1966, 145.

Appendix B: A Seventeenth-Century Midwife's Oath

From a *Book of Oaths* 1649 (Anon.) (administered by a bishop or his chancellor).

You shall sweare, First, that you shall be diligent and faithfull, and readie to helpe every Woman labouring of Childe, as well the poore as the riche; and that in time of nessitie[sic], you shall not forsake or leave the poore woman, to go to the Rich.

2. Item, Yee shall neither cause nor suffer any woman to name, or put any other Father to the childe, but onely him which is the very true Father thereof indeed.

3. Item, you shall not suffer any woman to pretend, faine, or surmize herselfe to be delivered of a Childe, who is not indeed; neither to claime any other womans Childe for her owne.

4. Item, you shall not suffer any Womans Childe to be murdered, maymed, or otherwise hurt, as much as you may; and so often as you shall perceive any perill or jeopardie, either in the Woman, or in the Childe, in any such wise, as you shall bee in doubt what shall chance thereof, you shal thenceforth in due time send for other Midwifes and expert women in that facultie, and use their advice and counsell in that behalfe.

5. Item, that you shall not in any wise use or exercise any manner of Witchcraft, Charme; or Sorcery, Invocation, or other Prayers than may stand with Gods Laws and the Kings.

6. Item, you shall not give any counsell, or minister any Herbe, Medicine, or Potion, or any other thing, to any Woman being with Childe whereby she should destroy or cast out that she goeth withal before her time.

7. Item, You shall not enforce any woman being with childe by any paine, or by any ungodly wayes or meanes, to give you any more for your paines or labour in bringing her a[to] bed, then they would otherwise do.

8. Item, you shall not consent, agree, give, or keepe counsell, that any woman be deliverd secretly of that which she goeth with, but in the presence of two or three lights readie.

9. Item, you shall be secret, and not open any matter appertaining to your Office in the presence of any man, unless necessity or great urgent cause do constrain you so to do.

10. Item, if any childe bee dead borne, you yourselfe shall see it buried in such secret place as neither Hogg nor Dogg, nor any other Beast may come unto it, and in such sort done, as it may not be found or perceived, as much as you may; And that you shall not suffer any such childe to be cast into the Jaques or any other inconvenient place.

11. Item, if you shall know any Midwife using or doing any thing contrary to any of the premisses, or in any other wise than shall be seemely or convenient, you shall forthwith detect open to shew the same to me [the bishop] or my chancellor for the time being.

12. Item, you shall use yourself in honest behaviour unto the woman being lawfully admitted to the roome [station, rank] and Office of a Midwife in all things accordingly

13. Item, That you shall truly present to myselfe, or my Chancellor, all such women as you shall know from time to time to occupie and exercise the roome

of a Midwife within my foresaid Diocesse and jurisdiction of A.[name of diocese] without my License and admission.

14. Item, you shall not make or assigne any Deputie or Deputies to exercise or occupie under you in your absence the Office or roome of a Midwife, but such as you shall perfectly know to be of right honest and discreet behaviour, as also apt, able, & having sufficient knowledge and experience to exercise the said roome and Office.

15. Item, you shall not be Privie, or consent, that any Priest, or other partie, shall in your absence, or in your companie, or of your knowledge or sufferance, Baptise any child, by any Masse, Latine Service, or Prayers, then such as are appointed by the Lawes of the Church of Englande; neither shall you consent, that any child, born by any woman, who shall be delivered by you, shall be carried away without being Baptised in the Parish by the Ordinarie Minister, where the said child is borne unless it be in the case of necessitie, Baptised privately, according to the Booke of Common Prayer: but you shall forthwith upon understanding thereof, either give knowledge thereof to me the said Bishop, or my Chancellour for the time being. All of which Articles and Charge you shall faithfully observe and keepe, so help you God and by the contents of this Booke [the Bible].[a]

A sixteenth-century midwife's license, issued by John Aylmer in 1588, contains only the first fourteen items, in language typical of the sixteenth century, but otherwise identical to the text of the seventeenth-century oath and license.[b]

The same fifteen items with very minor variations in language were incorporated into the license issued to Ellen Perkins of St Martins in the Fields in 1686 by the Bishop of London.[c]

[a]This oath is reprinted by kind permission of Yale University Press, from Thomas Forbes, *The Midwife and the Witch*, New Haven, Conn.: Yale University, 1966, 146–7.
[b]Christopher Charlton, ed. "A Midwife's Certificate," *Local Population Studies* 4 (1970): 56–8.
[c]James Hitchcock "A Sixteenth Century Midwife's License," *Bulletin of the History of Medicine* 41 (1967): 75–6.

Midwife's oath, 1713 (Canterbury). *Source*: LPL vx1a/11 no. 80. This oath is reproduced by kind permission of Lambeth Palace Library.

Appendix D: Midwives' Testimonial Certificates

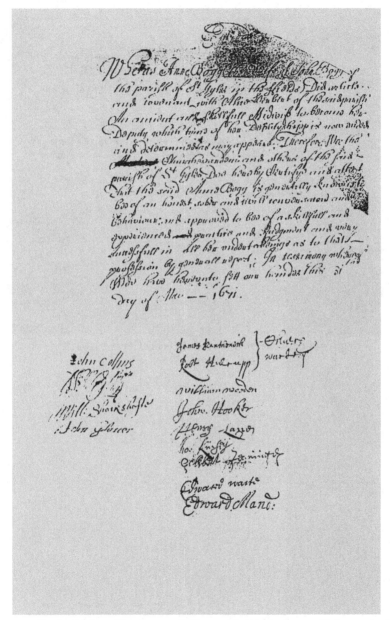

Testimonial certificate, 1671 (Bishop of London). *Source:* GL10, 116/7. This testimonial is reproduced by kind permission of Guildhall Library, Corporation of London.

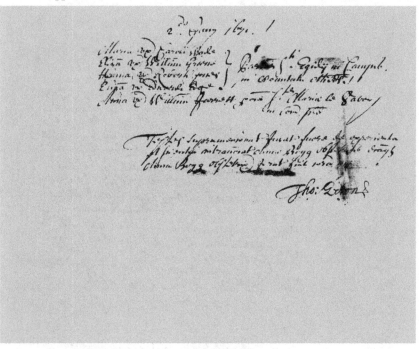

Testimonial certificate, 1671 (Bishop of London). (*cont.*)

Testimonial certificate, 1685 (Canterbury). *Source:* LPL vx 1a/11 no. 33. This testimonial is reproduced by kind permission of Lambeth Palace Library.

Appendix E: Probate Inventory for Elizabeth Heron, 1667

An inventory of the Goods and Chattels of Elizabeth Heron late of the pish of St Giles in the Fields in ye county of Middx. widd. Taken that 24th day of April 1667.

Impns   In the Fore Garrett
one old Table foure stools
Two chaires one table and Bedstead   xxs
Coard @ matt and flocke bed & bolster and straw bolster four old
Trunks and old hamper & and old desk

In the back Garrett
one bedstead, mat @ Coard one fether bed bolster. Blankets curtains &   xxs
vallances. Table & some old stools

In ye Chamber backward 2 pair of stairs
one bolster matt @ Cord. Curtaines
vallens & tester. one fether bed. bolster two pillowes one flock bed. three   ls
blankets one rugg and table seavon old chaires and stooles the hangings
about the room one pr of fire irons and andirons tonges and shovell

In ye fore room 2 pair of stairs
one bedstead mat @ Cord. Curtins vallens @ tester. Stript hangings   lvs
about ye room. one bolster bed two bolsters three blankets. one rugge
one table. two cowch cupbords
Tenn chaires @ stooles fire irons shovell @ tonges.   xvs

In ye Chamber backward one pair stairs
one bedstead, mat cord. tester, curtaines @ vallons. one fether bed bolster   lxxs
and pillow three blankets and rugg foure peires of tapestry hangings
Tenn chaires @ stools. 2 tables one pre of andirons shovell tonges bel-
lowes @ 2 strypt carpets   xxs

In the parlor backward
one setlebed and trundlebed two bolster beds two flock beds three bol-   lxxs
sters four blankets. 2 coverlids. two pillows

one chest one Engg. four pillows
old hangings about the room fire irons doggs. two shovells one fork   xxs
tonges pot iron one Jack four spitts
five chaires @ stools wth some other Lumber

Nyne pair of sheets three dozen of napkins and some other smale linin   lxxs
with some woollen cloathes

two old bras kittles two bras potts   xxs
one warming pan slice skinner and ladle. two bras skillets one bras morter

one hundred and eight pounds   ivLxs
halfe of pewter at 9p ye pound

In the low room Forward
one setlebed one tester bed @bolster blankets @ coverlid two tables five   xxxs
chaires @ stooles five irons tonges @ shovell frying pan, skillet

The partitions about the room with some other Lumber therein	xxs
In the kitchen Two iron potts. one old cupboard three old stooles one andiron one rack one pair of pott racks	vs
In the Cellar Eight barrells of Beer and Stavings	ivL vs
In the room in the yard Two tables four formes five old stooles 2 pair of pott racks	xiis
In ready money	xls
In desperate notes	xii L
The lease of the house & back house	ivL
Sum totall	C iiiL xvii s

Passed by whose names are heer under subscribed the day & year before written [signed] Georg Nelson, F – Munt

Source: (GL MS 9174/19)

Appendix F: Senior Midwives and Their Associates/Deputies

Senior Midwife	Associate/Deputy
Adams, Anne	Lucas, A(u)drey
Annett, Elizabeth	Charles, Bridgett
Atkins, Elizabeth	Wood, Mary
Austen, Frances	Alkin, Anne, Bacon, Alice, Field, Mary
Alkin, Anne	Carpin, Eliz., Lestocart, Eliz.
Bacon, Elizabeth	Thornton, Sara, Wynn, Eliz.
Bacon, Alice	Lamb, Katherine
Belson, Margaret	Cooper, Eliz., Bird, Anne, Blackett, Sarah
Benton, Alice	Walker, Elizabeth
Berrisford, Barbara	Churchwell, Margaret
Best, Elizabeth	Lewys, Eliz., Vesey, Eliz.
Bett, Katherine	Burton, Mary
Biggs, Mary	Langton, Charity
Bink, Elizabeth	Sinclair, Joan
Bissick, Elizabeth	Alkin, Anne
Blackmore, Ms.	Digborow, Margaret
Bolte, Deborah	Yates, Eliz.
Boshier, Ms.	Fletcher, Eliz.
Botts, Katherine	Burton, Mary
Boulton, Elizabeth	Newman, Judith
Boycot, Elizabeth	Hunt, Eliz., Geary, Katherine,
Bradley, Anne	Mason, Alice
Brampton, Dorothy	Best, Elizabeth
Broadgate, Christian	Swanley, Susan
Brownlow, Susanna	Pauley, Sara
Carpender, Katherine	Parsons, Mary
Challenyse, Mary	Towers, Eleanor, Grymes, Martha
Chappell, Francis	Johnson, Rebecca
Charnack, Sara	Jackman, Mary
Chesmore, Ursula	Bright, Elizabeth
Cleeter, Elizabeth	Sault, Susan
Coates, Joan	Read, Eliz.
Cole, Grace	Woodward, Eliz.
Collins, Elizabeth,	Wharton, Eliz.
Cozens, Elizabeth	Nollhaus, Ursula
Crocksall, Ann	Buskill, Mary
Crouch, Elizabeth	Nash, Eliz.
Dansey, Elizabeth	Sampson, Mary, Wicks, Elizabeth
Darley, Mary	Toller, Isobel
Davis, Alice	Whyte, Eliz.
Davis, Elizabeth	Glover, Debora
Davis, Jane	Coles, Rachel
Dawes, Francis	Johnson, Jane
Dawes, Frances	Gill, Ann, Lucas, A(u)drey

Senior Midwife	Associate/Deputy
Dickenson, Eleanor	Allcroft, Ann, Coleman, Eliz.
Edwards, Mary	Cooke, Mary dau. of Edwards
Elder, Elizabeth	Adams, Anne, Fletcher, Eliz.
Ellin (Allen)	Mary Trip, Sarah
Elyot, Elizabeth	de la Roche, Jaqueline
Faure, Catherine	Desormeaux, Mary
Field, Mary	Allen, Hanna
Fields, Prudence	Mason, Alice
Fletcher, Elizabeth	Turner, Anne
Flood, Elizabeth	Ward, Jane
Forsher, Elizabeth	Sherwood, Mary
Foster, Mary	Richards, Eleanor
Green, Mary	Budden, Susan
Gillam, Elizabeth	Cockson, Joan
Griffin, Sarah	Williscott, Margaret
Hainsworth, Ann	Ferris, Frances
Hales, Elizabeth	Corney, Margaret, Mason, Alice
Hales, Susanna	Syrett, Eliz.
Hall, Margaret	Wiggins, Rebecca
Harris, Elizabeth	Blackborrow, Bridgitte
Hatton, Ms	Duckett, Mary
Herbert, Alice	Adams, Anne, Wigby, Gertrude, Lucas, Audrey, Venable, Marg., Bogg, Anne, Martin, Eliz., Dobson, Anne
Heron, Elizabeth	Van Hatten, Mary
Hobbs, Katherine	Johnson, Jane
Hodgkinson, Mary	Howell, Katherine
James, Elizabeth	Harris, Elizabeth
Jennings, Mary	Ward, Jane
Johnson, Elizabeth	Leigh, Isabel
Keackwig, Elizabeth	Burton, Mary
Kenton, Anne	Baxter, Anne
Kilbury, (H)Esther	Lucas, Audrey, Venable, Marg., Martin, Eliz., Chappell, Frances
King, Abigail	Davis, Eliz.
Lamb, Ann	Smith, Rebecca, Warren, Eleanor
Laramitt, Hester	Burnham, Mary
Laselles, Mary	Pattison, Beatrix
Lawes, Elizabeth	Buskill, Mary
Laywood, Elizabeth	Coster, Isobel
Lee, Isobel	Hobson, Mabel
Leverett, Mary	Cooke, Margaret
Mabbs, Frances	Collins, Eliz.
Martin, Elizabeth	Tomlinson, Mary, Deane, Mary, Walford, Mary
Mason, Hannah	Johnson, Ann

Senior Midwife	Associate/Deputy
May (Meye), Alice	Ellis, Isobel
Melsome, Mary	Langton, Charity
Millie, Jane	Hunt, Elizabeth
Moore, Anne	Johnson, Margaret
Morecooke, Elizabeth	Pinnock, Alice
Orme, Helen	Foster, Phoebe, Penney, Hester (daughter of Orme)
Pendleton, Elizabeth	Cooper, Sara
Penn, Ann	Annett, Alice
Perkins, Sarah	Coale, Katherine
Plumer, Ms.	Newman, Judith
Potter, Phoebe	Carter, Elizabeth
Pratt, Temperence	Fendele, Anne, Stokes, Ursula, Lewis, Joan
Rampton (Wright), Anne	Stanton, Anne, Warren, Eleanor, Lamb, Ann (dau. of Rampton)
Richardson, Mary	Snead, Mary
Rogers, Sarah	Day, Catherine
Rowley, Joan	Board, Joan
Saywell, Ms.	Rickes, Eliz.
Seeley, Jane	Richards, Eleanor
Slicer, Sara	White, Mary
Smith, Elizabeth	Wright, Susan
Smith, Hannah	Linicomb, Margaret
Snape, Francis	Snead, Mary
Somner (Sumner), Anne	Davis, Eliz.,
Somner, Eliz.	Dickenson, Eleanor, Glover, Debora
Sowden (Soedin), Mary	Corney, Margaret (also taught by her mother)
Stanfro, Eleanor	Laramitt, Hester
Stannard, Frances	Dowke, Eliz.
Stone, Martha	King, Elizabeth
Swanley, Susan	Rickes, Eliz., Kilbury, Esther, Broadgate, Christian
Sweatman, Isabel	Light, Eliz.
Sydey, Sara	Sherwood, Mary
Syrett, Elizabeth	Hales, Susanna
Townes, Elizabeth,	James, Elizabeth
Terry, Margaret	Grymes, Martha
Tracee, Elizabeth	Sinclair, Joan
Troone, Mary	Thomas, Elizabeth
Veere, Anne	Morse, Margaret, Briscoe, Susan
Waite, Mary	Flowers, Anne
Ward, Jane	Cloys, Frances
Watson, Ann	Welch, Mary
Wharse, Margaret	White, Lucy
Wheeler, Joan	Rickes, Eliz.
Whithington, Mary	Dickenson, Eleanor

Senior Midwife	Associate/Deputy
Wickes, Elizabeth	Robinson, Elizabeth
Winchurst, Elizabeth	Thomas, Eliz.
Winchester, Hanna	White, Mary Ann
Wooden, Joan	Dunstall, Elizabeth
Yarwood, Joan,	Stanton, Anne

Sources: GL MSS 10,116, 25,598/2; LPL MS VX1A/11.

Appendix G: Quaker Midwives

The following names were taken from Quaker birthnotes, PRO RG 6/26,27,28. Aside from midwives Boulton, Gabird, and Wigan, who were London residents, the remaining women may or may not have been settled in London parishes, but since they were offering their services to London inhabitants, they are listed here. Included are those women named *two* or more times in the documents in the place where the midwife's name usually appeared. The most active was Anne Heariford, who delivered at least twenty-six London women between 1698 and 1701.

Albrighton, Anne	Gabird, Elizabeth	Mackly, Sarah
Boulton, Alice	Gale, Dorothy	Markland, Elizabeth
Caterbancke, Anne	Galladine, Alice	Peake, Mary
Chapman, Jane	Guernall (Juernell), Mary	Percival, Marsh
Clapham, Amy	Ann	Poore, Anne
Coal, Margery	Harrison, Margaret	Sparrow, Margaret
Cock, Rebecca	Hartley, Hephzia	Stuart, Sarah
Dixon, Mary	Heariford, Ann	Whellen (Whelten)
Draper, Mary	Holton, Mary	Whyte, Elizabeth
Dyer, Mary	Howell, Mary	Wigan, Margaret
Fly, Elizabeth	Lacey, Elizabeth	Wilson, Hannah

Note: For a list of midwives licensed by the Church of England who delivered Quaker women, see Chapter 3.

Appendix H: London Parishes

Parishes Within the Wall

1	Allhallows Barking	45	St Lawrence Pountney
2	Allhallows Bread Street	46	St Leonard Eastcheap
3	Allhallows the Great	47	St Leonard Foster Lane
4	Allhallows Honey Lane	48	St Magnus the Martyr
5	Allhallows the Less	49	St Margaret Lothbury
6	Allhallows Lombard Street	50	St Margaret Moses
7	Allhallows London Wall	51	St Margaret New Fish Street
8	Allhallows Staining	52	St Margaret Pattens
9	Christ Church	53	St Martin Ironmonger Lane
10	Holy Trinity the Less	54	St Martin Ludgate
11	St Alban Wood Street	55	St Martin Orgar
12	St Alphage	56	St Martin Outwich
13	St Andrew Hubbard	57	St Martin Vintry
14	St Andrew Undershaft	58	St Mary Abchurch
15	St Andrew by the Wardrobe	59	St Mary Aldermanbury
16	St Anne and St Agnes Aldersgate	60	St Mary Aldermary
17	St Anne Blackfriars	61	St Mary Bothaw
18	St Antholin	62	St Mary le Bow
19	St Augustine	63	St Mary Colechurch
20	St Bartholomew by the Exchange	64	St Mary at Hill
21	St Benet Fink	65	St Mary Magdalen Milk Street
22	St Benet Gracechurch	66	St Mary Magdalen Old Fish Street
23	St Benet Paul's Wharf	67	St Mary Mounthaw
24	St Benet Sherehog	68	St Mary Somerset
25	St Botolph Billingsgate	69	St Mary Staining
26	St Christopher le Stocks	70	St Mary Woolchurch
27	St Clement Eastcheap	71	St Mary Woolnoth
28	St Dionis Backchurch	72	St Matthew Friday Street
29	St Dunstan in the East	73	St Michael Bassishaw
30	St Edmund Lombard Street	74	St Michael Cornhill
31	St Ethelburga	75	St Michael Crooked Lane
32	St Faith under St Paul's	76	St Michael Queenhithe
33	St Gabriel Fenchurch	77	St Michael le Querne
34	St George Botolph Lane	78	St Michael Paternoster Royal
35	St Gregory by St Paul's	79	St Michael Wood Street
36	St Helen	80	St Mildred Bread Street
37	St James Duke's Palace	81	St Mildred Poultry
38	St James Garlickhithe	82	St Nicholas Acons
39	St John the Baptist	83	St Nicholas Cole Abbey
40	St John the Evangelist	84	St Nicholas Olave
41	St John Zachary	85	St Olave Hart Street
42	St Katherine Coleman	86	St Olave Old Jewry
43	St Katherine Cree	87	St Olave Silver Street
44	St Lawrence Jewry	88	St Pancras Soper Lane

Parishes Within the Wall (*cont.*)

89	St Peter Westcheap	94	St Stephen Walbrook
90	St Peter Cornhill	95	St Swithin
91	St Peter Paul's Wharf	96	St Thomas the Apostle
92	St Peter le Poor	97	St Vedast
93	St Stephen Coleman Street		

Parishes Outside the Wall

98	St Andrew Holborn	109	St Sepulchre
99	St Bartholomew the Great	110	Whitefriars Precinct
100	St Bartholomew the Less	111	St Giles in the Fields
101	St Botolph without Aldersgate	112	St Martin in the Fields
102	St Botolph without Aldgate	113	St Clement Danes
103	St Botolph without Bishopsgate	114	St Leonard Shoreditch
104	St Bride	115	St Mary Matfellon/Whitechapel
105	Bridewell Precinct	116	St Mary Savoy
106	St Dunstan in the West	117	St James Clerkenwell
107	St Giles without Cripplegate	118	St Paul Covent Gardens
108	St Olave Southwark	119	St Mary Isligton

Appendix I: London and Area Midwives' Directory for the Seventeenth Century*

For the following directory, the numbering of parishes has been adapted from Tai Liu to include the areas outside of the City where a number of midwives were licensed (see Figure I.1). Where the year of licensing is known, it has been included; the year of licensing was established by testimonial certificates and/or bishops and archbishops' registers. If the midwife was identified only through a visitation, this is indicated by "v" after the date. Where the parish or date is unknown, it is indicated by n.p., or n.d. Senior midwives are shown as *s.m.w.* Duplications and omissions are inevitable because of incomplete records, remarriage, and inconsistencies in spelling. In some cases, the midwives lived, and probably carried out most of their deliveries, at a distance from London. Their licences, however, were issued by the archbishop (and in some cases, the bishop) to encompass London, hence their inclusion in the directory.

In addition to those midwives licensed by the Church, midwives identified in James Alexander's thesis are marked (a); midwives' names that Peter Earle and Jennifer Melville have found in court depositions and kindly shared with me are marked (b) and (c), respectively. In two cases, Quaker midwives who appeared in Quaker birth notes and one other source have been included and designated as "Q." For a more complete list of Quaker midwives, see Appendix G.

*The relatively small number of eighteenth-century midwives licensed by the Church have been included. Many of these would have begun their apprenticeship with senior midwives in the seventeenth century.

Abbott, Mrs. 111; 1664 v.
Aberell(?) Mrs. 8; 1637 v.
Adams, Elizabeth (Ambrose) Kensington; 1715
Adams, Frances (Matthew) Richmond, Surrey; 1679
Adams, Mary (Thos.) St Margaret Westminster; 1705
Ad(d)ams, Anne (Thos.) 112; 1661 *s.m.w.*
Addams, Anne (Thos.) 17; 1636
Albrit(t)tain², Ann 28; fl. 1683–95 (Q)
Alcroft, Anne (Thos.) 112; 1690
Aleworth, Margaret 113; 1672
Alkin, Anne (Francis) 15; 1670 *s.m.w.*
Alkins, Eliz. 112; 1680 v.
Allen, Hannah (Wm.) 114; 1679
Allen, Winnifred (John) 15; 1662
Allin, Mrs. 1; 1680 v.
Allred, Grace (Thos.) 98; 1617.
Alvey^c, Rebecca (Robert) St James Westminster; (fl. 1687)
Annett, Alice (Nicholas) 39; 1676 *s.m.w.*
Anson, Anne West Ham, Essex; 1679
Appleby, Joan (Richard) St Mary Newington
Arderne, Jane (fl. 1672) *s.m.w.*
Arnett, Eliz. (Wm.) 91; 1616
Ashley, Mrs. 112; 1669 v.
Ashley, Eliz. (Thos.) 116; 1664
Ashwell, Anne 54; 1633
Askew, Anne 17; 1637 v.

Askew, Eliz., Stepney, formerly Shadwell; 1680 v.
Askew, Ramath 113; 1685
Aster, Sara (Nathaniel) 1; 1709
Asterley, Mary (Thos.) 65; 1687
Atkins, Eliz. *s.m.w.*
Atkinson, Priscilla (Gregory) 93; 1619.
Atkinson, Sara 103; 1637 v.
Atkinson, Anne (John) 98; 1662
Austen, Andrea (Robert) 3; 1628
Austen, Francis (John)? 98? (fl. 1670s) *s.m.w.*
Awcett, Eliz. (Wm.) 119; 1619
Aynsworth, Civil (Robert) 114; 1616
Ayre, Eliz. 107; 1664

Bacon, Alice (Robert) Edmonton; 1676 *s.m.w.*
Bacon, Eliz. (Wm.) 85; (fl. 1697) *s.m.w.*
Bacon, Mary Edmonton; 1680 v.
Bagster^b, Margaret Stepney (fl. 1695)
Baker, Anne (Andrew) 107; 1704
Baker, Rebecca (Nathaniel) 112; 1675
Baldwin, Ann 113; 1664 v.
Banbury, Jane 99; 1640
Banks, Jane 111; 1701
Banton, Eleanor (Robt.) Chelsea; 1669?
Barford, Anne 117; 1686
Barnett, Eliz. (Richard) 102; 1662
Barr, Mrs. 104; 1680 v.
Bartlett, Eliz. (John) 98; 1627

Barrett, Rebecca, 112; 1700
Barwick, Mrs. 118; 1669 v.
Basure, Mrs. 118; 1669 v.
Bateman, Rose (John) Herbill, Midds.; 1664
Bates, Mrs. 114; 1669 v.
Baunton (Banton), Eleanor (Robert) Chelsea, Midds.; 1669
Baxter, 112; 1669 v.
Baxter, Anne 113; 1663
Beadle, Mary (Thos.) 17; 1703
Beadnell, Hannah 106; 1694
Bedford, Anne (Edward) 101; 1664 v.
Beikcon, Margaret 118; 1692
Belford, Mrs. 115; 1669 v.
Bell, Ann (Wm.) 112; 1677
Bell, Jane (John) 86; 1686
Belson, Margaret (Thos.) 112; 1663 *s.m.w.*
Bendskin, (Benskin) Mrs. 31; 1669 v.
Benet, Sarah (John) 106; 1675
Benner, Grace 109; 1637 v.
Bennet, Frances (John) 115; 1697
Bennett, Mary 42; 1690
Benson, E. 112; 1664 v.
Benson, Mary (John) 106; 1664
Bent, Sara 111; 1663
Benton, Alice 109 *s.m.w.*
Beranger, Elizabeth 92; 1674
Berrisford, Barbara Chelsea? (fl. 1702) *s.m.w.* Q?
Best, Elizabeth (John) 102; 1667 *s.m.w.*
Best[a], Mrs. 30 (fl. 1700)
Bett, Katherine *s.m.w.*
Bevis, Mary 98; 1662
Bickerstaffe, Eliz. (James) 87; 1679
Bigges, Mary 3; 1664 v. *s.m.w.*
Bigg, Eliz. 112; 1719
Bignell, Anna Mary (Wm.) 111; 1719
Bingham, Mrs. 84; 1637 v.
Bink, Eliz. *s.m.w.*
Birch, Eliz. 76/57?; 1668
Bird, Anne (Richard) 109
Bird, Anne (Ouswele?) 98; 1672
Bishop, Mrs. 101; 1680 v.
Bissick, Eliz. 113 (fl. 1670) *s.m.w.*
Black, Mary 115; 1685
Blackborow, Bridgette 102; 1690
Blackett, Sara (John) 112; 1680
Blackman, Alice (Samuel) 1; 1706
Blackmore, Mrs. *s.m.w.*
Blague, Sarah 101; 1690
Blake, Mrs. 48; 1695
Blehemier, Eliz. 12; 1676
Bleyart, Martha (Anthony) 102; 1639
Board, Joan (Richard) 109; 1662
Bogg, Anne (John) 111; 1671
Bolte, Debora (John) 113; 1674 *s.m.w.*
Bolton, Eliz. 102; 1680 v.

Bont, Catherine (Jonas Morise) Stepney; 1688
Booker, Hester 98; 1634
Boone, Mrs. 14; 1637 v.
Booth, Jane (Thos.) 103; 1699
Booth, Winnifred (Edward) St Ann Soho; 1692
Boshier, Mrs. *s.m.w.*
Botts, Katherine (Richard) Shadwell, Stepney; 1669
Boulton, Eliz. 1; 1670 *s.m.w.*
Boycott, Eliz. (John) 109; 1636 *s.m.w.*
Boyer[c], Sara (Thos.) 69 (fl. 1692)
Bracewell, Grace (Robert) 113; 1637 v.
Bradford, Anne (Wm.) 106; 1672
Bradley, Anne n.p., n.d. *s.m.w.*
Bradley, Anne (Langley) St Mary Pattens; 1715
Brampton, Dorothy 102; (fl. 1669) *s.m.w.*
Brand, Edy (John) Cheshunt; 1724
Brandin, Eliz. 93; 1680 v.
Brasier, Mary (Thos.) Much Baddow; 1689
Brayne (Brian), Joan (Wm.) 54; 1631
Brenton, Mrs. 111; 1664 v.
Bridge, Eliz. (Samuel) 102; 1671
Bright, Eliz. (Wm.) 103; 1698
Briscoe, Susan (Frances) n.p.; 1690
Broadgate, Christiana Stepney; 1669 *s.m.w.*
Brokley, Mrs. 104? (fl. 1700)
Bromfield, Debora (Wm.) 98; 1662
Bromlow (Brownlow?), Mrs. 3; 1664 v. (see Susanna Glover)
Brooker, Joan (Edward) 111; 1620
Broughton, Eyton (Samuel) Lambeth, Surrey; 1686/1700
Brown, Ann or Alice 109; 1637
Browne, Mrs. 112; 1680 v.
Browne, Elizabeth (Henry) Chiswick; 1711
Browne, Mary (Adam) 98?; 1704
Brown, Mary (Joseph) 14: 1680
Buckley, Mary (John) 104; 1719
Budden, Susan 98; 1691
Bulc, or Budd Martha 51; 1662 *s.m.w.*
Bumstead, Mrs. 104; 1637 v.
Bunce, Mary (Matthew) 103; 1687
Bunworth, Alice 98; 1671
Burnham, Mary (Thos.) widow Stepney; 1674
Burrell, Alice (Wm.) 106; 1686
Burrows, Eliz. 103; 1712
Burton, Ellenor (John) Lambeth, Surrey; 1677
Burton, Mary 109; 1633
Burton, Mary 115; 1672
Bush, Eliz. Croydon; 1679
Bushar(er)[b], Mary (John) 99; 1712 (fl. 1719)
Bushell, Lucy 112; 1685
Busie, Ann 111; 1637 v.
Buski(e)ll, Mary 115; 1664
Butcher, Margaret 111; 1637 v.
Butterfield, Mary 112; 1675

Byers, Mary (Wm.) Walton, Surrey; 1685
Byrd, Alice 109; 1637 v.
Bysey, Eliz. (Thos.) n.p.; 1618

Cakewood, Eliz. (Bartholomew) 109; 1666
Cardiffe, Jane (Charles) Lambeth, Surrey; 1685
Carlington, Eliz. 54; 1637 v.
Carnaby, Alice 106; 1637
Carnell, Alice (Frances) 106; 1629
Carpender, Catherine 115; 1663 *s.m.w.*
Carpin, Eliz. (Francis) widow 17; 1680
Carroll, Joan 114; 1637 v.
Carson, or Carter, Frances 102; 1676
Carter, Mrs. 106; 1680 v.
Carter, Eliz. 113; 1664 v.
Carter, Mary (John) 98; 1674
Carter², Mary 47; (fl. 1700)
Carter, Mirabella (Edward) 34; 1687
Caulson, Eliz. 101; (1670–3)
Cavere, Dorothy 79; 1671
Cavette, Mrs. 98; 1637 v.
Cayford, Emma 113; 1661
Ceeley, Anne (George) 113; 1622
Cellier, Eliz. (Peter) 113; n.d.
Challenyse, Mary *s.m.w.*
Chamberlain, Eliz. 111; 1697
Chamberlain or Chambers, Susan (Robert) 42; 1662
Chambers, Dorothy (Edward) 109; 1608
Champion, Joan 113; 1637 v.
Chanon, Joan 54; 1611
Chaplin, Jane 107?; 1674 v.
Chappele, Margaret South Minster; 1680 v.
Chappell, Frances (Jonathan) 111; 1671
Charles, Bridgett (John) 112; 1673
Charles, Edith Stepney; 1637
Charneck, Sara 107; *s.m.w.*
Cheney, Susannah (John) 29; 1667
Chesmore, Ursula (Edmund) 103; 1677 *s.m.w.*
Child, Eliz. (John) 107; 1694 (1672–3 v.)
Child, Susanna (Francis) 9; 1715
Churchwell (Churchill), Margaret (Andrew) Chelsea; 1702
Clapton², Francis 16; (fl. 1700)
Clare, Mrs. 101; 1680 v.
Clark, Eliz. (Wm). Isleworth Midds.; 1697
Clarke, Anne (Wm.) 111; 1622
Clarke, Anne 92; 1673
Clarke, Eliz. (Wm.) 31; 1673
Claybrook, Audree 44; 1611
Clayton, or Clapton 76; 1680 v.
Cleaver, Mrs. 115; 1669 v. 1680 v
Clifton, Anne (Kellem) 87; 1619
Cloys, Francis 102; 1666
Coale, Katherine (John) Shadwell; 1681
Coates, Joan *s.m.w.*

Cockrey, Dorothy (James) 86; 1633
Cockson, Joan (Thos.) 106; 1661
Coggs, Cecilia 107; 1669
Cole, Grace Kingston *s.m.w.*
Coleman, Eliz. 112; 1690
Coles, Rachel (Benjamin) 112; 1662
Coleston, Sarah (John) Chelsea; 1664
Collier, Alice (Richard) 111; 1674
Collier, Eliz. (Samuel) 73; 1715
Collins, Eliz. (Thos.) 98; 1662
Collop, Barbara (Lawrence) 111; 1697
Combes, Mrs. Hendon; 1680 v.
Conay, Sara 113; 1664 v.
Cooke, Eliz. (Robert) 3; 1698
Cooke, Jane (John) 106; 1684
Cooke, Juliana (John?) 15; 1636, (1637 v.)
Cooke, Margaret Chelsea; 1664
Cooke, Mary (Richard) 115; 1669
Cooper, Eliz. (Charles) Stepney; 1724
Cooper, Margaret (John) 103; 1616
Cooper, Anne (John) 111; 1675
Cooper, Eliz. (Richard) 17; 1636
Cooper, Eliz. (Wm.) 112; 1663
Cooper, Hannah (Robert) 104; 1710
Cooper, Mary alias Holland 112; 1637 v.
Cooper, Sarah (Daniel) 107; 1676
Cope, Joanna (John) 113; 1719
Cope, Margaret 111; 1675
Cope, Mrs. 115; 1669 v.
Coppniger, Mrs. 103; 1669 v.
Cornelius, Anne (Thos.) 111; 1705
Corney, Margaret 91; 1661
Cornwall², Mrs. Chancery Lane, (fl. 1699)
Coster, Isobel (Robert) 111; 1661
Costin, Eliz. (Wm.) Newington Butts, Surrey; 1685
Cotton, Francis Bermondsey; 1700
Could, Mrs. 5; 1637 v.
Courthope, Anne (James) 106; 1719
Cowlwell, Anne (Owen) 83; 1622
Coxe, Ann (Henry) 15; 1613
Coxon, or Croxon, Catherine 47; 1633
Cozens, Eliz. (Wm) 3; (fl. 1663) *s.m.w.*
Cradle, or Cridle, Lucy 112; 1637 v.
Cranford, or Crawford, Eliz. (John) 113; 1629
Cranwell, Alice (Chidley) 92; 1663
Creed, Margaret (Frances) 98; 1619
Crocher, Anne (Thos.) 82; 1673
Crocksall, Anne *s.m.w.*
Crockwell, Mary St James Westminster; 1703
Crofford, Mrs. 85; 1664 v.
Crompton, Mrs. 111; 1637 v.
Crosley, Deborah 114; 1665
Crosley, Eliz. (Robert) 103; 1673
Crouch, Eliz. *s.m.w.*
Crowch, or Crouch, Ann 42; 1680 v.

Crowd, or Croud, Barbara (Michael) 59; 1619
Cuddon, Sarah (Elias) 114; 1671
Culpepper, Alice Stepney; 1665
Cumber, Rose (Roger) 104; 1610
Cunny, Eliz. 115; 1671
Curry, Sara, 115; 1611
Curtis, Mary (John) Edmonton; 1697

Dans(z)ey, Eliz. 111; 1697 *s.m.w.*
Darby 107; 1671 v.
Dards, Anna, Lamborne; 1685
Davies, Joan (Wm.) 119; 1694
Davis, Alice Stepney; 1663 *s.m.w.*
Davis, Eliz. (Thos.) 43; 1662
Davis, Jane 112; 1664 v. *s.m.w.*
Dawes, Francis (fl. 1664) *s.m.w.*
Dawling, Susan n.p.; 1674 *s.m.w.*
Dawson, Catherine (Richard) 113; 1686
Day, Ann 12; 1695
Day, Catherine Chelsea; 1664
de la Roche, Jaqueline 112; 1678
Deacon, Anne 109; 1637 v.
Deale, Rebecca (John) 9; 1680
Dean, Maryann 112; 1680 v.
Deane, Eliz. (Richard) St James Weston; 1688
Deane, Mary (John) 76; 1622
Deane, Mary 111; 1680
Deane, Sarah 62; 1677
Dennis, Alice (in Aveling)
Dennis, Margaret (Wm.) 111; n.d.
Desborow, or Digborow, Margaret (Thos.) 70 or 71; 1662
Desormeaux, Mary (Daniel) 111; 1680
Desser, Katherine 109; 1673
Dickenson, Elizabeth (Edward) 112; 1725
Dickenson, Ellenor 112; 1669 *s.m.w.*
Dickinson, Mrs. 118; 1669 v.
Dickinson, Margaret 113; 1719
Dikes[a], Mrs. 109; (fl. 1700)
Dixon, Mary (Henry) 114; 1700
Dobson, Anne (Wm.) 111; 1676
Dodd, or Dodson, Anne 98; 1688
Dodson, Margaret (Thos.) 109; 1638
Doman, or Dorman, Emma (Richard) 102; 1664
Doggett, Mary (Thos.) 112; 1671
Donne, Joan (John) 112; 1640
Dorell, Mrs. 113; 1680 v.
Dorrington, Faith 107; 1671 v. (deputy m.w.)
Doubleday, Isobel 106; 1611
Douglas, Sibil (Edwin) 98; 1618
Dowdall, Mary (Nathaniel) Chipping Barnett, Hartford; 1664
Dowke, Eliz. 99; 1661
Downs, Eliz. 104; 1677
Drake, Katherine (John) 104; 1677
Drake, Rose (George) 85; 1607

Duckett, Mary (John) 106; 1669
Dunsley, Mary Barking; 1706
Dunstall, Eliz. (John) 16; 1664

Eagleston, Eliz. 113; 1699
Eaton, Anne (Edward) 116; 1698
Edwards[b], Alice (Ralph) 102; 1690 (1700)
Edwards, Mary (fl. 1669) *s.m.w.*
Edwards, Susan (Wm.) 104; 1674
Elder, Eliz. 113; *s.m.w.*
Eldridge, Alice (Richard) 109; 1667
Ellin, Mary *s.m.w.*
Elliot, Eliz. (Peter) Hampton; 1715
Ellis, Mrs. 98; 1669 v.
Ellis, Isobel 112; 1664; 98; 1669 v.
Ellsworth, Jane (Marmaduke) 113; 1723
Elmes, Mrs. 45; 1680 v.
Elsey, or Ollsey, Joan Enfield; 1687
Elyot, Eliz. *s.m.w.*
Emerson[c], Anna 112; (fl. 1692)
Emery, Isobel (Thos.) 113; 1610
Evans, Eliz. (Richard) 98; 1691
Evans, Eliz. (John) 114; 1705
Evans, Helenora (Thos.) 103; 1639
Evans, Mary (Robert) St James in the Fields; 1689
Everard, Margaret (George) Chelsea; 1684
Everet, Mary (Wm.) 103; 1701
Excel(l), Mary (Wm.) St James in Fields; 1703

Farewell, Mrs. 106; 1680 v.
Farmer[a], Eliz. 79; (fl. 1700)
Faure, Katherine 111; (fl. 1680) *s.m.w.*
Fendele, Anne (Thos.) 115; 1679
Ferris, Francis 107; 1674
Field, Jane 104 or 109; 1637 v.
Field, Eliz. (Benjamin) Hexton, Herts; 1697
Field, Mariam 107?; 1673 v.
Field, Mary (James) 107; 1674 *s.m.w.*
Field, Prudence 109; 1662; *s.m.w.*
Fish, Sarah (Robert) Enfield; 1697
Fisher, Eliz. 43; 1662
Fisher, Francis (Edward) Isleworth; 1664
Fletcher, Susan (Robt.) 74; 1626
Fletcher, Eliz. (Leonard?) 111; 1665 *s.m.w.*
Flewelling, Alice 92; 1687
Flood, Mrs. 68; 1637 v. *s.m.w.*
Flowers, Ann (James) 112; 1690
Floyd, Mary 89; 1666
Ford, Jane (John) 102; 1699
Ford[c], Thomasina (Richard) 98; (fl. 1676)
Forgy[b], Catherine (fl. 1707)
Forrest, Eliz. (Samuel) Chelsea, 1690
Forshaw, Eliz. (Thos.) 21; 1684
Forster, Phobe 109; 1662
Fortte, Anne (Edward) 112; 1618

Harwood, Ann 112; 1680 v.

Harwood, Alice (Robert) Kensington; 1663

Harwood[b], Eliz. (Lawrence) Q. (fl. 1705)

Hasleton, Mary 112; 1664 v. (lic.)

Hassell[a], Eliz. 35; (fl. 1700)

Hastrick, Frediman 112; 1676

Hatton, Mrs. 49; 1637 v.(deputy) (fl. 1669) *s.m.w.*

Hatton, Mrs. 110; 1680 v. *s.m.w.*

Haw, Mary 56; 1715

Hawkins, Anne 111; 1670

Hawkins, Ann Kensington; 1688

Hawkins, Mary (James) 113; 1632

Hawley, Alice 112; 1631

Haynsworth, Anne (Richard) 111; 1667

Haywood, Eliz. (Joseph) 98;1725

Heale, Mary 111; 1637 v.

Healeing, Mrs. 104; 1680 v.

Heap, Jane? (John) 11; 1618

Heath, Katherine (Henry) 98; 1674

Heldar, Eliz. 113; 1664 v.

Hendrick, Ann 102; 1667

Henley, Mary (Robert) 104; 1673

Henly, Sara (Wm.) St Saviours Southwark; 1685

Henry, Margaret (James) 112; 1719

Hensman, Mrs. (Wm.) 31; 1669 v.

Herbert, Alice 111; 1664 *s.m.w.*

Herbert, Catherine 113; 1637 v.

Heron, alias Mekins, Eliz. *s.m.w.*

Hicks, Eliz. St Pancras Midds.; 1676

Hide, Anne 119; 1678

Higdon, Mary 103; 1680

Higginson, Anne (Lawrence) 54; 1611

Hill, Anne 84; 1700

Hill, Eliz. 79; 1667/68

Hill, Sarah (Wm.) Lymes end, Stebenheath; 1669

Hilles, alias Nores, Alice (Peter) Wapping; 1630

Hilliard, Mrs. 98; 1680 v.

Hillman, Sara (Henry) Liberty of Norton Holgate, Midds.; 1691

Hillyard, Eliz. (Richard) 101; 1678

Hoare, Catherine (Joshua) 113; 1719

Hobbs, Katherine 44; 1663 *s.m.w.*.

Hobby, Mrs. 106; 1664 v.

Hobson, Mabella (George) 111; 1664

Hodges, Eliz. (James) Isleworth; 1697

Hodgkinson, alias Osgood Mary (Thos.) 15/98; 1669 *s.m.w.*

Hollansby, Barbara (Christopher) 107; 1618

Hollingshead, Mrs. 106

Holmes, Sarah (Peter) 111; 1697

Holt, Rebecca 114; 1681

Honiborne, Margaret (John) 102; 1673 (1637 v.)

Hopkins, Margaret (John) Edmonton; 1670

Hopkins, Mary (Wm.) Westham, Essex; 1639

Hopkins, Mary 15; 1680 v. *s.m.w.*

Hopper, Anne St James in the Fields; 1690

Horner, Katherine (Joshua) 15; 1619

House, Mary Shadwell, Stepney; 1674

How, Sara (Thos.) 102; 1715

Howell, Eliz. (Samuel) 103; 1632

Howell, Katherine (Peter) 104; 1678

Hubbard, Mary (John) 104; 1641

Hubbard, Sarah (Edward) 111; 1669

Hubberd, Eliz. 73; 1637 v.

Huddlestone, Mary 98; 1700

Hughes, Mrs. 112; 1680 v.

Hughes, Mary (Richard) 35; 1615

Hull, Katherine 101; 1663

Humton, Mrs. 42; 1680 v.

Hunt, Eliz. 98; 1661

Hunt(sman)[c], Elinor (George) 107; 1683 (1700)

Hurle, Margaret, Chiswick; 1675

Hutchins, Margery (John) St James Westminster; 1704

Hutchins, Mary 104 (fl. 1696)

Hutchinson, Alice 109; 1637 v.

I (E) ngarson, Eliz. 98; 1674

Ireland, Dina 104; 1638

Ives, Ann (Wm.) St John Hackney; 1691

Jackman, Eliz. (Francis) 54; 1683

Jackman, Mary (Robert) 112&113; 1689 *s.m.w.*

Jacks, Martha 112; 1673

Jackson, Mary 98; 1674

Jackson, Mrs. 109; 1680 v.

Jake, Bridgid (Jacob) 114; 1609

James[c], Eliz. (John) 103; 1678 *s.m.w.*

James, Mary (Robert) 113&112; 1686

James, Susan (Albani) 109; 1628

Jeanes, or Jones, Alice 114; 1637 v.

Jeffery, Rebecca (Richard) 102; 1662

Jeffreys, Eliz. (Thos.) St Anne Westminster; 1719

Jekel, Eliz. (Robert) St Paul Shadwell; 1716

Jennings, Mary *s.m.w.*

Jermyn (German), Bridgid (Robert) 54; 1632

Jewell, Philido (John) 99; 1632

Jey, or Jay, Margaret 42; 1661

Jo(a)nes, Joan (Edward) 102; 1611

Johns, Charity 113; 1664 v.

Johns, Eliz. (Robert) St George, Southwark; 1697

Johnson, Alice 23; 1637 v.

Johnson, Ann (Edmund) Bethnal Green; 1692

Johnson, Eliz. 103; 1669 v. *s.m.w.*

Johnson[c], Frances 112; 1670 (fl. 1684)

Johnson, Grace (Robert) St John Wapping; 1708

Johnson, Jane 38; 1661

Johnson, Margaret (Henry) 113; 1661

Johnson, Mary 83; 1637 v.

Johnson, Mary (Roger) 66; 1929

Johnson, Rebecca (Henry) 119; 1676

Jones, Alice (Richard) 114; 1631
Jones, Anne (David) 19; 1618
Jones, Mrs. 7; 1680 v.

Keackwig, (Keckwich) Eliz. 5 *s.m.w.*
Keene, Eliz. (Wm.) 73; 1663
Kelch, Mrs. 19; 1680 v.
Kelsall, Hannah (James) 112; 1723
Kempton, Susan (Thos.) Cheshunt, Herts.; 1694
Kemwell or Remwell Anne 98; 1616
Kendall², Martha 103; (fl. 1700) (Q)?
Kensey, Eliz. 103; 1637 v.
Kent, Susanna 29
Kenton, Anne *s.m.w.*
Kettle, Mary (Alexander) Wivenhoe; 1707
Keyfar, Eliz. 102; 1611
Keymer, Sara 88; 1669
Kidd, Eliz. (Francis) 103; 1639
Kidder, Susanna (Edward) 113; 1700
Kikhimer, Rachel 101; 1672
Kilbury, Hester (Wm.) 111; 1664 *s.m.w.*
Kilfoe, Elianor 112; 1680 v.
King, Abigail (Thos.) 106; n.d. *s.m.w.*
King, Andrea or Abigail (John) 104; 1638
King, Eliz. Chipping Ongar; 1706
King, Margery (Jeffrey) widow Chipping Ongar;
   1696
King, Susan; 1634
Kist, Ann (John) 103; 1690
Kitchen, Mrs. 111; 1637 v.
Knapp, Eliz. 102; 1672
Knell, or Krell, Ann 111; 1667
Kneyton, Eliz. 112; 1680 v.
Knott, Mary (Richard) 104; 1663
Knowles, Catherine (Thos.) 102; 1668
Korkin, Eliz. (in Willughby)

Labany, Mrs. (in Aveling)
Lamb, alias Rampton, Anne 112; 1678 *s.m.w.*
Lamb, Eliz. (Richard) Cheshunt; 1691
Lambe, Katherine (Richard) Edmonton; 1687
Lambert, Mary (Francis) Evesham, Surrey; 1686
Lane, Rebecca 112; 1637 v.
Langley, Mary 112; 1671
Langton, Charity 12; 1663
Langton, Eliz. 111; 1718
Laramitt (Lermitt), Hester 114; 1671 *s.m.w.*
Larchin, Anne Chelsea; 1704
Larking, Eliz. (Timothy) n.p.; 1695
Lasselles, Mary (Don) 104; 1663 *s.m.w.*
Lattyn (Latin), Mrs. 86? (fl. 1649)
Laurence, Mary (Wm.) 54; 1634
Lawes, Eliz. Wapping; (fl. 1664) *s.m.w.*
Laywood, Eliz. 113; 1662 *s.m.w.*
Le Double, Mary 112; 1719
Leaber, Mrs. 109; 1669 v.
Leape, Christian (John) 11; 1618

Lee, Eleanor 30; 1637 v.
Lee, Joan 5; 1619
Lee, Mary Woodford, Essex; 1685
Lee, Sibill (Isobel) 111; 1665 *s.m.w.*
Leefs, Mary (Abraham) Tottenham; 1715
Leigh, Isobel (George) 113; 1678
Lemmyham, Mrs. 3; 1637 v.
Lemon, Anne (Wm.) 113; 1622
Lendall, Sara 80; 1611
Lestocart, Eliz. (John) 17; 1700
Leverett, Mary Chelsea; (1631?) *s.m.w.*
Lewis, Joan (Roger) 1; 1687
Lewis, Mary (David) 107; 1692
Lewys, Eliz. (Charles) 20; 1677
Light, Eliz. 119; 1688
Lindsay, Mary (Thos.) 57; 1637
Linicomb, Margaret St Windsor, Berks.; 1698
Linsey, Mrs. 43; 1637 v.
Lisle, Sarah (Nicholas) n.p.; 1667
Lister, Margaret (John) St James Westminster;
   1724
Littleboy, Mary (Robert) 109; 1687
Livingston, Christiana (Thos.) 112; 1639
Lloyd, Katherine (David) 112; 1668
Lodge, Alice (Henry) 103; 1609
Lodge, Lucy (John) 114; 1663
Long, Mary 113; 1682
Love, Eliz. (Edward) 117; 1663
Lovedon, Mary 111; 1671
Lovell, Mrs. 54; 1637 v.
Lovelock, Margaret (George) Woodham; 1671
Lowe, Ellen 112; 1669
Lucas, Adry (Henry) 98; 1667
Lucas, Jane 10; 1700
Lucas, Mary, 109; 1637 v.
Lucy, Mrs. 95/61; 1680 v.
Lyndsey, Mrs. 57; 1637 (1664 v.)

Mabbs, Frances (Wm) 102 (fl. 1662) *s.m.w.*
Maddiford𝑐, Anne St Margaret Westminster (fl.
   1680)
Maddison, Anne St John Wapping; 1703
Mainwaring, Sara (Thos.) 106; 1680 & 1690
Malam, Ann 88; 1673
Male, Mrs. 114; 1680 v.
Mallet, Alice (John) 115; 1612
Man, Margery (John) Stepney; 1704
Mannering, Francis 113; 1685
Mannersley, Catherine 98; 1634
Manning, Mrs. 104; 1680 v.
Manslawe, Mary 59; 1637 v.
Markham, Eliz. 74; 1619
Markham, Jane Hampstead; 1680 v.
Markinson, Alice (Wm.) Chigwell; 1715
Marriott, Margaret *s.m.w.*
Marshall, Mrs. 114; 1669 v.
Martin, Anne (Thos.) 111; 1719

Martyn, Eliz. (Wm.) 111; 1669 *s.m.w.*
Mason, Alice (Charles) 112 (Marybone); 1662
Mason, Blanch (Henry) 107; 1634
Mason, Hannah (John) Stepney Stebenheath
Mason, Hannah (John) 114; 1679 *s.m.w.*
Mason, Jane 113; 1640
Mason, Joan (John) 112; 1637
Massey[b], Jane 111 (fl. 1716)
Masters, Mary (Martin) Epping; 1676
Mathers, Rebecca (Wm.) 102; 1697
Mathews, Alice (Edmond) 115; 1609
Matin, Rebecca 101; 1715
Matthews, Isobel (Richard) 102; 1628
Matthews 107; 1667 v.
Maynard, Avis (John) 35; 1708
Mayne, Mrs. 1; 1680 v.
Maynell, Margaret (Gerard) 103; 1684
Mayott[b], Esther (fl. 1718)
Maxey, Joan (Simon) Hammersmith, Fullam 1666
Megon, Joyce (James) 106; 1616
Melsom, Mary 96; 1626 *s.m.w.*
Mercer, Eliz. 116; 1666
Mercer, Margaret (Aveling)
Mercey, Mrs. 112; 1669 v.
Merry, Mary (Thos.) Stepney; 1674
Meynes, Agnes (Robert) 109; 1609
Middleton, Mary (James) Eltham; 1669
Miles, Eliz. (Richard) 44; 1678
Millar, Joan (Henry) Hampstead; 1665
Miller, Joan. 49; 1637 v.
Miller, Anne 1; 1706
Millie, Jane, n.p. (fl. 1662) *s.m.w.*
Minchell, or Mitchell, Isobel (John?) 98; 1611
Mitchell, Jane (Peter) 8; 1616 (v. 1637)
Mitchell, Joan (Wm.) 111; 1610
Mitchell, Margaret 112; 1685
Mitchell[b], Mary 111; 1719 (fl. 1710)
Mitchelson, Mrs. 1; 1637 v.
Monger, Eliz. (John) 113; 1677
Montfort, Anne 113; 1699?
Moor, Rebecca St Anne Westminster; 1724
Moore, Anne 101; 1660
Moore[c], Jane 112; 1680 (fl. 1684)
Moore, Mrs. 109; 1680 v.
Moors, Eliz. Rayleigh, Midds.; 1664
Mordant[a], Eliz. 18 (fl. 1700)
More, Ann 103; 1637 v.
More[a], Eliz. 96; (fl. 1700)
More, Jane (Ralph) 9; 1664
Morecooke, Eliz. *s.m.w.*
Morgan, Eliz. 101; 1663
Morgan, Mrs. 112; 1680 v.
Morgan, Sybil (John) 107; 1703
Morgan, Ursula 107; 1667 v.
Morris, or Marris, Margaret 96; 1614
Morris, Eliz. (Thos.) Chigwell; 1715

Morris, Gertrude, Chelsea; 1705
Morse, Margaret 109; 1697
Motts, or Matts, Eleanor, Enfield; 1675
Mountford, Eliz. (Thos.) 102; 1678
Mourdion, Judith Poplar, Stepney; 1664
Mugg[c], Margaret Tottenham (fl. 1678)
Mullett, Alice (Wm.) 113; 1624
Mullett, Mrs. 1; 1637 v.

Nash, Eliz. (John) 114; 1692
Neams, Anne (George) 48; 1619
Neave, Susannah (Richard) 112; 1697
Needs, Mary (Wm.) 112; 1712
Nelmes, 3; 1664 v.
Newman, Judith (Wm.) 5; 1661
Nicholson, Sarah (Henry) 112; 1680
Nicholson 1; 1637 v.
Nicoll, Mary (Henry) 112; 1725
Nobb, Joane, (John) 43; 1613
Nollhaus, Ursula (John?) 3; 1664
Noone, Francis (Robert) 43; 1636
North, Mary Hackney, Midds.; 1677
Northall[b], Rebecca St Paul Shadwell; (fl. 1715)
Norton, Eliz. (Edmond) 113; 1705
Norton, Jane 107; 1693
Norton, alias Desborow, Margaret 70/71; 1680 v.
Norton, Ruth 104 /106; 1700
Nott, Joan (John) 42; 1637 v.
Nuthall, Mary (James) 113; 1685

Okes, Mary 74; 1622
Okey, Anne Stepney; 1663
Ollee, Mary Finchingfield; 1707
Orme[c], Eliz. (John) St James Westminster (fl. 1698)
Orme, (H)Ellen (James) 97; 1636 *s.m.w.*
Orme, Martha (Robert) 101; 1700
Osborne, Sara (John) 111; 1665
Osling, Mrs. 98; 1669 v.
Osmond[b], Elizabeth (fl. 1699)

Paddington, Mrs. 118; 1669 v.
Page, Mary (Wm.) 102; 1617
Page, 14; 1637 v.
Palmer, Alice (Edward) Stepney; 1612;(5; 1619)
Palmer, Francis (Henry) 109; 1619
Parkehurst, Eliz. 37; 1637 v.
Parker, Anna 112; 1686
Parkes, Mrs. (James) 84; 1638
Parnell, Fandrell (James) 114; 1619
Parrott, Anne (John) 113; 1671
Parsons, Margaret (John) 114; 1670
Parsons, Mary (John) 115; 1668
Partridge, Abigail (Abraham) New Brentford; 1686
Pattison, Beatrix 118; 1663

Pauley, Sara (Wm.) St Salvator, Southwark; 1687
Paulson, Eliz. 102; 1670
Paxton, Eliz. (Wm.) 98; 1684
Pead, Mrs. 7; 1664 v.
Pedro, Alice St Paul's, Shadwell; 1696
Peele, Alice (John) 54; 1611
Peerte, alias Bayley, Elizabeth (Peter) 104; 1608
Pell, Eliz. 18; 1689
Pendleton, Eliz. (Edmund) 107; 1670 *s.m.w.*
Penn, Ann 107; 1670
Penney, Hester (John) 117; 1669 *s.m.w.*
Pennyell, Eliz. St Margaret, Westminister; 1686
Pepper, Aurora (Richard) 101; 1663
Peppett, Pricilla (Robert) 112; 1685
Perkins, Ellen (Richard) 112; 1686
Perkins, Sara (Philip) St Paul's Shadwell (fl. 1681)
Pestle, Anne (John) 9; 1633
Pettingale, Margaret 104; 1637 v.
Philips[c], Tabitha (Richard) 102; (fl. 1684)
Phillips, Anne (Christopher) 115; 1628
Phillips, Sibill 112; 1637 v.
Pickard, Dorothy (Francis) 54; 1673
Pierce, Eliz. (Wm.) 93; 1713
Pierson, Anne (Christopher) 12; 1700
Pinchon, Katherine 57; 1663
Pink, Mary 49; 1677
Pinnock, Alice (Thos.) Shadwell; 1673
Plummer, Joan (John) 101; 1687
Ponsam (Penson), Eliz. (Thos.) 107; 1663
Pooke[c], Eliz. 31, (fl. 1694)
Poole, Anne Spitalfields, Stepney; 1700
Pope, Margaret 111; 1676
Porter, Barbara (John) 117
Porter, Barbara 104; 1612
Porter[b], Eliza (fl. 1708)
Poston, Sara (Timothy) 109; 1711
Pratt, Temperance 102; 1664 *s.m.w.*
Pratten, Margaret (James) 113; 1662
Preston, Mary (Edward) Hackney, Midds.; 1697
Price, Mary (Richard) 112; 1720
Price, Susan (Thos.) Acton. Midds.; 1698
Pritchard, Francis (Robert) Lancaster?; 1666
Pye, Dorothy 112; 1678

Quant, Mary (Edward) 112; 1697
Quelch, Mrs. (Wm.) 111; n.d.

Ramscall, Thomasina (Thos.) 109; 1666
Ramsey[c], Eliz. (Henry) 14; 1696
Ramton (Ramsay), Ann 85; 1611
Ranckle, Margaret (Richard) 67; 1637
Ranew, Martha 109; 1686
Ranger, Sara 114; 1680 v.
Ratcliffe, Jane 98; 1625
Rathbone, Joan (John) 49; 1625

Rathborne, Mary (Randall) 112; 1685
Raven, Dorothy (John) 112; 1619
Rawbone, Eliz. 101; 1677
Rawlins, Catherine (Robert) 99/100?; 1614
Rawlins, Mrs. 103; 1680 v.
Read, Brigid 49; 1637 v.
Read, Eliz. (John) 102; 1672
Read, Mrs. 119; 1637 v.
Reade, Joan (John) 115; 1639
Redding, Mary (Henry) St James in the Fields; 1695
Reekes, Mary (John) 115; 1667
Relkin, Mrs. 112; 1680 v.
Reyley, Mrs. 66; 1680 v.
Reynolds, Sara (James) St Anne in the Fields; 1695
Reysar, Tymothea (John) 111; 1612
Rhodes, Jane or Joan Poplar; 1663
Richards, Eleanor 3; 1663
Richardson, Mary *s.m.w.*
Richardson, Sara (Richard) 113; 1685
Rickes, Eliz. (Edmond) Stepney 1664
Roberts, Alice (Wm.) 107; 1634 (12; 1664 v.)
Roberts, Barbara 115; 1686
Roberts, Hannah (Robert) 103; 1669
Roberts, Susanna (Henry) 102; (d. 1610)
Roberts, Katherine 50; (fl. 1724)
Robinson, Eliz. (Wm.) 109; 1674
Rogers, Eliz. (John) 83; 1689
Rogers, Eliz. (Wm.) 9; 1631
Rogers, Mary (Edward) 79; 1690
Rogers, Sarah 9; 1637 v. *s.m.w.*
Rogers, Ursula (Thos.) 113; 1664 v. *s.m.w.*
Rose, Mrs. 114; 1669 v.
Rosewell, Francis (Joshua) 112; 1678
Ross, Sara 107; 1672
Rosson, Dorothy (Henry) 111; 1692
Rowden, Mary (Frances) 113; 1617 (1637 v.)
Rowe, or Reve, Judith (John) 96; 1610
Rowley, Joan (Thos.) 113; 1632 *s.m.w.*
Royston, Sara 111; 1682
Rudge, Sara 63; 1637 v.
Russell, Mary Tottenham High Cross Midds.; 1697, 1680 v.
Russell, Mary (Edward) 112; 1664 *s.m.w.*
Rutter, Ann 102; 1661

Salmon, Mary (John) 115; 1693
Sampson, Mrs. 118; 1669 v.
Sam(p)son, Phillipa 113; 1677
Sampson, Mary (Henry) 113; 1697
Sampson, Mrs. 112; 1680 v.
Sanders, Mrs. 101; 1680 v.
Sandiman, Jane (Charles) 112; 1692
Sandys, Eliz. 98; 1703
Sare, Emmett 107; 1662
Sarney, Hester 49; 1637 v.(deputy)

Saule, Marjorie (Edward) 33; 1621
Sault, Sara (Richard) 92; 1696
Saunders, Eliz. n.p.; 1619
Saunders(on), Ann (Wm) 112; 1697
Saxton, Eliz. 112; lic. 1719 (Giffard)
Saywell, Mrs. Limehouse, (fl. 1664) *s.m.w.*
Scattergood, Esther (Roger) 9; 1717
Scott, Hanna (Thos.) 117; 1676
Seale, Eliz. 1; 1619
Sedgewick, Barbara 107; 1674
Seeley, Eliz. (George) 106 (113); 1622
Seeley, Jane 35; (fl. 1663) *s.m.w.*
Seigmor, or Seymour, Mary; 106; 1663
Sell, Mrs. Hampstead; 1666
Semcoe, or Semcott, Eliz. (George) 103; 1673
Semor, Mrs. 41; 1637 v.
Senior, Mary (Wm.) 117; 1623
Sension, Joan 87; 1627
Sessions, Margaret 112; 1637 v.
Shaw, Eliz. 113; 1664 v.
Shaw, Mrs. Hester 1; 1637 v.
Shaw, Mrs. 109; 1680 v.
Sheffield, Margaret (Joseph) 112; 1689
Shelton, or Skelton, Mary 111; 1665
Sherman, Frances (Charles) 105; 1700
Sherwood, Mary (Ralph) 56; 1676
Shipley, Eliz. 73; 1637 v.
Shipley, Sara (Dean & Chap of St Paul's); 1669 v.
Shorter, Ann 87; 1680 v.
Shute, Christian (George) 43; 1631
Siverthorn, Susan Tottenham High Cross; 1705
Simmonds, Mary (Stephen) Wapping, Stepney; 1697
Sinclair, Joan (George) 112; 1684
Simpson, Rebecca (Richard) 98; 1700
Skelton, Susanna? 112; 1680 v.
Skidmore[b], Jane (Robert) Southwark (fl. 1711)
Slarke, Rebecca (John) 59; 1664
Slater, Eleanor (Richard) Kensington; 1697
Slicer, Sarah (Joseph) 104; 1684
Smith, Joyce 90; 1637 v.
Smith, Ann 103; 1700
Smith, Eliz. (Thos.) 103; 1621
Smith[c], Eliz. (Thos) 112 (fl. 1679)
Smith, Eliz. (Henry) 103; 1693?
Smith, alias Webb, Eliz. (Anthony) 104; 1664
Smith[a], Emma (John) 102 (d. 1615)
Smith, Frances, 113; 1664 v.
Smith, Hanna (David) 68; 1685 *s.m.w.*
Smith, Joanne (Thos.) 112; 1681
Smith, Mary (George) Miles End, Stepney; 1663
Smith, Mrs. 111; 1637 v.
Smith, Rebecca 111; 1682
Smith, Sara 21; n.d.
Smith, Tabitha (George) 102; 1678
Smithson, Sara (Francis) 116; 1662

Smorthwayte, Margaret 113; 1673
Smyth, Anna (John) 75; 1636
Snape, Frances *s.m.w.*
Snead, Mary (Wm.) 119; 1677, 1680 v.
Soedin, or Sowden Mary *s.m.w.*
Solines, or Somes, Jane 102; 1663
Somner, or Sumner Anne (Samuel) 112; (fl. 1669) *s.m.w.*
Somner, Eliz. (Wm.) 106; 1639 *s.m.w.*
Southen, or Sowden, Frances (Wm.) 56; 1686
Spalding, Sara (Robert) Lambeth
Sparks, Mrs. 84; 1637 v.
Sparks, Mrs. 113; 1637 v.
Spinner, Ellinor 15; 1615
St John, Anne (James) 51; 1664
Stainsmore 107; 1669 v.
Stanchroft 114; 1680 v.
Stanfro, or Stamprow, Eleanor (Edward) 114; 1663 *s.m.w.*
Stannard, Francis (John) 109; 1661
Stansmore, Ellen (Joseph) 41; 1670
Stanton[c], Anne (Nicholas) 112; 1665 (fl. 1673)
Stanton 107; 1671 v.
Stanworth, Ann (Wm) 112; 1700
Staufer, Mrs. 114; 1669 v.
Stevens, Margaret (John) 104; 1663
Stokes, Katherine n.p.; 1628
Stokes, Ursula (Eliz.?) (John) Stepney; 1677, 1680 v.
Stone, Martha Chipping Ongar? (fl. 1706)
Storke, Anne (Thos.) 104; 1617
Stourton, or Strutton, Anne 115; 1661
Strange, Sara (Thos.) Stepney ; 1697
Streete, Frances 58; 1637 v.
Strowbridge, Mary 113; 1697
Stuart, Mary 112; 1662
Styles, Mrs. 114; 1669 v.
Sumers, Charity? 112; 1680 v.
Sute, Mrs. 43; 1637 v.
Sutton, Julian 47; 1611
Swanley, Susan Shadwell, Stepney; 1669 *s.m.w.*
Sweatman, Isabel 98; 1688 *s.m.w.*
Sydey, Sara (Waldegrave) 31; 1663
Symonds, Abigail 106; 1667
Syrett, Eliz. (Edward) 111; 1690

Tanfield, Sara (Solomon) 17; 1636 & 1637 v.
Tatham, Anne (John) 113; 1712
Taylor, Anne (Thos.) 114; 1675
Taylor, Anne Mary (Thos.) 107; 1698
Taylor, Catherine 28; 1677
Taylor, Katherine, 9; 1637 v.
Taylor, Mary (James) Fulham; 1664
Taylor, Mary (Thos.) 87; 1661
Taylor, Winnifred (Thos.) 119; 1692
Tellier, Esther 101/109; 1715
Terry, Anne, (Wm.) Stepney; 1619

Whyte, Eliz. (Humphrey) St Paul Shadwell; 1675

Wickes[b,c], (Weekes) Eliz. (Edward) 117; 1673 s.m.w. (1698)

Wicks, Catherine (Richard) 106; 1630

Wicks, Eliz. 112; 1692 s.m.w.

Wicks, Mrs. 113; 1680 v.

Wiggens Rebecca (Richard) 112; 1664

Wigly, or Wigby, Gertrude (Thos.) 111; 1662

Wilder, Hanna (Henry) 103; 1683

Wilkes, Dorcas (Roger) 43; 1684

Wilkins, Mrs. (in Willughby)

Wilkins, Sarah (Robert) 54; 1682

Wilkinson, Isabel (Lynton) 98; 1609

Willcox, Eliz. (John) 98; 1687

Williams, Mary (Thos.) 107; 1697

Williams, Mary 107; 1672

Williams, Mrs. 102; 1637 v.

Williams, Susanna (Edward) Watcliffe, Stepney; 1608

Willis, Margaret (Gregory) 115; 1631

Williscott, Margaret 103; 1666

Willoughby, Margaret 112; 1639

Wills, Eliz. (Thos.) Stepney; 1663

Willson, Anne 113; 1663

Wilson, Debora 104; 1677

Wilson, Mary (George) 68; 1637 v.

Wilton, Catherine 37; 1630, 1637 v.

Winchester, Hannah (Daniel) 104; 1699 s.m.w

Winchurch, or Winchurst Eliz. (Walter?) Stepney; 1663 s.m.w.

Winckles, Jane (Jonathan) 35; 1679

Withers, Eliz. n.p.; 1673

Wolverston, Mrs. (fl. 1689)

Wood[a], Eliz. 105; (fl. 1700)

Wood, Mary 112; 1685

Wooden, Jone (James) 109; 1664 s.m.w.

Woodford, Sara (John) 7; 1684

Woodward, Eliz. (Joseph) Kingston on Thames, Surrey; 1684

Woole, Anne (John) 112; 1680

Woolsey[b], Anne (fl. 1722)

Wright, Anne (John) Acton; (fl. 1665) s.m.w.

Wright, Barbara (Edward) 98; 1690

Wright, Mary (Thos.) 112; 1671

Wright, Sara 49; 1664 v.

Wright, Susan 115; 1698

Wynn, Eliz. (Wm.) Hampton; 1697

Yarwood, Joan s.m.w.

Yarrow[c], Mrs. (fl. 1692)

Yates, Eliz. (Robert) 47; 1685

Yates, Phillis (Wm) Navestock; 1664

Young, Dionitia (Dennys) Enfield; 1675

Younger, Hannah (Alexander) 60; 1676

BIBLIOGRAPHY

PRIMARY SOURCES

Manuscript Sources

Bodleian Library, Oxford

Midwife's Account Book, Rawlinson MS. D 1141.

Corporation of London Record Office

Hearth Taxes: Box 41.15 (1670); Box 25.9/5, 15, 20, 22, 27, 34, 36 (1672?).
Marriage Tax Assessments 1695.
Parish and ward tithe rate assessments: Box 20.6(1673); Box 41.15a, 17, 23 (1671); Box
    45.11,17 (1675, 1671); Box 46.12, 13, 15, 19 (1671–1688); Box 16.11; Box 5.7 (1671);
    Box 29.10 (1673) 24 (1673/4); Box 32.6 (1673); Box 7.7 (1680); Box 31.12 (1688);
    Box 7.8 (1690); Box 40.8 (1693/4).
Poll taxes: Box 20.13 (1690); Box 33.17 (1688); Box 33.2 (1692); Box 14.21 (1693); Box
    20.6 (1672); 12 (1690); Box 11. 6,4 (1677–8), Box 67.10 (1978); Box 67.4 (1678); 68.3
    (1678); Box 11.24 (1678); Box 11.12 (1678); Box 15.21 (1690); Box 33.2 (1692).
Royal and additional aids: Box 18.1 (1666); Box 66.3 (1666); Box 56.8 (1666); Box 66.12
    (1666); Box 56.22 (1667); Box 71.13 (1668); Box 65.3 (1668); Box 57.19 (1671); Box
    16.1 (1673); Box 34.6 (1674); Box 19.6 (1674); Box 6.13 (1688); Box 15.21 (1690).
Window Tax Box 14.26 (1696).

Cumbria Record Office

MS. WD/Cr Kendal Midwife's Diary.

Greater London Record Office

Consistory Court, Vicar General's Registers, volumes 10–16 (1607–1685) MSS. DL/C/
    339–45
Minutes of the Lying in Hospital for Married Women in Brownlow St near Longacre,
    GLRO MSS. H14/BLI/A1/1; H14/BLI/A3/1

Minute Book of The City of London Maternity Hospital 1750–54, MS. H10/CLM A1/1.
Records of the New Westminster Lying-in Hospital, MS. H1/ST/K10/23; H1/GLI/A3/1.

Guildhall Library

Account Books of Overseers of the Poor: St Andrew Wardrobe, MS. 2089/1–2 (1613–95); St Dunstan in the West, MS. 2999/1; St Katherine Coleman MSS. 1145/1–2; St Olave Silver Street, MS. 1262/1.

Assessment for cost of army, navy and militia: St Dunstan in the West, MS. 2969/1–4 (1654–80).

Bishop of London Registers vol. 9531 (1634).

Bishop of London Visitation Registers: MSS. 9537/14–22 (1636–80).

Churchwardens' Account Books: Allhallows the Less, MS. 823/1; St Dunstan in the West, MSS. 2968/1–6 (1596–1699); St Bartholomew at the Exchange, 4383/1; St Gregory by St Paul's, MS. 1337/1; St Ethelburga, MS. 4241/1–2; St John the Baptist, MSS. 577/1–2, 7619 (collections as a result of appeals in church); St Katherine Coleman, MS. 1124/1; St Martin Outwich, MS. 1194/1; St Mary Aldermanbury, MSS. 3556/2–3; St Olave Silver Street, MSS. 1257/1–8.

"Citizens of London 1641–1643." Unpublished typescript by T. C. Dale, 1936.

Clerk's Memoranda Book St Botolph Aldgate, MS. 9234/7–8.

Commissary Court of London, will registers 9050, 9051, 9052, 9168, 9171, 9172, 9174.

List of Householders who lost property in the Great Fire of 1666, MS. 14819.

Lists of Parish Officials, St Katherine Coleman, MS. 1125/1.

"Members of the City Companies in 1641 as set forth in the returns for the Poll Tax." Unpublished typescript, Society of Genealogists, 1935.

Midwives' Testimonial Certificates, MSS. 10,116/1–14, 25, 598 (1661–1700).

Orphan Tax assessment: St Dunstan in the West, MS. 2998/1–3 (1695,1698).

Parish Assessments, miscellaneous: MS. 823/1–2 (1630–42); MS. 2961/1 (1658–61); MS. 2969/2–4 (1661–80); MS. 3556/2–3; MS. 2188 (1674); MS. 7619.

Poll Tax MSS. 7770 (1689) 7769, 1692, and 1694, St Andrew Wardrobe and St Anne Blackfriar, MS. 9801 (1674)

Reassessment : navy, garrisons, etc., St Dunstan in the West. MS. 3015 (1699).

Scavenger Rates: St Martin Outwich, MS. 11395; St Dunstan in the West, MS.3783.

Tithe assessments: St Andrew Wardrobe and St Anne Blackfriars (1674), MS. 9801/ 1; St Mary Aldermanbury, MS. 9801/2. St Olave Silver Street, MS. 9801/3; St Gregory by St Paul's MS. 9801/2

Trophy Tax assessment, St Dunstan in the West: MS. 3014/1–2 (1689, 1696).

Parish Registers: St Dunstan in the West, MS. 10,342–48 (1558–1739); Parish Registers St Andrew Wardrobe, MSS. 4502, 4507, 4503 (1558–1850).

Vestry Minute Books: Allhallows the Less, MS. 8241/1; St Dunstan in the West, MSS. 3016/1–2 (1587–1695); St Gregory by St Paul's, MS. 1336/1; St Mary Aldermanbury, MS. 4880; St Botolph Bishopsgate, MS. 4526/1.

Visitation Records of the Peculiar of the Dean and Chapter of St Paul's: MSS. 25,533/1–2 (1667–74).

Lambeth Palace Library

Catalogue of Inhabitants of London, MS. 272 (1638).
Institution Act Book (1663–73).
Process Books D1960 case No. 8596 (1665).
Midwives' Testimonial Certificates, MS.VX 1A/11/1–82 (1669–1700).
Registers of Archbishop Richard Bancroft (1604–10).
Registers of Archbishop George Abbott (1611–33), vols. 1–3.
Registers of Archbishop William Laud (1633–45).
Registers of Archbishop Gilbert Sheldon vol. 2 (1663–77).
Registers of Archbishop William Sancroft vol. 2 (1678–90).
Registers of Archbishop William Juxon (1660–63).
Registers of Archbishop John Tillotson (1691–94).
Registers of Archbishop Thomas Tenison vols. 1–2 (1695–1715).
Will Register VH95 (1705).

Public Record Office, London (Chancery Lane)

Chancery Proceedings, MS. 25,625/4 (1686–87) Francis Alkin
Hearth Taxes E 179/252/15, 32, 28. (1645, 1666, 1687).
Lay Subsidy Assessments, MS. E 179/147/491, 492, 494, 497, 577; E 179/252/4, 7, 15, 17;
    179/143/349, 351, 365; E 179/253/19; E 179/186/437 (various dates).
Prerogative Court of Canterbury, probate registers, Prob.11/ 50, 120, 133, 153, 217, 222,
    312, 322, 340, 343, 344, 350, 351, 432, 456, 485.
Quaker Birth Notes RG 6.

Royal College of Gynaecologists

Minute Books of the Royal Maternity Charity.

Toronto Public Library

Parish Registers of St Andrew Wardrobe and St Anne Blackfriars (microform).

Middlesex Hospital Archives

Middlesex Hospital Fair Minute Books 1747–54.

Printed Sources

Aitken, John. *Principles of Midwifery or Puerperal Medicine*. London: 1685.
Anon. *An Account of the British Lying in Hospital for Married Women, Situated in Brownlow St,
    Long Acre from its institution in Nov. 1749 to Lady Day, 1756*. London: 1756.
*Articles to be Inquired of, in the First Metropoliticall Visitation of the Most Reverend Father: Richard
    Archbishop of Canterbury*. London, 1605; reprint edition, Amsterdam: Theatrum Orbis
    Terrarum, 1975.

Astry, Diana. "Diana Astry's Recipe Book." Bette Stitt ed., *The Publications of the Bedford-shire Historical Record Society* 37 (1957): 83–169.

The Book of Oaths, and the severall forms thereof, both Antient and Modern. London, 1649; Thomason E 1129.

Bannerman, Bruce, ed. *The Registers of St. Mary Aldermanbury* parts 1&2. London: Harleian Society Publications vols. 61–2, 1932.

The Registers of St. Martin Outwich, London. London: Harleian Society, vol. 32, 1905.

Briggs, William, ed. *The Register Book of St. Nicholas Acons, London 1539–1812.* Leeds: Walker & Laycock, 1890.

C. R. *The Complete Midwives Practice Enlarged.* London: 1680.

Cellier, Elizabeth. *To Dr. . . . an answer to his queries.* London: 1688; Wing C1457(3).

———. *A Scheme for the Foundation of a Royal Hospital, and raising a Revenue of Five or Six Thousand Pounds a Year, by and for the Maintenance of a Corporation of skilful Midwifes, and such Foundlings, or exposed Children, as shall be admitted therein.* London: 1687; Printed in Somner's Tracts, vol. 9 1813, pp. 248–53.

Chamberlen, Peter. *A Voice in Rhama: or, The Crie of Women and Children.* London: 1646.; Thomason E 1181 (8).

Chapman, Edmund. *A Treatise on the Improvement of Midwifery chiefly with regard to the Operator.* London: 1735.

Chester, J. L. *The Parish Registers of St. Michael Cornhill, London.* London: 1882.

Cooke, James. *Mellificium Chirurgiae.* London: 1648.

Culpeper, Nicholas. *A Directory for Midwives: or A Guide for Women, in their Conception, Bearing and Suckling their Children.* London: 1651; Thomason E 1340 (1).

The Directory Containing an Alphabetical List of the Names and Places of Abode of the Directors of Companies, Persons in Public Business, Merchants etc. and Places of Abode of Companies, Persons in Public Business, Merchants etc. London: 1736.

Dorset Folk Remedies of the 17th and 18th Centuries. Edited by J. Stevens Cox. Dorchester: The Dorset Natural History and Archeological Society.

Fell, Sarah. *The Household Account Book of Sarah Fell of Swarthmoor Hall.* Edited by Norman Penney. Cambridge: Cambridge University Press, 1920.

Frere, W. H. and Kennedy, William, eds. *Visitation Articles and Injunctions of the Period of the Reformation* vol.2. London: Longmans, Green & Co., 1910.

Freshfield, Edwin. *The Vestry Minute Books of the Parish of St. Bartholomew Exchange in the City of London 1567–1676.* London: Rixon and Arnold, 1890.

Gardiner, Dorothy, ed. *The Oxinden Letters 1607–1642.* London: Constable and Company, 1933.

Giffard, William. *Cases in Midwifry.* London: B. Motte and T. Wotton, 1734.

Goodall, Charles. *The Royal College of Physicians of London. An Account of their proceedings against empirics.* London: 1684; Wing G 1091.

Guillimeau, James. *Child-Birth, or, The Happy Deliverie of Women.* London: 1612; reprint ed. Amsterdam: Theatrum Orbis Terrarum, 1972.

Hartlib, Samuel. *Ephemenides.* London: 1650

Harvey, William. *Anatomical Exercitations, Concerning the Generation of Living Creatures. To which are added Particular Discourses of Births, and of Conceptions etc.* London: 1655; Thomason E 1435.

Hinton, Sir John. *Memoirs of Sir John Hinton, Physitian in ordinary to His Majesties Person 1679.* London: T. Bentley, 1814.

Hoby, Lady Margaret. *Diary of Lady Hoby.* Edited by Dorothy Meads. Boston and New York: Houghton Mifflin Co., 1930.

Jocelin, Elizabeth. *The Mother's Legacy to her Unborn Child.* London: 1864; Wing J 756.

Josselin, Ralph. *Diary of Ralph Josselin 1616–1683.* Edited by Alan MacFarlane. London: Oxford University Press, 1976.

Lake, Rev. Edward. *Diary of the Rev. Edward Lake (1641–1704).* London: Camden Society, 1847; reprint ed. New York: Johnson Reprint Corporation, 1968.

Latham, Robert and Matthews, William, eds. *The Diary of Samuel Pepys.* Berkeley and Los Angeles: University of California Press, 1970.

Leake, John. *A Syllabus of Lectures or the Theory and Practice of Midwifery.* London: 1776.

Lestrange, Roger. *A Collection of the Names of the Merchants Living in and about the City of London; Very useful and Necessary.* London: 1677; Wing C 5204.

Loftis, John, ed. *The Memoirs of Ann, Lady Halkett and Ann, Lady Fanshawe.* Oxford: Clarendon Press, 1979.

Manningham, Richard. *The Institution and Oeconomy of the Charitable Infirmary for the Relief of Poor Women Labouring of Child and during their Lying-in.* (1739) Reprinted in *An abstract of midwifery for the use of the Lying-in Infirmary.* London: 1744.

Marriage Licenses Westminister 1658–1669 Canterbury 1660–68. 23 London: Harleian Society, 1886.

M.B. *The Ladies Cabinet Enlarged and Opened.* London: 1654; Wing B135.

Massarius, A. *De Morbeis Foeminis. The Womans Counsellour or The Feminine Physician.* Translated by R. T. London: 1657; Thomason E 1650.

The Midwives Just Petition or a Complaint of divers good Gentlewomen of that Faculty. London: 1643; Thomason E 86(14).

Maubray, John M.D. *The Female Physician.* London: 1724.

Morrison, J. H. *Prerogative Court of Canterbury Register "Scroope" (1630).* London: J. H. Morrison, 1934.

Nicholls, F. *The Petition of the Unborn Babes to the Censors of the Royal College of Physicians of London.* London: 1751.

Nicholson, Marjorie Hope, editor. *Conway Letters: the correspondence of Anne, Viscountess Conway, Henry More, and their friends, 1642–1648.* Oxford: Oxford University Press, 1930.

Nihell, Elizabeth. *A Treatise on the Art of Midwifery.* London: 1760.

Pechey, William. *Compleat Midwives Practice Enlarged.* London: 1698; Wing P 220 (7).

Philiatros, F. *Nature Exenterata: or Nature Unbowelled by the most Exquisite Anatomizers of Her.* London: 1655.

The Registers of the Church of St. Ethelburga The Virgin within Bishopsgate. London: Press of the Church of St. Ethelburga, Bishopsgate, 1915.

Rosselin, E. *The Byrth of Mankynde.* Translated by Thomas Raynold. London: 1540; S.T.C. No. 21154.

Rueff, Jacob. *The Expert Midwife, or an Excellent and most necessary Treatise of the generation and birth of Man.* London: E. Griffen, 1637; S.T.C. No. 1004.

Sadler, John. *The Sick Woman's Private Looking Glass.* London: 1636; reprint ed. Amsterdam: Theatrum Orbis Terrarum, 1977.

Searle, Arthur, ed. *Barrington Family Letters 1628–1632.* London: Offices of the Royal Historical Society, University College, 1983.

Sermon, William. *The Ladies Companion or the English Midwife*. London: 1671; Wing S 2628.

Sharp(e), Jane. *The Midwives Book*. London: 1671; reprint ed. New York and London: Garland Publishing Inc. 1985.

Smellie, William. *Treatise on the Theory and Practice of Midwifery*. London: 1752.

Starkey, George. *Nature's explication and Helmont's Vindication or a short and sure way to a long and sound life*. London: 1656; Thomason E, 1635.

Sterne, Laurence. *The Life and Opinions of Tristram Shandy*. Harmondsworth, Middlesex: Penguin, 1967.

Stephen, Margaret. *The Domestic Midwife*. London, 1795.

Stone, Sara. *A Complete Practice of Midwifery*. London, 1737

T. C. et al. *The Compleat Midwife's Practice, in the most weighty and high Concernments of the Birth of Man*. London: 1656; Thomason 1588(3).

Thicknesse, Philip. *Man Midwifery Analysed*. London: 1764.

Thornton, Alice. *The Autobiography of Mrs. Alice Thornton of East Newton, Co. York (1627–1707)*. Edited by C. Jackson. Durham: Andrew and Company, 1875.

Twysden, Isabella. "The Diary of Isabella, Wife of Sir Roger Twysden, Baronet of Royden Hall, East Peckham, 1645–1651." Edited by F. W. Bennett. *Archeologica Cantiana*. 51 (1939): 113–36.

Vauguion, La. *A Compleat Body of Chirurgical Operations Containing the Whole Practice of Surgery with Observations and Remarks on each case Amongst which are inserted, the several ways of Delivering Women in Natural and Unnatural Labours*. London: 1707.

Verney, Frances P. and Verney, M. M. *The Verney Memoirs* 2 vols. London: Longmans, Green and Co., 1925.

W. M. *The Queen's Closet Opened*. London: 1655.

Walker, Anthony W. *The Holy Life of Mrs. Elizabeth Walker*. London: 1690; Wing W 305.

Ward, Rev. John. *Diary of the Rev. John Ward A.M.: Vicar of Stratford-Upon-Avon 1648–79*. Edited by C. Severn. London: Henry Colborn Pub., 1839.

White, Charles. *A Treatise on the Management of Pregnant and Lying-in Women*. London: 1773.

White, J. *A Rich Cabinet with Variety of Inventions*. London: 1651.

Willughby, Percival. *Observations in Midwifery*. Edited by H. Blenkinsop, 1863; reprint ed., East Ardley, Wakefield: SR Publishers, 1972.

SECONDARY SOURCES

Abbott, Mary. *Life Cycles in England 1560–1720*. London: Routledge, 1996.

Alexander, James. "The economic and social structure of London c. 1700." Ph.D. dissertation, University of London, 1989.

Allen, Phyllis. "Medical Education in 17th Century England." *Journal of the History of Medicine* 1 (1946): 115–43.

Amussen Dwyer, Susan. *An Ordered Society*. Oxford: Basil Blackwell, 1988.

Anderson, Bonnie and Zinsser, Judith. *A History of Their Own: Women in Europe From Prehistory to the Present*. New York: Harper and Row, 1988.

Anon. "Celebrated Midwives of the 17th and Beginning of the 18th Centuries: with a short account of the present position of midwives." *St. Thomas's Hospital Gazette* vol.53 (March 1895): 33–6.

Anon. *Laws, Rules and Orders for the Government of the Westminster Lying-in Hospital.* London: 1802.

Arons, Wendy. translator. *When Midwifery Became the Male Physician's Province: The Sixteenth Century Handbook "The Rose Garden for Pregnant Women and Midwives, Newly Englished."* Jefferson, N.C. and London: McFarland & Co. Inc., 1994

Arthure, Humphrey. "Early English Midwifery." *Midwife, Health Visitor & Community Nurse.* 2 (1975): 187–90.

Aveling, James H. *English Midwives, Their History and Prospects.* London: 1872; reprint ed., London: Hugh K. Elliott Ltd., 1967.

——. *The Chamberlens and the Midwifery Forceps.* London: J.& A. Churchill, 1882.

Aveling, J. C. H. *The Handle and the Axe: The Catholic Recusants in England from Reformation to Emancipation.* London: Blond and Briggs, 1976.

Axtell, James. "Education and Status in Stuart England: the London Physician." *History of Education Quarterly* 10 (1970): 141–59.

Barkai, Ron. "A Medieval Hebrew Treatise on Obstetrics." *Medical History* 33 (1988): 96–119.

Beaven, A. B. *The Aldermen of the City of London.* London: The Corporation of the City of London, 1908.

Beier, A. L. and Finlay, Roger, eds. *London 1500–1700.* London: Longman, 1986.

——. "The Significance of the Metropolis." In *London 1500–1700,* pp. 1–33. London: Longman, 1986.

Bell, E. Moberley. *Storming the Citadel; the rise of the woman doctor.* London: Constable, 1953.

Benedek, Thomas G. "The Changing Relationship between Midwives and Physicians during the Renaissance." *Bulletin of the History of Medicine* 51 (1977): 550–64.

Bennett, G. V. *The Tory Crisis in Church and State 1688–1630.* Oxford: Clarendon, 1975.

Biller, Peter. "Childbirth in the Middle Ages." *History Today* 36 (August 1986): 42–9.

Blackman, Janet. "Seventeenth Century Midland Midwifery – a comment." *Local Population Studies* 9 (1972): 47–8.

——. "Lessons from the history of maternal care and childbirth." *Midwives Chronicle* 90 (March 1977): 46–9.

Bloom, J. Harvey and James, R. Rutson. *Medical Practitioners in the Diocese of London, Licensed under the Act of 3 Henry VIII, C.11.* Cambridge: Cambridge University Press, 1935.

Borst, Charlotte. *Catching Babies: The Professionalization of Childbirth, 1870–1920.* Cambridge, Mass.: Harvard University Press, 1995.

Boss, B. and Boss, J. "Ignorant midwives – a further Rejoinder." *The Society for the Social History of Medicine* Bulletin 33 (December 1983): 71.

Bossy, John. *The English Catholic Community 1570–1850.* London: Darton, Longman and Todd, 1975.

Boulton, Jeremy. *Neighbourhood and Society: A London Suburb in the Seventeenth Century.* Cambridge: Cambridge University Press, 1987.

Brett-James, Norman G. *The Growth of Stuart London.* London: George Allen & Unwin Ltd., 1935.

Brockbank, W. "Mrs. Jane Sharp's advice to midwives." *Medical History* 2 (1958): 153–5.

Brody, Steven A. "The Life and Times of Sir Fielding Gould: man midwife and master physician." *Bulletin of the History of Medicine* 52 (1978): 228–50.

Buer, Martin. *Health, Wealth and Population.* London: Routledge, 1926.

Bullough, Vern L. "Medieval Medical and Scientific Views of Women," *Viator*, vol. 4 (1973): 485–501.

Burch, Brian. "The Parish of St. Anne's Blackfriars, London, to 1665." *The Guildhall Miscellany* 3 (October, 1969): 1–55.

Burke, J. B. *A Genealogical History of the Dormant, Abeyant, Forfeited and Extinct Peerages of the British Empire*. London: Harrison, 1883.

Burn, Richard. *The Ecclesiastical Law*. 2, London: 1842.

Burtch, Brian. *Trials of Labour: The Re-emergence of Midwifery*. Montreal & Kingston: McGill-Queen's University Press, 1994.

Burton, Elizabeth. *The Jacobeans at Home*. London: Secker & Warburg, 1962.

Bynum, W. F. and Porter, Roy, eds. *Medical Fringe and Medical Orthodoxy 1750–1850*. London: Croom Helm, 1987.

Cannings, Ralph. *The City of London Maternity Hospital: a Short History*. London: J. S. Forsaith and Son, 1922.

Cardwell, Edward. *Documentary Annals of the Reformed Church of England* vol. 1. Oxford: University Press, 1844.

Carter, E. H. *The Norwich Subscription Books: A Study of the Subscription Books of the Diocese of Norwich 1637–1800*. London: Thomas Nelson and Sons Ltd., 1937.

Carter, M. "The Royal Midwives." *Midwives Chronicle* 90 (1977): 300–1.

Cash, Arthur. "The Birth of Tristram Shandy: Sterne and Doctor Burton." In *Sexuality in eighteenth-century Britain*, pp. 198–224. Edited by P. A. Bouce. Manchester: Manchester University Press, 1982.

Chaber, Lois A. " 'This Affecting Subject': An 'Interested' Reading of Childbearing in Two Novels by Samuel Richardson." *Eighteenth-century Fiction* vol. 8, 2, (January 1996): 193–250.

Charlton, Christopher. "A Midwives Certificate, London, 1686." *Local Population Studies* 4 (1970): 56–8.

Chartres, John. "Food Consumption and Internal Trade." In *London 1500–1700*, pp. 168–96. Edited by A. L. Beier and Roger Finlay. London: Longman, 1986.

Clark, Alice. *Working Life of Women in the Seventeenth Century*. London: Frank Cass and Co. Ltd., 1919; reprint ed., Fairfield, N.J.: Augustus M. Kelley, 1978.

Clark, Sir George. *A History of the Royal College of Physicians of London* vol. 1. Oxford: Clarendon Press, 1964.

Cockburn, J. S., editor. *Western Circuit Assize Orders 1629–1648*. London: Butler & Tanner, 1976.

Code, Lorraine. *What Can She Know: Feminist Theory and the Construction of Knowledge*. Ithaca & London: Cornell University Press, 1991.

Cohen, Shay D. "Menstruants and the Sacred." In *Women's History and Ancient History*, pp. 273–299. Edited by Sarah B. Pomeroy. Chapel Hill: University of North Carolina Press, 1991.

Coleman, D. C. *The Economy of England 1450–1750*. Oxford: Oxford University Press, 1977.

Cooke, Harold. *The Decline of the Old Medical Regime in Stuart London*. Ithaca: Cornell University Press, 1986.

———. "The Regulation of Medical Practice in London under the Stuarts, 1607–1704." Ph. D. thesis, University of Michigan, 1981.

Cox, J. Charles. *The Parish Registers of England*. Totowa, N.J.: E.P. Publishing, Ltd., 1974.

Crawford, Patricia. "The construction and experience of maternity in seventeenth-century England." In *Women as Mothers in Preindustrial England*, pp. 3–38. Edited by Valerie Fildes. London: Routledge, 1990.

———. "Printed Advertisements for Women Medical Practitioners in London, 1670–1710." *The Society for the Social History of Medicine* Bulletin 35 (December 1984): 66–9.

———. "Attitudes toward Menstruation in Seventeenth-century England." *Past and Present* 91 (May 1981): 47–73.

Cressy, David. *Birth, Marriage and Death: Ritual, Religion and the Life-Cycle in Tudor and Stuart England*. Oxford and N.Y.: Oxford University Press, 1997.

———. "Purification, Thanksgiving and the Churching of Women in Post-Reformation England." *Past and Present*, 141 (1993): 104–46.

———. *Literacy and the Social Order*. Cambridge: Cambridge University Press, 1979.

Cunnington, Phillis and Lucas, Catherine. *Occupational Costume in England from the Eleventh Century to 1914*. London: Adam and Charles Black, 1967.

Dale, T. C. *The Inhabitants of London in 1638*. London: Society of Genealogists, 1931.

Davis, Margaret. *The Enforcement of English Apprenticeship 1563–1642*. Cambridge: Harvard University Press, 1956.

Davis, Natalie Zemon. "City Women and Religious Change." In *Society and Culture in Early Modern France*, pp. 65–95. Edited by Natalie Zemon Davis. Stanford: Stanford University Press, 1975.

De Vries, Raymond, G. *Making Midwives Legal: Childbirth, Medicine and the Law*, 2nd ed. Columbus: Ohio State University Press, 1996.

Dickson, P. G. M. *The Financial Revolution in England*. London: St. Martin's Press, 1967.

Dictionary of National Biography. London: Oxford University Press, 1964.

Ditchfield, Peter H. *The Parish Clerk*. New York: E. P. Dutton & Co., 1907.

Donegan, Jane. *Women and Midwives, medicine, morality and misogyny in Early America*. Westport, Conn. and London: Greenwood Press, 1978.

Donnison, Jean. "The Development of the Occupation of Midwife: a Comparative View." In *Midwifery is a Labour of Love*, pp. 38–52. Vancouver, B.C.: Maternal Health Society, 1981.

———. *Midwives and Medical Men*. London: Heinemann, 1977.

———. "Medical Men and Lady Midwives: a case study in medical and feminist politics." *Society for the Social History of Medicine* Bulletin 18 (1976): 9–11.

Dowell, Stephen. *A History of Taxation and Taxes in England*, 4 vols. London: 1884; reprint ed., London: Frank Cass and Co., 1965.

Durston, Christopher. *The Family in the English Revolution*. Oxford: Basil Blackwell.

Earle, Peter. *A City Full of People: Men and Women of London 1650–1750*. London: Methuen, 1994.

———. "The female labour market in London in the late seventeenth and early eighteenth centuries." *Economic History Review*, XLII, 3 (1989): 328–53.

———. *The Making of the English Middle Class*. London: Methuen, 1986.

Eccles, Audrey. *Obstetrics and Gynaecology in Tudor and Stuart England*. London: Croom Helm, 1982.

Ehrenreich, B. and English, D. *Witches, Midwives and Nurses: a history of women healers*. 2nd ed., Old Westbury, New York: Feminist Press, 1973.

Emmison, F. G. *Morals and the Church Courts*. Chelmsford: Essex County Council, 1973.

Erickson, Robert A. "The books of generation: some observations on the style of the British Midwife books 1671–1764." In *Sexuality in eighteenth-century Britain*, pp. 74–94. Edited by P. A. Bouce. Manchester: Manchester University Press, 1982.

Evenden, Doreen A. "Gender Differences in the Licensing of Male and Female Surgeons in Early Modern England," *Medical History* (April, 1998): 194–216.

———. "Mothers and their midwives in seventeenth-century London." In *The Art of Midwifery*, pp. 9–26. Edited by Hilary Marland. Routledge: London, 1993.

Evenden, Kristin. " 'The "Popish Midwife': Printed Representations of Elizabeth Cellier and Midwifery Practice in Late Seventeenth-Century London." *Racar*, XX, i–2, 1993: 44–59.

Evenden-Nagy. "Seventeenth-century London Midwives: their training, licensing and social profile." Ph.D. dissertation, McMaster University, 1991.

———. *Popular Medicine in Seventeenth-century England*. Bowling Green, Ohio: Bowling Green State University Press, 1988.

Ewald, William B. *The Newsmen of Queen Anne*. Oxford: Blackwell, 1956.

Filippini, Nadia Maria. "The Church, the State and childbirth: the midwife in Italy in the eighteenth century." In *The Art of Midwifery*, pp. 152–75. Edited by Hilary Marland. London: Routledge, 1993.

Finlay, Roger. *Population and Metropolis: The Demography of London 1580–1650*. Cambridge: Cambridge University Press, 1981.

——— and Shearer, Beatrice. "Population growth and suburban expansion." In *London 1500–1700*, pp. 37–57. London: Longman, 1986.

Fitch, Marc. *Index to Testamentary Records in Archdeaconry Courts of London*, 2. London: British Record Society, 1985.

Fletcher, Anthony. *A Country Community in Peace and War: Sussex 1600–1660*. London and New York: Longman, 1975.

Forbes, Thomas R. "Weaver and Cordwainer: Occupations in the Parish of St. Giles without Cripplegate, London, in 1654–1693 and 1729–1743." *Guildhall Studies in London History* vol. 4, no. 3 (1980): 119–32.

———. *Chronicle from Aldgate*. New Haven and London: Yale University Press, 1971.

———. *The Midwife and the Witch*. New York: AMS Press, 1966.

———. "The Regulation of London Midwives in the Sixteenth and Seventeenth Centuries." *Medical History* 8 (1964): 235–44.

———. "Midwifery and Witchcraft." *Journal of the History of Medicine and Allied Sciences* 16 (1962): 264–82.

Fraser, Antonia. *The Weaker Vessel*. London: Methuen, 1984.

French, R. K. and Wear, Andrew, eds. *The Medical Revolution of the Seventeenth Century*. Cambridge: Cambridge University Press, 1989.

Fuhrer, Charlotte. *The Mysteries of Montreal: Memoirs of a Midwife*. Vancouver: University of British Columbia Press, 1984.

Gallagher, Catherine and Laqueur, Thomas, eds. *The Making of the Modern Body: Sexuality and Society in the Nineteenth Century*. Berkeley: University of California Press, 1987.

Gelbart, Nina. "Midwife to a Nation: Mme du Coudray serves France." In *The Art of Midwifery*, pp. 131–51. Edited by Hilary Marland. London: Routledge, 1993.

Gélis, Jacques. *History of Childbirth*. Translated by Rosemary Morris. Boston: Polity Press, 1991.

George, Margaret. *Women in the First Capalist Society: Experiences in Seventeenth-Century England*. Urbana & Chicago: University of Illinois Press, 1988.

Giardina Hess, Ann. "Midwifery Practice among the Quakers in southern rural England in the late seventeenth century." In *The Art of Midwifery*, pp. 49–76. Edited by Hilary Marland. London: Routledge, 1993.

———. "Community Case Studies of Midwives from England and New England c. 1650–1720." Ph.D. dissertation, Cambridge University, 1993

Gibson. *Codex Juris Ecclesiastici*. 2, Oxford: Clarendon Press, 1761.

Glass, D. V. "Socio-economic status and occupation in the City of London at the end of the seventeenth century." In *The Early Modern Town*, pp. 216–32. Edited by Peter Clark. New York: Longman, 1976.

———. *London Inhabitants Within the Walls 1695*. London: London Record Society, 1966.

Gordon, J. Elise. "Mrs. Elizabeth Cellier – 'the Popish Midwife' of the Restoration." *Midwife, Health Visitor & Community Nurse*, 2 (May 1975): 139–42.

———. "Some Women Practitioners of Past Centuries." *Practitioner* 208 (1972): 561–7.

Graham, Harvey. *Eternal Eve*. New York: Doubleday, 1951.

Greilsammer, Myriam. *L'envers du Tableau: Mariage and Maternité en Flandre Médiévale*. Paris: Armand Colin, 1990.

Grundy, Isobel. "Sara Stone: Enlightenment Midwife." In *Medicine in the Enlightenment*, pp. 128–44. Edited by Roy Porter. Amsterdam: Rodopi, 1995.

Guy, John. "The Episcopal Licensing of Physicians, Surgeons and Midwives." *Bulletin of the History of Medicine* 56 (1982): 528–42.

Gwynn, R. D. "The Distribution of Huguenot Refugees in England, II; London and its Environs." *Proceedings of the Huguenot Society of London* 22 (1976): 509–68.

Hamilton, Bernice. "The Medical Professions in the Eighteenth Century." *The Economic History Review* Second Series, 4 (1951): 141–69.

Hanawalt, Barbara A. *Women and Work in Pre Industrial Europe*. Bloomington: Indiana University Press, 1986.

Hands, A. P. and Scouloudi, Irene. *French Protestant Refugees Relieved Through the Threadneedle Street Church, London 1681–1687*. London: Huguenot Society of London, 1971.

Hanlon, Sister Joseph Damien. "These Be But Women." In *From the Renaissance to the Counter Reformation*, pp. 371–400. Edited by Charles H. Carter. New York: Random House, 1965.

Harley, David. "The scope of legal medicine in Lancashire and Cheshire, 1600–1760." In *Legal Medicine in History*, pp. 45–63. Edited by Michael Clark and Catherine Crawford. Cambridge University Press, 1994.

———. "Provincial midwives in England: Lancashire and Cheshire 1660–1760." In *The Art of Midwifery*, pp. 27–48. Edited by Hilary Marland. Routledge: London, 1993.

———. "English Archives, Local History, and the Study of Early Modern Midwifery," *Archives* 21 (October 1994): 145–54

———. "Historians as Demonologists: The Myth of the Midwife-witch." *Social History of Medicine* 3 (April 1990): 1–27.

———. "Ignorant Midwives–a persistent stereotype." *The Society for the History of Medicine Bulletin* 28 (June 1981): 6–9.

Harris, George. "Domestic Everyday Life, Manners, and Customs in this Country, from the Earliest Period to the End of the Eighteenth Century." *Transactions of the Royal Historical Society* 9 (1881): 224–53.

Harvey, Elizabeth. *Ventriloquized Voices: Feminist Theory and English Renaissance Texts.* London: Routledge, 1992.

Harvey, W. J. *List of Principal Inhabitants of the City of London 1640.* Isle of Wight: Pinhorns, 1886.

Herlan, Ronald W. "Poor Relief in London During the English Revolution." *Journal of British Studies* 28 (1979): 30–51.

———. "Poor Relief in the London Parish of Dunstan in the West during the Revolution." *Guildhall Studies in London History* 3, no.1 (1977): 13–36.

———. "Social Articulation and the Configuration of Parochial Poverty in London on the Eve of the Restoration." *Guildhall Studies in London History* 11 (1976): 43–53.

Hill, Bridget. *Women, Work and Sexual Politics in Eighteenth-Century England.* Oxford: Basil Blackwell, 1989.

Hill, Christopher. *Change and Continuity in Seventeenth-Century England.* London: Weidenfeld and Nicholson, 1974.

Hobby, Elaine. *Virtue of Necessity.* London: Virago Press, 1988.

Houlbrooke, Ralph A. *The English Family 1450–1700.* London: Longman, 1984.

———. *Church Courts and the People During the English Reformation 1520–1570.* Oxford: Oxford University Press, 1979.

Howell, Martha C. *Women, Production and Patriarchy in Late Medieval Cities.* Chicago: University of Chicago Press, 1986.

Hughes, Muriel Joy. *Women Healers in Medieval Life and Literature.* Freeport, N.Y.: Books for Libraries Press, 1943.

Hull, Suzanne W. *Chaste, Silent and Obedient: English Books for Women 1475–1640.* San Marino: Huntingdon Library, 1982

Hunter, Richard and MacAlpine, Ida, eds. "The Diary of John Causabon." *Proceedings of the Huguenot Society of London* 21 (1966): 31–57.

Hurd-Mead, Kate Campbell. *A History of Women in Medicine.* Haddam, Conn.: Haddam Press, 1938.

Illich, Ivan. *Limits to Medicine.* Toronto: McClelland & Stewart, 1976.

Jackson, Mark. "Developing Medical Expertise: Medical Practitioners and the Suspected Murders of New-Born Children." In *Medicine in the Enlightenment*, pp. 145–65. Edited by Roy Porter. Amsterdam: Rodopi, 1995.

Johnstone, R. W. *William Smellie: The Master of British Midwifery.* Edinburgh and London: E.& S. Livingstone Ltd., 1952.

Jones, Emrys. "London in the Early Seventeenth Century: An Ecological Approach." *London Journal* 6 (1980): 123–33.

Jones, P. E. and Judges, A. V. "London Population in the Late Seventeenth Century." *Economic History Review* 6 (1935–6): 45–63.

Jordan, W. K. *The Charities of London 1480–1660.* London: George Allen and Unwin Ltd., 1960.

Kamm, Josephine. *Hope Deferred: Girl's Education in English History.* London: Methuen, 1965.

Keene, Derek. "A New Study of London before the Great Fire." *Urban History Year Book* (1984): 11–21.

Kennedy, W. P. M. "List of Visitation Articles and Injunctions 1604–1715." *English Historical Review* 40 (1925): 586–92.

———. *Visitation Articles and Injunctions of the Period of the Reformation.* vol. 2, 1636–1658. London: Longmans Green & Co., 1910.

King, Helen. " 'As if none Understood the Art that Cannot Understand Greek': The Education of Midwives in Seventeenth-Century England." In *The History of Medical Education in Britain,* pp. 184–98. Edited by Vivian Nutton and Roy Porter. Amsterdam: Rodopi, 1995.

———. "The politick midwife: models of midwifery in the work of Elizabeth Cellier." In *The Art of Midwifery,* pp. 115–30. Edited by Hilary Marland. London: Routledge, 1993.

King, Howard. "The Evolution of the Male Midwife, with some Remarks on the Obstetrical Literature of Other Ages." *American Journal of Obstetrics* vol.77 (February, 1918): 177–86.

Kirk, R. E. G. and Kirk, Ernest F., eds. *Returns of Aliens Dwelling in the City and Suburbs of London: part one 1523–1571.* Aberdeen: Huguenot Society of London, 1900; reprint ed., 1969.

Kramer, Stella. *The English Craft Guilds and the Government.* London: 1905. Reprint ed., New York: AMS, 1968.

Lake, Rev. Edward. *Diary of the Rev. Edward Lake (1641–1704).* Camden Miscellany ser. 1 vol.39. London: Camden Society, 1847; reprint ed., New York: Johnson Reprint Corporation, 1968.

Lane, Joan. "Provincial Medical Apprentices and Masters in Early Modern England." *Eighteenth-Century Life* 12 (November 1988): 14–27.

———. "The Medical Practitioners of Provincial England in 1783." *Medical History* 28 (1984): 353–71.

———. "The Provincial Practitioner and his Services to the Poor, 1750–1800." *Society for the History of Medicine* Bulletin 31 (1982): 10–13.

Laslett, Peter, Oosterveen, Karla and Smith, Richard, eds. *Bastardy and its Comparative History.* Cambridge, Mass.: Harvard University Press, 1980.

Leavitt, Judith Walzer. *Brought to Bed: childbearing in America, 1750–1950.* New York and Oxford: Oxford University Press, 1986.

Le Fanu, W. R. "A North-Riding Doctor in 1609." *History of Medicine* 5 (1961): 178–88.

Linebaugh, Peter. "The Tyburn Riot against the Surgeons." In *Albion's Fatal Tree,* pp. 67–117. Edited by Douglas Hay, P. Linebaugh, J. Rule, E. P. Thompson, and C. Winslow. London: Pantheon Books, 1975.

Liu, Tai. *Puritan London.* Newark, N.J.: University of Delaware Presses and Associated University Presses, 1986.

Logan, Onnie Lee. *Motherwit: An Alabama Midwife's Story.* As told to Katherine Clark. New York: E. P. Dutton, 1989.

Loudon, Irvine, ed. *Childbed Fever: a documentary study.* New York and London: Garland, 1995.

———. "Some international features of maternal mortality, 1880–1950." In *Women and Children First: International Maternal and Infant Welfare 1870–1945,* pp. 5–28. Edited by Valerie Fildes. London: Routledge, 1992.

———. "Deaths in Childbed from the Eighteenth Century to 1935." *Medical History* 30 (1986): 1–41.

————. *Medical Care and the General Practitioner 1750–1850*. Oxford: Clarendon Press, 1986.

MacFarlane, Stephen. "Social Policy and the Poor in the Later Seventeenth Century." In *London 1500–1700*, pp. 252–77. Edited by A. L. Beier and Roger Finlay. London: Longman, 1986.

Marland, Hilary. " 'Stately and Dignified, Kindly and God-fearing': midwives, age and status in the Netherlands in the eighteenth century." In *The Task of Healing: Medicine, religion and gender in England and the Netherlands 1450–1800*, pp. 271–305. Rotterdam: Erasmus, 1996.

————, "The *'burgerlijke'* midwife: the *stadsvrouw* of eighteenth-century Holland." In *The Art of Midwifery*, pp. 192–213. Edited by Hilary Marland. London: Routledge, 1993.

————, translator. *"Mother and Child were Saved": The memoirs (1693–1740) of the Frisian Midwife Catharina Schrader*. Amsterdam: Rodopi, 1987.

Matthews, A. G. *Calamy Revised*. Oxford: Clarendon Press, 1988.

McCambell, Alice E. "The London Parish and the London Precinct 1640–1660." *Guildhall Studies in London History* 2 (October 1976): 107–24.

McMurray, William. "London: its population in 1631." *Notes and Queries* 11 (May 1910): 426.

Michel, Robert H. "English Attitudes Towards Women, 1640–1700." *Canadian Journal of History* 13 (April 1978): 35–60.

Moore, J. S., ed. *The Goods and Chattels of Our Forefathers*. London and Chichester: Phillimore, 1976.

Morrison, J. H. *Prerogative Court of Canterbury Letters of Administration 1620–30*. London: J. H. Morrison, 1935.

Munk, William. *The Roll of the Royal College of Physicians of London: comprising biographical sketches*. 2nd ed. London: The College, 1878.

Oakley, Anne. *The Captured Womb*. Oxford: Basil Blackwell, 1984.

Oldham, James C. "On Pleading the Belly: A History of the Jury of Matrons." *Criminal Justice History* 6 (1985): 164.

Ortiz, Teresa. "From hegemony to subordination: midwives in early modern Spain." In *The Art of Midwifery*, pp. 95–114. Edited by Hilary Marland. London: Routledge, 1993.

Pantin, C. G. "A Study of Maternal Mortality and Midwifery on the Isle of Man, 1882–1961." *Medical History* 40 (1996): 141–65.

Parry, Noel and Parry, Jose. *The Rise of the Medical Profession*. London: Croom Helm, 1976.

Parton, A. G. "The Hearth Tax and the distribution of population and prosperity in Surrey." Guildford: *Surrey Archeological Society* 75 (1984): 55–60.

Paster, Gail Kern *The Body Embarrassed: Drama and the Disciplines of Shame in Early Modern England*. Ithaca: Cornell University Press, 1993

Patten, John. "The Hearth Taxes, 1662–1689." *Local Population Studies* 7 (1971): 14–27.

Peachey, George C., ed. *The Life of William Savory (surgeon) of Brightwalton*. London: J. J. Keliher & Co. Ltd., 1903.

————. *A Memoir of William and John Hunter*. Plymouth: Wm Brendon and Son Ltd., 1924.

Pearl, Valerie. "Change and Stability in seventeenth-century London." *London Journal* 5 (1979): 3–34.

Pelling, Margaret. "Appearance and reality: barber-surgeons, the body and disease." In

London 1500–1700, pp. 82–112. Edited by A. L. Beier and Roger Finlay. London: Longman, 1986.

———. "Medicine and Sanitation." In *William Shakespeare: His World, His Work, His Influence*, vol. 1, pp. 75–84. Edited by John F. Andrews. New York: Scribner, 1985.

———. "Occupational Diversity: Barbersurgeons and the Trades of Norwich, 1550–1640." *Bulletin of the History of Medicine* 56 (1982): 484–511.

Perkins, Wendy. "Midwives versus Doctors: The case of Louise Bourgeois." *The Seventeenth Century* 3 (1988): 135–57.

———. *Midwifery and Medicine in Early Modern France: Louise Bourgeois*. Exeter: University of Exeter Press, 1996.

Petrelli, Richard. "The Regulation of French Midwifery during the Ancient Regime." *Journal of the History of Medicine and Allied Sciences* 26 (1971): 276–92.

Phelps Brown, E. H. and Hopkins, Sheila V. "Seven Centuries of Building Wages." *Economica* 22 no. 87 (August 1955): 195–206.

Phillimore. *Phillimore's Ecclesiastical Law*. 2, 2nd ed. London: 1895.

Pinchbeck, Ivy and Hewitt, M. *Children in English Society*. London: Routledge and Keegan Paul, 1969.

Porter, Roy. *Patients and Practitioners: Lay Perceptions of Medicine in Pre-Industrial Society*. Cambridge: Cambridge University Press, 1985.

——— and Porter, Dorothy. *In Sickness and in Health: the British Experience 1650–1850*. London: Fourth Estate, 1988.

———. *Patient's Progress: Doctors and Doctoring in Eighteenth-century England*. Cambridge: Polity Press, 1989.

Power, Sir D'Arcy. "The Birth of Mankind or the Woman's Book: A Bibliographical Study." *The Library*, fourth series, 8 (June 1927): 1–37.

Power, M. J. "The Social Topography of Restoration London." In *London 1500–1700*, pp. 199–223. Edited by A. L. Beier and Roger Finlay. London: Longman, 1986.

Poynter, F. N. L. "Nicholas Culpeper and His Books." *Journal of the History of Medicine*. 17 (1962): 152–67.

Prior, Mary. "Reviled and crucified marriage: the position of Tudor bishop's wives." In *Women in English Society 1500–1800*, pp. 118–48. Edited by Mary Prior. London: Methuen, 1985.

Prokter, Adrian and Taylor, Robert. *The A to Z of Elizabethan London*. Lympne Castle, Kent: Harry Margary, 1979.

Purvis, J. S. *An Introduction to Ecclesiastical Records*. London: St. Anthony's Press, 1953.

Raach, John. *A Directory of English Country Physicians 1603–1643*. London: Dawsons of Pall Mall, 1962.

———. "Medical Licensing in the Seventeenth Century." *Yale Journal of Biology and Medicine* 16 no.4 (1944): 267–88.

Ramsay, Michael. *Professional and Popular Medicine in France 1770–1830*. Cambridge: Cambridge University Press, 1988.

Rawcliffe, Carole. *Medicine and Society in Later Medieval England*. Stroud, Gloucestershire: Alan Sutton, 1995.

Reader, D. A. "Keeping up with London's Past." *Urban History Year Book* 1977: 48–54.

Rhodes, Philip. *Dr.John Leake's Hospital*. London: Davis Poynter, 1977

Richardson, R. C. *Puritanism in North-west England*. Manchester: Manchester University Press, 1972.

Richardson, Ruth. *Death, Dissection and the Destitute*. Harmondsworth, Middlesex: Penguin, 1989.

Riden, Philip, ed. *Probate Records and the Local Community*. Stroud, Gloucester: Alan Sutton, 1985.

Roberts, R. S. "Medicine in Tudor and Stuart England: part 2 London." *Medical History* 8 (1964): 217–34.

Rowland, Beryl. *Medieval Woman's Guide to Health*. Kent, Ohio: The Kent State University Press, 1981.

Rowlands, Marie B. "Recusant Women 1560–1640." In *Women in English Society 1500–1800*, pp. 149–80. Edited by Mary Prior. London: Methuen, 1985.

Savona-Ventura, C. "The Influence of the Roman Catholic Church on Midwifery Practice in Malta." *Medical History* 39 (1995): 18–34.

Sawday, Jonathan. *The Body Emblazoned: Dissection and the human body in Renaissance culture*. London and New York : Routledge, 1995.

Schama, Simon. *The Embarrassment of Riches*. New York: Alfred A. Knopf, 1987.

Schnorrenberg, Barbara Brandon. "Is Chilbirth any Place for a Woman? The Decline of Midwifery in Eighteenth-Century England." *Studies in Eighteenth-Century Culture* 10 (1981): 393–408

Schnucker, R. V. "The English Puritans and Pregnancy, Delivery and Breast Feeding." *History of Childhood Quarterly* (Spring 1974): 637–58.

Schofield, Roger. "Did the Mother's really die?" In *The World We Have Gained*, pp. 231–60. Edited by L. Bonfield. Oxford: Basil Blackwell, 1986.

———— and Wrigley, E. A. "Infant and child mortality in England in the late Tudor and early Stuart Period," in *Health, Medicine and Mortality in the Sixteenth Century*, pp. 61–95. Edited by Charles Webster. Cambridge: Cambridge University Press, 1979.

Scouloudi, Irene. *Returns of Strangers in the Metropolis 1593, 1627, 1635, 1639*. London: Huguenot Society of London, 1985.

Seaver, Paul. *Wallington's World*. Stanford: Stanford University Press, 1985.

Seligman, Stanley A. "The Royal Maternity Charity: The First Hundred Years." *Medical History* 24 (1980): 403–18.

Shorter, Edward. *A History of Women's Bodies*. New York: Basic Books, 1982.

Shute, Wallace B. "History of Obstetrical Forceps from 1750 to the present era." *Acta Belgica Historiae Medicinae* vol.5, (no.2, 1992): 65–9.

Smith, Hilda. "Gynecology and Ideology in Seventeenth-Century England." In *Liberating Women's History: Theoretical and Critical Essays*, pp. 97–114. Edited by Bernice A. Carroll. Urbana, Ill.: University of Illinois Press, 1976.

Smith, Lacey Baldwin. *This Realm of England*. Toronto: D. C. Heath, 1976.

Snell, K. D. M. *Annals of the Labouring Poor: Social Change and Agrarian England, 1660–1900*. Cambridge: Cambridge University Press, 1985.

Snell Smith, Donna. "Tudor and Stuart Midwifery." Ph.D. thesis, University of Kentucky, 1980.

Spencer, Herbert. *The History of British Midwifery from 1650–1800*. London: John Bale, Sons & Danielson, 1927.

Stone, Lawrence. *The Family, Sex and Marriage in England 1500–1800*. Abridged edition, Harmondsworth, Middlesex: Pengin, 1979.

Stow, John. *Survey of London.* Edited by C. L. Kingsford. London: J. M. Dent and Sons Ltd., 1912.

Tanner, J. R. *English Constitutional Conflicts of the Seventeenth Century 1603–1689.* Cambridge: Cambridge University Press, 1928.

Tate, W. E. *The Parish Chest.* Cambridge: Cambridge University Press, 1946.

Thomas, Henry. "The Society of Chymical Physitians." In *Science, Medicine and History* 2, pp. 55–71. Edited by E. Underwood. Oxford: Oxford University Press, 1953.

Thomas, Keith. *Age and Authority in Early Modern England.* London: The British Academy, 1976.

———. *Religion and the Decline of Magic.* Harmondsworth, Middlesex: Penguin, 1971.

Thornton, John L. "The First Printed English Edition of 'Observations in Midwifery' By Percival Willughby (1596–1685)." *Practitioner* 208 (1972): 295–7.

Towler, Jean and Bramall, Joan. *Midwives in History and Society.* London: Croom Helm, 1976.

Ulrich, Laurel Thatcher. *A Midwife's Tale.* New York: Alfred A. Knopf, 1990.

———. " 'The Living Mother of a Living Child': Midwifery and Mortality in Post-Revolutionary New England." *William and Mary Quarterly* 46 (January 1989): 27–48.

Upton, Eleanor. *Guide to Sources of English History from 1603–1660: Early Reports of the Royal Commission on Historical Manuscripts.* New York: Scarecrow Press, 2nd ed., 1964.

Van Lieburg, M. J. and Marland, Hilary. "Midwife Regulation, Education, and Practice in the Netherlands during the Nineteenth Century." *Medical History* 33 (1989): 296–317.

Vesluysen, Margaret Connor. "Midwives, medical men and 'poor women labouring of child': lying-in hospitals in eighteenth-century London." In *Women, health and reproduction,* pp. 18–49. Edited by Helen Roberts. Routledge and Keegan Paul, 1981.

Vicinus, Martha. *Independent Women: Work and Community for Single Women 1850–1920.* Chicago: University of Chicago Press, 1985.

Walzer Leavitt, Judith. *Brought to Bed.* New York, Oxford: Oxford University Press, 1986.

Webster, Charles. *Health, Medicine and Mortality in the Sixteenth Century.* Cambridge: Cambridge University Press, 1979.

Wiesner, Merry E. "The midwives of south Germany and the public/private dichotomy." In *The Art of Midwifery,* pp. 77–94. Edited by Hilary Marland. London: Routledge, 1993.

———. "Early Modern Midwifery: A Case Study." In *Women and Work in Pre Industrial Europe,* pp. 94–113. Edited by Barbara A. Hanawalt. Bloomington: Indiana University Press, 1986.

Willmott Dobbie, B. M. "An Attempt to estimate the true rate of maternal mortality, sixteenth to eighteenth centuries." *Medical History* 26 (1982): 79–90.

Wilson, Adrian. *The Making of Man-midwifery: Childbirth in England, 1660–1770.* Cambridge, Mass.: Harvard University Press, 1995.

———. "The ceremony of childbirth and its interpretation." In *Women as Mothers in Industrial England,* pp. 68–107. Edited by Valerie Fildes. London and New York: Routledge, 1990.

———. "Participant or patient? Seventeenth century childbirth from the mother's point of view." In *Patients and Practitioners: Lay Perceptions of Medicine in Pre-Industrial Society,* pp. 129–44. Edited by Roy Porter. Cambridge: Cambridge University Press, 1985.

————. "William Hunter and the Varieties of Man-midwifery." In *William Hunter and the eighteenth-century medical world*, pp. 343–69. Edited by W. F. Bynum and Roy Porter. Cambridge: Cambridge University Press, 1985.

————. "Childbirth in seventeenth and eighteenth-century England." Ph.D thesis, University of Sussex, 1983.

————. "Ignorant Midwives – a Rejoinder." *The Society for the Social History of Medicine* Bulletin 32 (June 1983): 46–9.

Woodhead, J. R. *The Rulers of London 1660–1689.* London: London and Middlesex Archeological Society, 1965.

Wrightson, Keith. "Infanticide in Earlier Seventeenth-century England." *Local Population Studies* 15 (1975): 10–22.

Wrigley, E. A. and Schofield, Roger. "English Population History from Family Reconstruction: Summary Results 1600–1799." *Population Studies* 37 (1983): 157–84.

Wrigley, E. A. "Explaining the rise in marital fertility in England in the 'long' eighteenth century." *Economic History Review* LI 3 (1998): 435–64

————. "A simple model of London's Importance in Changing English Society and Economy 1650–1750." *Past and Present* 37 (1967): 44–70.

Yeardsley, MacLeod. *Doctors in Elizabethan Drama.* London: John Bale Sons and Danielson Ltd., 1933.

Young, Sidney. *The Annals of the Barber Surgeons of London.* London: East & Blades, 1890; reprint ed. New York: A.M.S., 1978.

Zell, Michael. "The Social Parameters of Probate Records in the Sixteenth Century." *Bulletin of the Institute of Historical Research* 57 (1984): 107–13.

INDEX